# Paediatric Movement Disorders
## Progress in understanding

# Paediatric Movement Disorders
## Progress in understanding

*Editors:*
Emilio Fernández-Alvarez
Alexis Arzimanoglou
Eduardo Tolosa

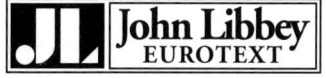

ISBN: 2-7420-0542-0

---

Éditions John Libbey Eurotext
127, avenue de la République, 92120 Montrouge, France
Tél. : 01 46 73 06 60
Editor : Maud Thévenin
Site internet : http://www.jle.com

John Libbey Eurotext
42-46 High Street
Esher, Surrey
KT10 9KY
United Kingdom

---

© 2005, John Libbey Eurotext

Il est interdit de reproduire intégralement ou partiellement le présent ouvrage sans autorisation de l'éditeur ou du Centre Français d'Exploitation du Droit de Copie, 20, rue des Grands-Augustins, 75006 Paris.

# List of Contributors

**Acosta Maria T.,** Department of Neurology, Children's National Medical Center, George Washington University School of Medicine and Health Sciences, Washington, DC, USA.

**Aicardi Jean,** Service de Neurologie pédiatrique et des Maladies métaboliques, Hôpital Robert Debré, 48 Boulevard Sérurier, 75935 Paris Cedex 19, France.

**Albanese Alberto,** Istituto Nazionale Neurologico Carlo Besta, Università Cattolica del Sacro Cuore, Via G. Celoria, 11, 20133 Milano, Italy.

**Arzimanoglou Alexis,** Child Neurology and Metabolic Diseases Dpt., University Hospital Robert Debré, 48 Boulevard Sérurier, 75935 Paris Cedex 19, France.

**Blau Nenad,** Division of Clinical Chemistry and Biochemistry, University Children's Hospital, Steinwiesstrasse 75, 8032 Zurich, Switzerland.

**Bottiglieri Teodoro,** Institute of Metabolic Disease, Baylor University Medical Center, Dallas, TX, USA.

**Cardoso Francisco,** Av Pasteur 89/1107, 30150-290 Belo Horizonte MG, Brazil.

**Chiriboga Claudia A,** Departments of Neurology and Pediatrics, College of Physicians and Surgeons of Columbia University, New York, NY, USA.

**Cif Laura,** Unité de recherche sur les mouvements anormaux, Département de Neurochirurgie pédiatrique, Centre Gui de Chauliac, 80 Avenue Augustin Fliche, 34295 Montpellier Cedex 5, France.

**Clayton Peter T,** Biochemistry Endocrinology and Metabolism Unit, Institute of Child Health at Great Ormond Street Hospital, University College London, United Kingdom.

**Coubes Philippe,** Unité de recherche sur les mouvements anormaux, Département de Neurochirurgie pédiatrique, Centre Gui de Chauliac, 80 Avenue Augustin Fliche, 34295 Montpellier Cedex 5, France.

**De Vivo Darryl C.,** Departments of Neurology and Pediatrics, College of Physicians and Surgeons of Columbia University, New York, NY, USA.

**Echenne Bernard,** Service de Neuropédiatrie, Hôpital Gui de Chauliac, 80 Avenue Augustin Fliche, 34295 Montpellier Cedex 5, France.

**El Fertit Hassan,** Unité de recherche sur les mouvements anormaux, Département de Neurochirurgie pédiatrique, Centre Gui de Chauliac, 80 Avenue Augustin Fliche, 34295 Montpellier Cedex 5, France.

**Elia Antonio E.,** Istituto Nazionale Neurologico Carlo Besta, Università Cattolica del Sacro Cuore, Via G. Celoria, 11, 20133 Milano, Italy.

**Fasano Alfonso,** Istituto Nazionale Neurologico Carlo Besta, Università Cattolica del Sacro Cuore, Via G. Celoria, 11, 20133 Milano, Italy.

**Fernández-Alvarez Emilio,** Servicio de Neuropediatria, Hospital Sant Joan de Déu, Carretera de Esplugas, s/n, 08034 Barcelona, Spain.

**Ford Blair,** Departments of Neurology and Pediatrics, College of Physicians and Surgeons of Columbia University, New York, NY, USA.

**Gaudin Daniel,** Unité de recherche sur les mouvements anormaux, Département de Neurochirurgie pédiatrique, Centre Gui de Chauliac, 80 Avenue Augustin Fliche, 34295 Montpellier Cedex 5, France.

**Gibson K. Michael,** Department of Molecular and Medical Genetics, Biochemical Genetics Laboratory, Oregon Health & Science University, 2525 S.W. 3rd Avenue, Mail Code MP-350, Portland, OR 97201, USA.

**Grattan-Smith Padraic,** Department of Neurology, Sydney Children's Hospital, High St Randwick, NSW 2031 Australia.

**Hemm Simone,** Unité de recherche sur les mouvements anormaux, Département de Neurochirurgie pédiatrique, Centre Gui de Chauliac, 80 Avenue Augustin Fliche, 34295 Montpellier Cedex 5, France.

**Hinton Veronica,** Departments of Neurology and Pediatrics, College of Physicians and Surgeons of Columbia University, New York, NY, USA.

**Hoffmann Georg F.,** Geschäftsführender Direktor/Chairman, Universitätsklinik für Kinder- und Jugendmedizin, Im Neuenheimer Feld 153, D-69120 Heidelberg, Germany.

**Hörster Friederike,** Universitätsklinik für Kinder- und Jugendmedizin, Im Neuenheimer Feld 153, D-69120 Heidelberg, Germany.

**Hyland Keith,** Institute of Metabolic Disease, Baylor University Medical Center, Dallas, TX, USA.

**Jakobs Cornelis,** Department of Clinical Chemistry, VU University Medical center, Amsterdam, The Netherlands.

**Jankovic Joseph,** Parkinson's Disease Center and Movement Disorders Clinic, Baylor College of Medicine, Department of Neurology, The Smith Tower, Suite 1801, 6550 Fannin, Houston, Texas 77030, USA.

**Lees Andrew J.,** National Hospital for Neurology and Neurosurgery, Queen Square, London WC1N 3BG, United Kingdom.

**Louis Elan D.,** Unit 198, Neurological Institute, 710 West 168th Street, New York, NY, 10032, USA.

**Mercimek-Mahmutoglu Saadet,** Department of Pediatrics, Vienna University, Währingergürtel 18-20, A- 1090 Vienna, Austria.

**Miotto Karen,** Department of Psychiatry and Biobehavioral Sciences, David Geffen School of Medicine at UCLA, University of California, Los Angeles, CA, USA.

**Moharir Mahendranath D.,** Department of Neurology, The Hospital for Sick Children, 555 University Avenue, Toronto, Ontario, Canada M 5 G 1 X 8.

**Nardocci Nardo,** Division of Child Neurology, Istituto Nazionale Neurologico « C. Besta », Via Celoria, 11, 20133 Milano, Italy.

**Ouvrier Robert,** T.Y. Nelson Department of Neurology and Neurosurgery, The Children's Hospital at Westmead, Locked Bag 4001, Westmead, NSW 2145, Australia.

**Paviour Dominic C.,** National Hospital for Neurology and Neurosurgery, Queen Square, London WC1N 3BG, United Kingdom.

**Pearl Phillip L.,** Department of Neurology, Children's National Medical Center, George Washington University School of Medicine and Health Sciences, Washington, DC, USA.

**Pons Roser,** Departments of Neurology and Pediatrics, College of Physicians and Surgeons of Columbia University, New York, NY, USA.

**Pranzatelli Michael R.,** National Pediatric Myoclonus Center, SIU-SOM, PO Box 19643, Springfield, IL 62794-9643, Illinois, USA.

**Roubertie Agathe,** Service de Neuropédiatrie, Hôpital Gui de Chauliac, 80 avenue Augustin Fliche, 34295 Montpellier Cedex 5, France.

**San Antonio Victoria,** Child Neurology and Metabolic Diseases Dpt., University Hospital Robert Debré, 48 Boulevard Sérurier, 75935 Paris Cedex 19, France.

**Schteinschnaider Ángeles,** Pediatric Neurology Department, Raúl Carrea Institute for Neurological Research (FLENI), Montañeses 2325, Buenos Aires, Argentina (C1428AQK).

**Serrat Stéphanie,** Unité de recherche sur les mouvements anormaux, Département de Neurochirurgie pédiatrique, Centre Gui de Chauliac, 80 Avenue Augustin Fliche, 34295 Montpellier Cedex 5, France.

**Sharma Radhakant,** Institute of Metabolic Disease, Baylor University Medical Center, Dallas, TX, USA.

**Stöckler-Ipsiroglu Sylvia,** Department of Pediatrics, Vienna University, Währingergürtel 18-20, A-1090 Vienna, Austria.

**Surtees Robert,** Neurosciences Unit, Institute of Child Health, University College London, 30 Guilford Street, London WC1N 1EH, United Kingdom.

**Temudo Teresa,** Serviço de Pediatria, Hospital Geral de Santo António, Largo Abel Salazar, 4099-001 Porto, Portugal.

**Tolosa Eduardo,** Hospital Clinical I Provincial de Barcelona, Villarroel, 170, 8036 Barcelona, Spain.

**Vayssière Nathalie,** Unité de recherche sur les mouvements anormaux, Département de Neurochirurgie pédiatrique, Centre Gui de Chauliac, 80 Avenue Augustin Fliche, 34295 Montpellier Cedex 5, France.

**Wallis Denise D.,** Department of Neurology, Children's National Medical Center, George Washington University School of Medicine and Health Sciences, Washington, DC, USA.

# Foreword

For the last two decades, disorders of movement have represented a major field in adult neurology. Several comprehensive books and a huge number of journal articles have dealt with the semiology, classification, mechanisms and treatment of Parkinson disease and related disorders. Conversely, movement disorders in childhood have not received much attention and the paediatric literature on this topic has remained rather limited. With the exception of Tourette's syndrome, only rare books have been specifically dedicated to this important area. Yet, childhood movement disorders, with their variable expressions, frequently confront child neurologists as they represent a major clinical manifestation of a large number of neurological diseases.

Keen to expand our knowledge on clinical expression, underlying mechanisms and treatment strategies in this exciting field, we created a few years ago an informal European Study Group on Movement Disorders in Children. It became rapidly evident that, as child neurologists, we would enormously benefit from the experience and knowledge of our adult neurology colleagues, particularly in what concerned the functions and dysfunctions of the basal ganglia and related structures. Similarly, the specific expertise of child neurologists in such fields as metabolic disorders or early onset neurodegerative diseases and other disorders of the developing nervous system would permit fruitful exchanges of ideas between adult and child specialists and broaden the scope of both fields of neurology.

The present book is not aimed to be an exhaustive and comprehensive review of the paediatric movement disorders. It represents the outcome of an International Workshop, organized for the first time as a forum for exchange between both adult and child neurologists, specialists in this rapidly expanding field. The workshop took place in Barcelona on February 2004, with the collaboration of the *Movement Disorders Society*, the *Société Européenne de Neurologie Pédiatrique*, the *Paediatric Neurotransmitter Association*, the *European Dystonia Federation* and the *Sociedad Espanola de Neurología Pediátrica*.

We are confident that the contributions selected for this book represent the state of the art in paediatric movement disorders and a source of thought for progress in further understanding.

As Editors we would like to express our gratitude to all authors and to all the participants at the *First International Symposium on Paediatric Movement Disorders*. We also sincerely thank the John Libbey Eurotext editions for their help and support in diffusing current knowledge in this field of child neurology.

**Emilio Fernández-Alvarez, Alexis Arzimanoglou, Eduardo Tolosa**

# Contents

Foreword
E. Fernández-Alvarez, A. Arzimanoglou, E. Tolosa ............................................. VII

Prevalence of paediatric movement disorders
E. Fernández-Alvarez ................................................................................... 1

Transient movement disorders of infancy and childhood
M.D. Moharir, R.A. Ouvrier, P. Grattan-Smith ............................................ 19

Early onset primary torsion dystonia
A. Fasano, A.E. Elia, A. Albanese ............................................................. 31

Focal and segmental dystonia in children
T. Temudo ................................................................................................. 57

Status dystonicus in children
N. Nardocci, T. Temudo, B. Echenne, A. Roubertie for: European Study Group
on Movement Disorders in Children .......................................................... 71

Deep brain stimulation in paediatric dystonia
L. Cif, H. El Fertit, N. Vayssière, S. Hemm, D. Gaudin, S. Serrat, P. Coubes..... 77

Essential tremor in children
E.D. Louis ................................................................................................. 87

Diagnostic considerations in juvenile parkinsonism
D.C. Paviour, A.J. Lees .............................................................................. 91

Benign hereditary chorea
Á. Schteinschnaider ................................................................................... 115

Opsoclonus-myoclonus-ataxia syndrome
M.R. Pranzatelli ........................................................................................ 121

Movement disorders in paediatric inherited ataxias
  A. Roubertie, B. Echenne .................................................................................. 137

Abnormal movements in alternating hemiplegia of childhood
  J. Aicardi .......................................................................................................... 147

Movement disorders in children and calcification of the basal ganglia
  V. San Antonio, A. Arzimanoglou ..................................................................... 159

Clinical, biochemical and molecular spectrum of aromatic L-Amino acid decarboxylase deficiency
  R. Pons, B. Ford, C.A. Chiriboga, P.T. Clayton, V. Hinton, K. Hyland,
  R. Sharma, D.C. De Vivo ................................................................................. 185

Tyrosine hydroxylase deficiency:
symptomatology, diagnosis, therapy and outlook
  F. Hörster, G.F. Hoffmann .............................................................................. 195

Dyskinetic features of succinate semialdehyde dehydrogenase deficiency, a GABA degradative defect
  P.L. Pearl, M.T. Acosta, D.D. Wallis, T. Bottiglieri, K. Miotto, C. Jakobs,
  K.M. Gibson .................................................................................................... 203

Tetrahydrobiopterin deficiencies and movement disorders
  N. Blau ............................................................................................................ 213

Cerebral creatine deficiency and movement disorders
  S. Mercimek-Mahmutoglu, S. Stöckler-Ipsiroglu ............................................. 223

Tourette syndrome: autoimmune mechanisms
  F. Cardoso ....................................................................................................... 231

Stereotypies in autistic and other childhood disorders
  J. Jankovic ....................................................................................................... 247

Functional (psychogenic) movement disorders in childhood
  R. Surtees ........................................................................................................ 261

# Prevalence of paediatric movement disorders

**Emilio Fernández-Alvarez**

*Neuropaediatric Department, Hospital Sant Joan de Déu, Barcelona, Spain*

Studying the movement disorders (MD) with paediatric onset, from an epidemiological perspective presents a few challenges. Diverse diagnostic entities with MD can begin at a paediatric age group and mostly include rare disorders. Abnormal movements can either be the main clinical problem or be ignored as a relative minor symptom (as occurs with the stereotypies often associated with autism or severe mental retardation) or as a late appearance symptom (as occurs in many severe neurometabolic or neurodegenerative disorders) of the syndrome component. Clinical examination in young children and in infants is often difficult, therefore an accurate syndromic identification of the abnormal movement can often be lacking. Moreover, till recently paediatric movement disorders have not received serious consideration and such cases frequently are not referred to neuropaediatric or neurological departments so it is difficult to have large enough series available for study. Despite these difficulties it is still important to study the incidence and prevalence of paediatric movement disorders (PMDs).

Epidemiology helps the clinician to organise a rational differential diagnosis and also offers a way to study both the public health impact and the global burden of the clinical entities [1].

Incidence and prevalence of overall PMDs have not been studied so far. Prevalence of specific PMDs has been studied in Tourette disease and in dyskinetic cerebral palsy. It can be broadly deduced in essential tremor but the remaining movement diseases are rare so epidemiological community based studies are lacking and their real prevalence is not known.

Accurate information about the general occurrence of medical disorders is obtained from community based epidemiological studies of specific disorders but when this type of information is lacking it is possible to turn to large clinical series even if random ascertainment, referral bias, and undefined populations are obvious problems. In this paper on the frequency of PMDs, we had to rely mainly on our own experience even if we are certain that the interpretation of these data is only a rough approximation to reality.

## ■ Population

We have studied the frequency of PMDs in subjects consulting at the Neuropediatric Department of the Hospital San Juan de Dios de Barcelona (Spain) between January 1$^{st}$, 1983 and January 1$^{st}$, 2004.

Inclusion criteria were:
1) age of onset of the abnormal movement before 18 years,
2) attended at consultation at the Neuropediatric Department of the Hospital San Juan de Dios de Barcelona (Spain) between January 1$^{st}$, 1983 and January 1$^{st}$, 2004.

Exclusion criteria were: 1) inadequate or insufficient data on the characteristics of the movement disorder, 2) dyskinetic forms of cerebral palsy (but delayed onset dystonia was included), 3) ataxia or cerebellar tremor as the only abnormal motor symptoms, 4) epileptic myoclonus, and 5) iatrogenic dyskinesias. Exclusion of subjects with cerebellar tremor or epileptic myoclonus have a rationale because by general consensus they are not included within MD. Iatrogenic dyskinesias are usually managed in emergency units and, except in some peculiar cases, a neurological consultation is not required. In our department overall cerebral palsy (including the dyskinetic type) is diagnosed and managed in another unit and, as occurs with iatrogenic dyskinesias, are not usually referred to our unit. Inclusion in this series of the few cases referred would bias the comparative figures.

## ■ Definition of terms

According to the abnormal movement type the cases were classified as: rigid-hypokinetic syndrome, dystonia, tremor, chorea, myoclonus, tics, stereotypies and, complex movement disorder. The standard criteria for these types of abnormal movements have been used [2]. Ballismus was included in the chorea group and athetosis in the dystonic group. Complex movements is a term that has been used when several types of abnormal movement without clear predominance of a given type coexist and/or when no clear definition of the movement(s) was possible.

From the aetiological point of view movement disorders are usually classified as *primary* (idiopathic, essential) and *secondary*. But there is no clear consensus on the meaning of these terms. Marsden [3] identifies as "primary or idiopathic" the disorders in which no cause is found. But nowadays the progress in molecular genetics may suggest an aetiological factor in diseases that in the past would have been definitely considered as primary. A good example is the DYT1 torsion dystonia which even when the genetic defect and its defective protein are well known, is still included in the primary dystonia group. On the other hand, some authors classify [4] dystonias as *primary* when dystonia is the sole symptom, "*dystonia-plus*" when dystonia "is one of only two neurological conditions present, the other usually being myoclonus or parkinsonism", *heredodegenerative dystonias* when the dystonia is part of a more widespread neurodegenerative syndrome and *secondary* when they are caused by environmental insults such as strokes, tumours or infections. Using a similar classification Kamm [5] includes metabolic diseases in the secondary group but Németh does so in the neurodegenerative group.

In this chapter according to their aetiology the overall PMDs will be grouped in three categories: primary, syndromic and secondary.

The term primary will be used when the disease accomplishes the following criteria:

1) movement disorders are the only symptom;
2) no detectable structural abnormality of the CNS;
3) the movement disorder is presumed not to be causally related to environmental insults such as stroke, infection, tumours, drugs or toxins.

The category syndromic movement disorders will be used when a CNS lesion or other neurological symptoms in addition to abnormal movements can be demonstrated. Metabolic and heredodegenerative diseases are included in this group.

The term secondary will be applied when the abnormal movement is caused by environmental insults such as stroke, infection, tumours, drugs or toxins.

According to their evolution, PMDs should be separated into chronic, paroxysmal and transient. The term *chronic forms* has been applied to cases in which abnormal symptoms (from the onset) persist uninterrupted throughout lifetime. *Paroxysmal disorders* means diseases in which the disturbance is episodic (even if the episodes last several days) and between the episodes the patient is free of symptoms The term *transient* is used in both primary and syndromic cases when the disorder spontaneously disappears without lasting effects. By consensus in tics the term transient is used when they last less than a year.

A total of 964 subjects with movement disorders starting before age of 18 years of age were analysed.

## ■ Results

### General data

*Tables I-II and IV-VI* show absolute values and percentage in our series according to the type of abnormal movement, age of onset, male/female proportion according the type of movement disorder, aetiology of the disorder (primary, syndromic or secondary), and type of evolution (transient and chronic).

*Figure 1* indicates the percentage of cases according to the type of abnormal movement and *Figure 2* frequency of PMDs according their aetiology.

### Age of onset *(Table II, Figures 3-4)*

The mean age of onset of tics (n = 417) is 6.43 years (SD ± 2.61). The mean age of onset of PMDs other than tics (n = 476) was 3.83 years. If tics are excluded age of onset of more than a half of our PMDs cases was before three years. These figures are influenced by the high prevalence of transient cases in the overall PMDs. Transient PMDs are especially frequent in the first 2 years of life (see below). Mean age of onset of our Tourette syndrome cases *(Table III)* was similar to the figures reported in the literature [6-13].

Table I. Absolute values and percentage according to the type of abnormal movement (n = 964).

|  | Percentage (%)* | N° of cases |
|---|---|---|
| Tics | 43 | 417 |
| Dystonia | 23 (40) | 223 |
| Tremor | 16 (30) | 163 |
| Myoclonus | 6 (11) | 61 |
| Complex | 4 (7) | 40 |
| Chorea | 3 (6) | 31 |
| Stereotypies** | 2 (3) | 16 |
| Rigid hypokinetic syndrome | 1 (2) | 13 |
| Total |  | 964 |

\* (...) The number in parenthesis represents percentage if tics are excluded.
\*\* Stereotypies were included in the database only from January 2000.

Table II. Age of onset of 476 patients with movement disorders other than tics and 428 with tics.

|  | MD other than tics | Tics |
|---|---|---|
| New-born | 53 (11.1%) | 0 |
| 31d-1 yr | 132 (27.7%) | 2 |
| 1-1.99 yr | 51 (10.7%) | 6 |
| 2-2.99 yr | 41 (9.7%) | 16 |
| 3-3.99 yr | 17 (3.6%) | 27 |
| 4-4.99 yr | 15 (3.2%) | 54 |
| 5-5.99 yr | 19 (4.0%) | 62 |
| 6-6.99 yr | 17 (3.6%) | 59 |
| 7-7.99 yr | 22 (4.6%) | 67 |
| 8-8.99 yr | 21 (4.4%) | 42 |
| 9-9.99 yr | 15 (3.2%) | 37 |
| 10-10.99 yr | 12 (2.5%) | 25 |
| 11-11.99 yr | 10 (2.1%) | 7 |
| 12-12.99 yr | 20 (4.2%) | 6 |
| 13-13.99 yr | 12 (2.5%) | 10 |
| 14-14.99 yr | 7 (1.5%) | 1 |
| 15-15.99 yr | 2 (0.4%) | 0 |
| > 16 yr | 5 (1.1%) | 7 |

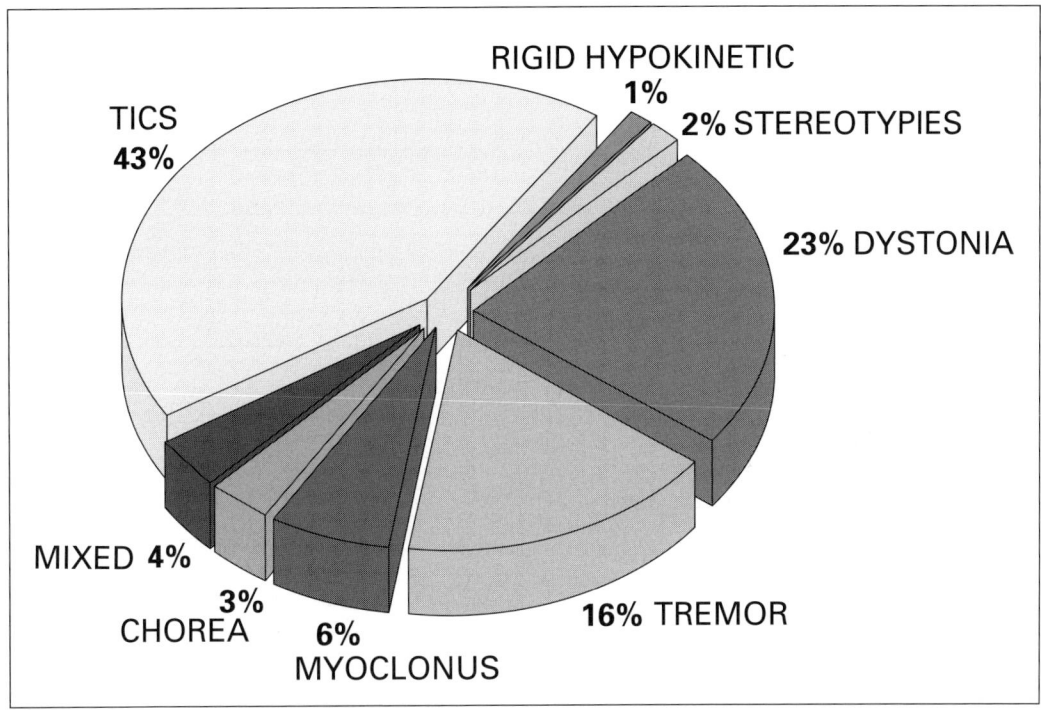

**Figure 1.** Percentage of 964 PMDs cases according to the type of abnormal movement.

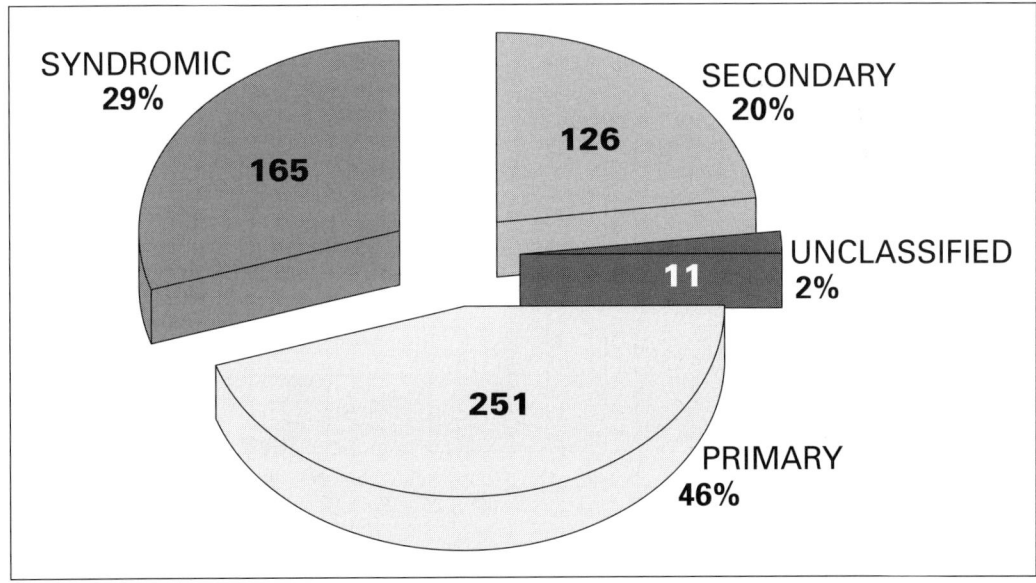

**Figure 2.** Absolute figures and percentage of 548 PMDs according to their aetiology. Tics not included.

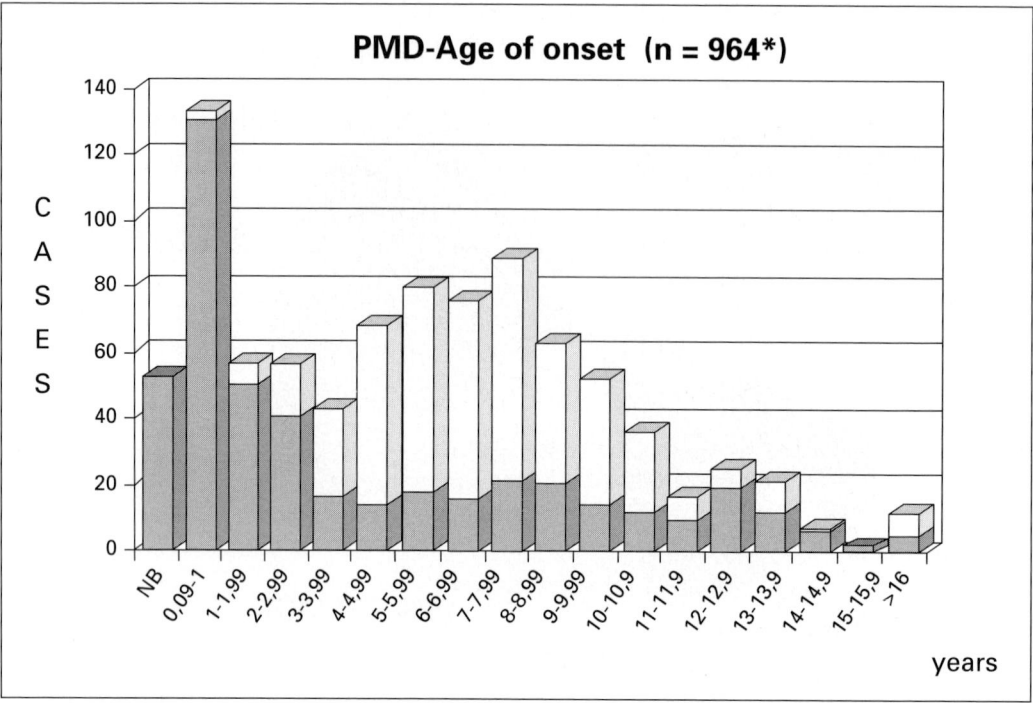

**Figure 3.** Age of onset of 904 PMDs cases (Iatrogenic and dyskinetic cerebral palsy excluded). Spotted bar = Non-tics cases.

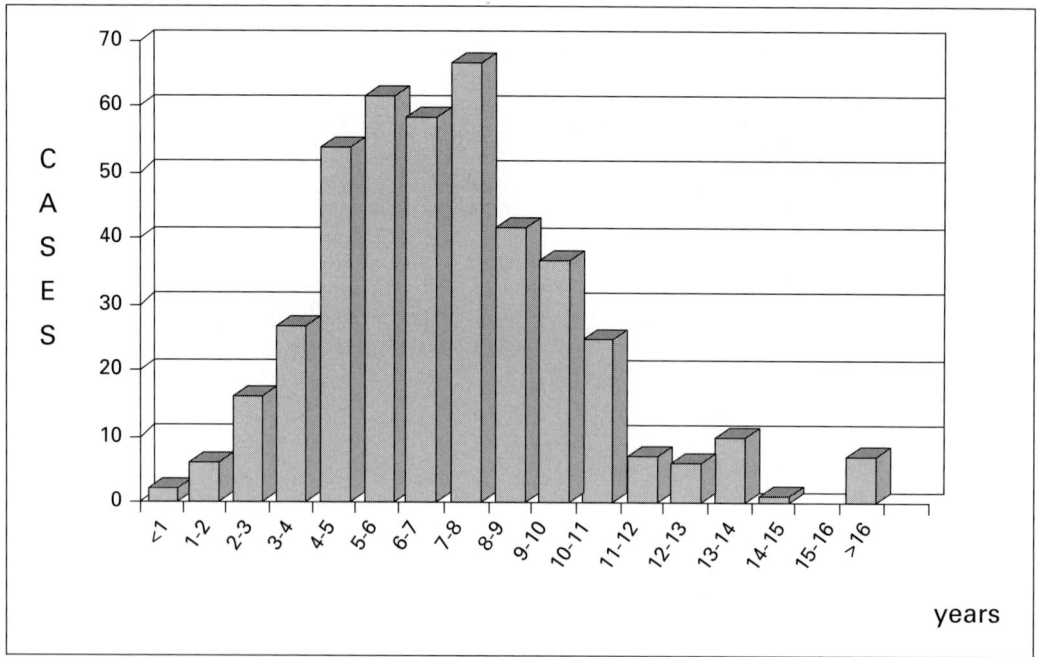

**Figure 4.** Tics: Distribution of a age of onset in 428 cases.

Table III. Mean age of onset in years of Tourette syndrome (Number of cases).

|  | N |  |
|---|---|---|
| Bruun, 1988 [10] | 5.8 | (350) |
| Erenberg et al., 1987 [9] | 6.3 | (200) |
| Freeman et al., 2000 | 6.4 | (3500) |
|  | male 6.3, female 6.6 | |
| Present series | male 6.40 (DS ± 2.49) (n = 248) female 6.54 (DS ± 2.99) (n = 79) total 6.44 (DS ± 2.62) (n = 327) | |
| Shapiro et al., 1988 | 6.7 | (661) |
| Comings and Comings, 1985 | 6.9 | (250) |
| Goldenberg et al., 1994 | 6.9 | (112) |
| Nee et al., 1980 | 7.0 | (50) |
| Lees et al., 1984 | 7.0 | (53) |

## Male/female proportion (Table IV)

The male predominance in tics is well known with a male-to-female ratio estimated around 4:1 [14]. Less known is the male predominance in paediatric cases with tremor. This male predominance is partially in consequence with the male predominance in essential tremor (ET). ET is the main disease causing paediatric non-cerebellar tremor [15-17]. In contrast to the association between male gender and paediatric ET, the prevalence of ET among adults is similar in both sexes in population-based studies as well as studies that ascertain their patients from medical centres [18]. But even excluding essential tremor there is also a male predominance in the remaining paediatric tremor cases (Table XI).

Table IV. Percentage of male/female according to the type of MD.

|  | Male | Female |
|---|---|---|
| Tics | 76 | 24 |
| Stereotypies | 69 | 31 |
| Tremor | 63 | 37 |
| Complex MD | 55 | 45 |
| Dystonia | 50 | 50 |
| Rigid-hypokinetic syndrome | 50 | 50 |
| Myoclonus | 42 | 58 |
| Chorea | 31 | 69 |

Female predominance is known in rheumatic chorea (9 of our eleven cases are female) and in the defect of GTP cyclohydrolase I or Segawa disease where the ratio female to male is 2.5:1 [19].

The factors that determine age of onset and sex distribution of PMDs are unknown. A role for cerebral steroids has been suggested on the basis of animal studies to explain male predominance in some autosomal inherited diseases [20].

## Percentage of primary, syndromic and secondary PMDs cases *(Table V)*

Almost a half of the PMDs cases are primary (the abnormal movement is the only symptom, no structural abnormality can be appreciated in the CNS and, the disorder is not related to acquired causes). 81 cases (33%) of the primary type are transient cases. More than a quarter of PMDs in our series are syndromic (genetic diseases where neurological symptoms are added to the abnormal movement or a CNS lesion can be demonstrated). Only 20 per cent of our PMDs cases can be classified as secondary.

Interestingly 59 cases (36% of the syndromic group) are metabolic diseases. In our series the most frequent metabolic disease is glutaric aciduria (23 cases) accounting for almost the 40 per cent of the metabolic cases and 14% of the total syndromic cases.

Table V. Percentage and number of PMDs cases according to aetiology (n = 547).

|  | Percent | Cases* |
|---|---|---|
| Primary | 46 | 246 |
| Syndromic | 29 | 165 |
| Secondary | 20 | 126 |
| Unclassified | 2 | 10 |

* Tics not included.

## Chronic vs transient PMDs *(Table VI)*

Chronic cases predominate over transient cases. The clear predominance of chronic versus transient cases (88 *versus* 12% and 84 *versus* 16% if tics are not included) is most probably influenced by the fact that our department is considered a reference center. However if tics are excluded the prevalence of transient cases is closely related to the age of onset of PMDs *(Table VII)*. The 40% of subjects with PMDs starting within the first year of age have transient disorder versus only 4% in the cases with onset at an older age. Of the 12 transient PMDs cases with onset after one year, 4 were benign palatal myoclonus.

Table VI. Percentage of 964 PMDs cases according to evolution.

|  | Cases* | % | All cases** | % |
|---|---|---|---|---|
| Chronic | 458 | 84 | 841 | 88 |
| Transient | 89 | 16 | 123 | 12 |

* Tics not included.
** Tics included.

Table VII. Chronic vs transient PMDs according to age of onset*.

|  | Chronic | % | Transient | % |
|---|---|---|---|---|
| New born period | 37 | 70 | 16 | 30 |
| 1 month to 1 year | 73 | 55 | 59 | 45 |
| > 1 year | 279 | 96 | 12 | 4 |

* Tics not included.

## Prevalence of tics

Almost half (43%) of our PMDs patients consulted because of tics. It is quite probable that the predominance of tics in the childhood population is even greater considering that mild to moderate cases often do not reach medical attention, are unrecognised or misdiagnosed. Frequently they are followed by a paediatric psychiatrist or psychologist and only the more severe cases are referred to the neuropediatrician. Frequency of tics according to the DSMIV classification is shown in *Table VIII*. It shows that two thirds of our patients had Tourette syndrome while only 8% of the cases had transient tics.

Table VIII. Frequency of tics according DSMIV classification.

|  | Male | Female | Total |
|---|---|---|---|
| Tourette syndrome | 215 | 60 | 275 (66%) |
| Chronic tics | 75 | 34 | 109 (26%) |
| Transient tics | 21 | 13 | 34 (8%) |

Because Tourette disease is better defined than transient or chronic tics and, usually last for a longer period, epidemiological studies are easier to realize [21]. The proteomorphic presentation, variable expressivity and the variation with age (highest severity reported between the ages of 9 and 14) [22] contribute to the difficulties for rigorous epidemiological studies. Other methodological difficulties are the fact that often symptoms diminish with age and, that male subjects are more likely to show tics [14].

Apparently, the prevalence seems to be similar regardless of ethnicity [23, 24], culture or geography. Prevalence figures in the general population, obtained in community based studies, are controversial *(Table IX)*. They range from 2,87 [25] to 1200 per 10000 [26] and they are about 8-9 times more frequent in males than in females. The prevalence of Tourette syndrome in psychiatric populations (especially in children with autism) is higher than in the general population [27-29]. As it can be seen in *Table IX* the figures of prevalence show important differences. Interestingly when the sample is larger and the population older [30, 31, 25] the figures of prevalence are

**Table IX. Epidemiological studies on the prevalence of Tourette syndrome in children.**

| Age | Sample size | Screening procedure | Prevalence per 10.000 | Country | Authors |
|---|---|---|---|---|---|
| 6-12 | 482 | Parent int | 1200 | USA | Lapouse et al., 1964 [26] |
| 9-12 | 1919 | Parent & teacher int | 400 | UK | Rutter et al., 1970 [27] |
| 9-12 | 95* | Parent & teacher int | 1800 | UK | Rutter et al., 1970 [27] |
| 6-16 | 1100 | Population sample | 770 | USA | Achenbach et al., 1978-9 [64, 65] |
| 6-18 | 140580 | Q | 5,2 (9, 3 m; 1 f) | USA | Burd et al., 1986 [30] |
| 5-18 | 142636 | Protocol | 2,87 | USA | Caine et al., 1988 [25] |
| 7-14 | 3034 | Classroom observat | 75,8 (105, 5 m, 13,2 f) | USA | Comings et al., 1990 [66] |
| 4-12 | 1218 | Mailing + tel int | 50 | Japan | Nomoto & Machiyama, 1990 [67] |
| 16-17 | 28037 | Armed forces | 4,2 (4,9 m, 3,1 f) | Israel | Apter et al., 1993 (31) |
| 9-15 | 35 | Personal interview + Parent Q | 490 | USA | Kurlan et al., 1994 [28] |
| 9-15 | 35** | Parent Q | 2190 | USA | Kurlan et al., 1994 [28] |
| 13-14 | 576 | Parent, teacher, pupil Q | 299 | UK | Mason et al., 1998 [68] |
| 13-14 | 918 | Q + Int + Exam | 76 to 185 | UK | Hornsey et al., 2001 [69] |
| 6-11 | 2347 | Teacher observation | 290 | Italy | Lanzi et al., 2004 [23] |
| 6-12 | 2000 | Q + Int + Score | 56 | Taiwan | Wang and Kuo, 2003 [24] |

* Psychiatric sample; ** Special classes.
Q, Questionnaire; Int, Interview; Exam, examination; tel, telephone; m, male; f, female.

ten or even twenty times lower than in the rest of the studies. Such data suggest a tendency towards a natural reduction in the frequency of tics after the age of 15 years.

When family members of affected people were directly interviewed, the frequency of tics for which no medical advice was sought was high [32]. Annual incidence of TD in a population-based study was 0,46 per 100,000 persons [33].

## Prevalence of dystonia

In general population prevalence of primary dystonias is between 11,3 and 29,5 per 100,000 [34-37] a figure similar in different countries.

In our series dystonia is the second more frequent PMDs after tics (Table I) and when tics are not included it represents 40% of the cases. Forty-four per cent (98) are primary cases, 35% (78) syndromic and the remaining 20% (46) secondary cases. Among the 78 syndromic cases, 47 are due to metabolic diseases. Glutaric aciduria type 1 is the most prevalent (23 cases) neurometabolic disease, with dystonia as the most prominent abnormal movement, followed by mitochondrial cytopathies (11 cases).

## Prevalence of tremor

Tremor is, in our series, the third MD in frequency after tics and dystonia. Although it is possible that the cerebellum or cerebellar pathways are involved in any type of tremor, only tremors not associated with cerebellar syndrome have been considered here. We considered as tremor a rhythmical oscillation of a part of the body around a fixed point or place resulting from alternating synchronous contractions of antagonist muscles reciprocally innervated [38]. With this definition slow cephalic tremors as observed in bobble head doll syndrome or in nodding head or less clear transient infant "tremors" such as jitteriness or shuddering spells were included in the tremor group *(Table X)*.

**Table X. Classification of paediatric non-cerebellar tremor.**

1. **Idiopathic**
    *1.1. Transient*
     – jitteriness
     – shuddering spells
     – essential palatal tremor
     – essential laryngeal tremor
     – *spasmus nutans*
    *1.2. Chronic*
     – enhanced physiological tremor
     – essential tremor
     – trembling of the chin

2. **Secondary**
    – parkinsonian (sometimes idiopathic)
    – essential-like associated
    – neuromuscular diseases
    – endocrinological disorders
    – metabolic diseases
    – drug induced
    – other disorders

The 16 percent (increasing to 30% if tics are not considered) of our PMDs cases show tremor as the main symptom *(Table I)*. Essential Tremor is the main cause (61/163 = 37%) of the childhood onset non cerebellar tremor. Jitteriness, shuddering spells, *spasmus nutans* and nodding head represents 24 cases (14% of the tremor cases). Interestingly 8 cases (5%) were functional (psychogenic). In 10 cases no definite cause of the tremor was found.

The prevalence of ET in childhood is unknown. Epidemiological studies in the adult populations, using community-based design, gave widely discrepant estimates of prevalence varying from between 4.1 to 39.2 per 1000 [18]. In community-based studies [39, 40] approximately 5% of new ET cases arise during childhood so we may to deduce that if the prevalence in the adult population is about 10/1000, in children the prevalence would be about 0,5/1000. But these figures can only be extrapolated with caution because there are basic differences concerning tremor in childhood and adults as for instance the male predominance in overall childhood tremor (Table IV), ET (see above) and also in non-ET childhood tremor (Table XI).

Table XI. Male/female percentage in paediatric non-cerebellar tremor.

|  | Male | Female |
|---|---|---|
| Essential tremor (n = 61) | 72 | 28 |
| No essential tremor (n = 92)* | 55 | 45 |
| All tremor cases (n = 163) | 63 | 37 |

\* 10 cases of tremor were not included because the evolution does not allow its classification.

## Prevalence of myoclonus

Differentiation between epileptic and non-epileptic myoclonus may sometimes be difficult. We consider non-epileptic myoclonus when an EEG paroxysm is not temporally linked with the clinical jerk and its electromyographic correlates. If tics are excluded, 11 per cent of our MPD had myoclonus as main movement disorder. Half (30) of the myoclonic cases were primary; 12 cases (20%) were syndromic and 19 (30%) were secondary. Caviness [41] in a general population study in Minnesota (USA) found an incidence of myoclonus of 1.3 cases for 100,000 person-years.

## Prevalence of chorea

As mentioned above ballismus is included in this group. In our series, as reported in the literature [42, 43], we found a female (69%) predominance. The main aetiology was rheumatic chorea (11/31 patients). Other causes included: lethargic encephalitis (2 cases), paroxysmal dyskinesia (2 cases) and some other disorders. No cause was found in 3 patients.

The mean age of onset in our 31 cases with chorea or ballismus as the predominant symptom was 4 years and did not differ with sex. The maximum prevalence of rheumatic chorea was between 7 and 12 years [44, 45]. In our series mean age of onset of rheumatic chorea was 8.33 years (range, 2.75 to 13 years). In rheumatic chorea there was a 2:1 female predominance but only after 10 years of age which suggests an influence of sex steroids [46]. In the literature a family history of chorea is found in 13 to 26% of cases [44] suggesting a genetic predisposition. After a marked decrease in incidence of rheumatic chorea in industrialised countries [47], even greater than that of rheumatic fever, recrudescence of chorea is being observed in the USA, United Kingdom and probably other developed countries [48, 49].

## Prevalence of rigid hypokinetic syndrome (RHS)

Rigid hypokinetic syndrome was the least frequent of our PMDs. Only 13 cases had rigid-hypokinetic syndrome as the main movement disorders symptom. None were primary cases. One was secondary to a subacute sclerosing panencephalitis. The 12 remaining were syndromic cases. There were no RHS primary cases in this cohort.

Aetiology in the syndromic group (12 patients) showed significant variability. Wilson disease (2 cases), Hallervorden-Spatz disease (3 cases), Huntington disease (1 case), GM2 (2 cases), neuronal intranuclear inclusion disease (2 cases), Gaucher disease (1 case), and an unidentified progressive leukoencephalopathy (1 case). The mean age of onset of the 13 RHS cases was 10.8 +/- 3,75 (range, 1 to 15) clearly higher than the mean age of onset (3,83 years) of the overall (excluding tics) cases of our series (n = 474). In the review of Pranzatelli et al. [50] based on 17 cases (6 personal cases) the main cause of secondary parkinsonism in children was encephalitis (6 cases), followed by hydrocephalus (4 cases).

## Prevalence of stereotypies

Stereotypies represent only 2% (16 cases) of our cases but their real prevalence is obviously higher. Several reasons justify this low figure. Firstly, stereotypies are commonly considered as a minor symptom when associated to severe pervasive disorders such as autism, mental retardation or sensory handicaps so, in many of these patients the stereotypies are not considered a reason for referral. Secondly, in our series stereotypies were only included in the database from January 2000 and moreover the stereotypies of Rett syndrome were excluded. Nine cases are primary cases, six syndromic and only 1 secondary (due to hydrocephalus).

Some primary stereotypies (also called physiologic) are frequent. Head banging occurs generally with the child in the prone position on all fours. It is observed in 5.1% [51] to 15.2% [52] of otherwise normal infants. It is more common in boys. Head rolling is a rhythmic oscillation of the head and it is also common in infants and young children (6.3 to 19.1%) [51].

In otherwise normal subjects stereotypies spontaneously disappear [53, 54] but in a small percentage (3% to 9% at age 5-8 years) [55, 56] will continue even in adolescence and adulthood [57].

## Prevalence of complex movement disorders

As previously mentioned the term "complex movements" has been applied when several types of abnormal movement, without clear predominance of any type, coexisted or when no clear definition of the movement was possible.

Forty cases (7%) in this series were included in this group. The "complex movement" group is a miscellaneous one, 40% being secondary and 37% syndromic.

## Prevalence of dyskinetic cerebral palsy

Prevalence of dyskinetic cerebral palsy has been deduced from the figures of all the cases of cerebral palsy. In industrialised countries the prevalence of cerebral palsy has been found to be around 25 per 10.000 live born infants [58] and dyskinetic cerebral palsy, which represents around 10% of the all subjects with cerebral palsy [59], so the prevalence of dyskinetic cerebral palsy should be around 3/10.000. This figure persists almost unmodified even if in more developed countries, where the prevalence of dyskinetic cerebral palsy secondary to Rhesus incompatibility is now very low [60].

As we previously mentioned cases of dyskinetic cerebral palsy have not been included in our series. However we have included the 16 cases of delayed onset dyskinesia [61].

## Prevalence of paediatric *versus* Adult movement disorders

The different prevalence between paediatric and adult patients according to the type of movement disorder is striking. In a large adult movement disorders series (2471 subjects) issued by a referral center, rigid-hypokinetic syndrome (parkinsonism) was the main group with 56.2%, tremor was the second with 23.1%, followed by dystonia only 8.3% and chorea 5.8% [62] (*Table XII*).

Table XII. Percentage of main MD types in 2471 adult cases *versus* 548 paediatric cases of our series. In both series tics are not included.

|  | Adult MD | PMDs |
|---|---|---|
| Rigid-hypokinetic | 56 | 2 |
| Tremor | 23 | 30 |
| Dystonia | 8 | 40 |
| Chorea | 5.8 | 6 |

Tremor (23.1% in the adult series *versus* 16% in our paediatric series) and chorea (5.8 *versus* 3% respectively) did not show significant differences. Even if the criteria used in the two series were not identical, differences between HR-S and dystonia cases with onset in adulthood and paediatric cases are so important that they overcome small methodological differences.

Factors that influence the predominance of some types of movement disorders in children as opposed to adults or their sex distribution are not known but, probably, neurotransmitters and the structures implicated in the complex process of movement are involved.

Of especial interest is the fact that when rigid-hypokinetic syndrome occurs at the paediatric age it is often associated with dystonia. It has been speculated that the same disorder of the basal ganglia that creates dystonia in childhood would produce parkinsonism in adulthood [63]. According to this theory, when Hallervorden-Spatz disease starts in the paediatric age, usually dystonia is the main abnormal movement but if the disease starts in the adult age parkinsonism predominates. Furthermore in early onset (before the age of 20 years) Parkinson's disease shows a high incidence of dystonia that sometimes precedes the appearance of parkinsonism.

## ■ Concluding remarks

The present series provides a relatively biased view of the frequency of paediatric movement disorders, as it may reflect the referral of more severe and complicated cases to a specialised child neurology centre. However, it also provides useful information on the predominance of movement disorders in children according to sexes, age at onset and evolution. It also allows comparison of relative frequency according to the predominant type of movement.

Paediatric Movement Disorders occur worldwide. However, differences between populations do exist, presumably because of different genetic and/or cultural characteristics or infectious conditions. This is well illustrated by the prevalence of rheumatic chorea, which is ten times higher in Brazil than in Europe, and the prevalence of conditions with acute necrosis of the thalamic structures, much more frequent in Japan.

The majority of our recruitment comes from the Mediterranean region. Even if during the last decade emigration mainly from South America and the North Africa countries increased considerably, the Spanish population remained quite stable. Consequently, it is still possible to dispose of a long term follow-up and an overall appreciation of the natural evolution of the various movement disorders in children.

The population included in this series is predominantly of Spanish origin. Consequently, differences due to ethnicity or culture are not represented, and this is a limitation to be taken under consideration. Similar studies in other regions are necessary.

# References

1. Unger JP, Dujardin J. Epidemiology's contribution to health service management and planing in developing countries: a missing link. *Bull World Health Organiz* 1992; 70: 487-97.
2. Fernández-Alvarez E, Aicardi J. *Movement disorders in children.* London: Mac Keith Press, 2001.
3. Marsden CD, Quinn NP. The dystonias. Neurological disorders affecting 20.000 people in Britain. *British Med J* 1990; 300: 139-44.
4. Németh AH. The genetics of primary dystonias and related disorders. *Brain* 2002; 125: 695-721.
5. Kamm T. Idiopathic torsion dystonia. *Orphanet encyclopedia*, May 2004.
6. Nee LE, Caine ED, Polinsky RJ, Elridge R, Eberth MH. Gilles de la Tourette syndrome: clinical and family study of 50 cases. *Ann Neurol* 1980; 7: 41-9.
7. Lees AJ, Robertson M, Trimble MR, Murray MMF. A clinical study of Gilles de la Tourette Syndrome in the United Kingdom. *J Neurol Neurosurg Psychiat* 1984; 47: 1-8.
8. Comings DE, Comings BG. Tourette syndrome: clinical and psychological aspects of 250 cases. *Am J Hum Genet* 1985; 37: 435.
9. Erenberg G, Cruse RP, Rothner AD. The natural history of Tourette syndrome: a follow-up study. *Ann Neurol* 1987; 22: 383-5.
10. Bruun RD. *The natural history of Tourette's syndrome.* In: Cohen DJ, Bruun RD, Leckman JF, eds. *Tourette's syndrome and tic disorders: clinical understanding and treatment.* New York: Wiley, 1988: 21-40.
11. Shapiro AK, Shapiro ES, Young JG, Fenberg TE. *Gilles de la Tourette Syndrome.* 2nd edition. New York: Raven Press, 1988.
12. Goldenberg JN, Brown SB, Weiner WJ. Coprolalia in younger patients with Gilles de la Tourette syndrome. *Mov Disord* 1994; 9: 622-5.

13. Freeman RD, Fast DK, Burd L, Kerbeshian J, Robertson MM, Sandor P. An international perspective on Tourette syndrome: selected findings from 3500 individuals in 22 countries. *Dev Med Child Neurol* 2000; 42: 436-47.
14. Tanner CM, Goldman SM. Epidemiology of Tourette syndrome. *Neurol Clin of NA* 1997; 15 (2): 395-402.
15. Fernández-Alvarez E, López-Casas J. *Essential tremor (ET) in childhood*. In: Arzimanoglou A, Goutières F, eds. *Trends in child neurology*. Paris: John Libbey Eurotext, 1996: 147-55.
16. Paulson GW. Benign essential tremor in childhood. *Clin Ped* 1976; 15: 67-70.
17. Louis ED, Dure L, Pullman S. Essential tremor in childhood. *Mov Disord* 2001; 16: 921-3.
18. Louis ED, Ottman R, Hauser WA. How common is the most common adult movement disorder? Estimates of the prevalence of essential tremor throughout the world. *Mov Disord* 1998; 13: 5-10.
19. Nygaard TG, Marsden CD, Duvoisin RC. Dopa-responsive dystonia. *Adv Neurol* 1988; 50: 377-84.
20. Loscher W, Blanke T, Richter A, Hoppen HO. Gonadal sex hormones and dystonia: experimental studies in genetically dystonic hamsters. *Mov Disord* 1995; 10: 92-102.
21. Pappert EJ, Goetz CG, Louis ED, Blasucci L, Leurgans S. Objective assessments of longitudinal outcome in Gilles de la Tourette's syndrome. *Neurology* 2003; 61: 936-40.
22. Leckman JF, Zhang H, Vitale A, et al. Course of tic severity in Tourette syndrome. The first two decades. *Pediatrics* 1998; 102: 14-9.
23. Lanzi G, Zambrino CA, Termine C, et al. Prevalence of tic disorders among primary school students in the city of Pavia. *Italy Arch Dis Childh* 2004; 89: 45-7.
24. Wang HS, Kuo MF. Tourette's syndrome in Taiwan: an epidemiological study of tic disorders in an elementary school at Taipei County. *Brain Develop* 2003; 25 (suppl 1): S29-S31.
25. Caine ED, McBride MC, Chiverton P, Bamford KA, Rediess S, Shiao J. Tourette's syndrome in Monroe County school children. *Neurology* 1988; 38: 472-5.
26. Lapouse R, Mank M. Behaviour deviation in a representative sample of children, variation by sex, age, race, social class and family size. *Am J Orthopsychiat* 1964; 34: 436-46.
27. Rutter M, Graham P, Yule W. *A neuropsychiatric study in childhood*. London: Spastic International Medical Publications, 1970.
28. Kurlan R, Whitmore BA, Irvine BS, McDermott MP, Como PG. Tourette's syndrome in a special education population: a pilot study involving a single school district. *Neurology* 1994; 44: 699-702.
29. Baron-Cohen S, Scahill VL, Izaguirre J, Hornsey H, Robertson MM. The prevalence of Gilles de la Tourette syndrome in children and adolescents with autism: a large scale study. *Psycholog Med* 1999; 29: 1151-9.
30. Burd L, Kerbeshian J, Wikenheiser M, Fisher WI. A prevalence study of Gilles de la Tourette's syndrome in North Dakota school-age children. *J Am Acad Child Psychiatry* 1986; 25: 552-3.
31. Apter A, Pauls DL, Bleich A, et al. An epidemiological study on Gilles de la Tourette's syndrome. *Israel Arch Gen Psychiatry* 1993; 50: 734-38.
32. Kurlan R. Tourette's syndrome: current concepts. *Neurology* 1989; 39: 1625-30.
33. Lucas AR, Behar CM, Rajput AH, Kurland LT. Tourette syndrome in Rochester, Minnesota (1968-79). In: Friedhoff AJ, Chase TN, eds. *Advances in Neurology*, vol. 35: Gilles de la Tourette Syndrome. New York: Raven Press, 1982: 267-9.
34. Nutt JG, Muenter MD, Aronson A, Kurland LT, Melton LJ. Epidemiology of focal and generalized dystonia in Rochester Minnesota. *Mov Disord* 1988; 3: 188-94.
35. Duffey POF, Butler AG, Hawthorne MR, Barnes MP. *The epidemiology of the primary dystonias in the North of England*. In: Fahn S, Marsden CD, De Lange M, eds. *Advance in neurology, dystonia 3*, vol 28. Philadelphia: Lippincott Raven, 1998: 121-5.
36. The epidemiological study of dystonia in Europe (ESDE) collaborative group. A prevalence study of primary dystonia in eight European countries. *J Neurol* 2000; 247: 787-92.

37. Matsumoto S, Nishimura M, Shibasaki H, Kaji R. Epidemiology of primary dystonias in Japan: comparison with Western countries. *Mov Disord* 2003; 18: 1196-8.
38. Jankovic J, Fahn S. Physiologic and pathologic tremors: diagnosis, mechanism, and management. *Ann Intern Med* 1980; 93: 460-5.
39. Hornabrook RW, Nagurney JT. Essential tremor in Papau New Guinea. *Brain* 1976; 99: 659-72.
40. Rajput AH, Offord KP, Beard CM, Kurland LT. Essential tremor in Rochester, Minnesota: a 45-year study. *J Neurol Neurosurg Psychiatry* 1984; 47: 466-70.
41. Caviness JN. *Epidemiology of myoclonus*. In: S. Fahn, ed. *Myoclonus and paroxysmal dyskinesias. Advances in Neurology*, vol. 89. Philadelphia: Lippincott Williams & Wilkins, 2002: 19-22.
42. Klawans HG, Brandaburg MM. Chorea in childhood. *Pediatr Annals* 1993; 22: 43-50.
43. Fernández-Alvarez E. Chorea in children. *Acta Neuropediatr* 1996; 2: 116-25.
44. Nausieda PA, Grossman BJ, Koller WC, Weiner WJ, Klawans HL. Sydenham chorea: an update. *Neurology* 1980; 30: 331-4.
45. Cardoso F, Eduardo C, Silva AP, Mota CCC. Chorea in fifty consecutive patients with rheumatic fever. *Mov Disord* 1997; 12: 701-3.
46. Bédard PJ, Langelier P, Dancova J. Estrogens, progesterone and the extrapyramidal system. In: Advances in Neurology, vol. 24, Poirier LJ, Sourkes TL, Bédard P, eds. *The extrapyramidal system and its disorders*. New York: Raven Press, 1979: 411-22.
47. Markowitz M. The decline of rheumatic fever: Role of medical intervention. *J Pediatr* 1985; 106: 545-50.
48. Kavey RE, Kaplan EL. Resurgence of acute rheumatic fever. *Pediatrics* 1989; 84: 585-6.
49. Philips S, Hogg J, Kurth M, Green J. A resurgence of Sydenham's chorea in children in West Texas with atypical presentations. *Neurology* 1992; 42 (suppl 3): 288.
50. Pranzatelli MR, Mott SH, Pavlakis SG, Conry JA, Tate ED. Clinical spectrum of secondary parkinsonism in childhood: A reversible disorder. *Pediatr Neurol* 1994; 10: 131-40.
51. Sallustro F, Atwell CW. Body rocking, head banging and head rolling in normal children. *J of Pediatr* 1978; 93: 704-8.
52. De Lissovoy V. Head banging in early childhood: a study of incidence. *J Pediatr* 1961; 58: 803-5.
53. Kravitz H, Boehm J. Rhythmic habit patterns in infancy: their sequence, age of onset and frequency. *Child Dev* 1971; 42: 399-413.
54. Ritvo ER, Ornitz EM, La Franchis S. Frequency of repetitive behaviours in early infantile autism and its variants. *Arch Gen Psychiat* 1968; 19: 341-7.
55. Abe K, Oda N, Amatomi M. Natural history and predictive significance of head-banging, head-rolling and breath-holding spells. *Dev Med Child Neurol* 1984; 26: 644-8.
56. Werry JS, Carlielle J, Fitzpatrick J. Rhythmic motor activities (stereotypes) in children under five: etiology and prevalence. *J Am Acad Child Psychiat* 1983; 22: 329-36.
57. Castellanos FX, Ritchie GF, Marsh WL, Rapoport JL. DSM-IV stereotypic movement disorder: Persistence of stereotypes of infancy in intellectually normal adolescents and adults. *J Clin Psychiatry* 1996; 57: 116-22.
58. Meberg A, Broch H. Etiology of cerebral palsy. *J Perinat Med* 2004; 32: 434-9.
59. Costeff H. Estimated frequency of genetic and nongenetic causes of congenital idiopathic cerebral palsy in West Sweden. *Ann Hum genet* 2004; 68: 515-20.
60. Paneth N. Etiologic factors in cerebral palsy. *Pediatr Ann* 1986; 15: 191, 194-95, 197-201.
61. Burke RE, Fahn S, Gold AP. Delayed-onset dystonia in patients with "static" encephalopathy. *J Neurol Neurosurg Psychiat* 1980; 43: 789-97.
62. Vazquez-Allen P, Perez-Gilabert Y, Mateo D, Gimenez-Roldan S. Estudio sobre una base de datos de 2.471 pacientes con enfermedad de Parkinson y trastornos del movimiento en el Área Sanitaria 1, de la Comunidad de Madrid. Cambios demográficos observados a lo largo de ocho años. *Rev Neurol* 2000; 30: 635-40.

63. Segawa M. Development of the nigrostriatal dopamine neuron and the pathways in the basal ganglia. *Brain Develop* 2000; 20: S1-S4.
64. Achenbach TM. The child behavior profile: I Boys aged 6-11. *J Consult Clin Psychol* 1978; 46: 478-88.
65. Achenbach TM, Edelbrock CS. The child behavior profile: II. Boys aged 12-16 and girls aged 6-11 and 12-16. *J Consult Clin Psychol* 1979; 47: 223-33.
66. Comings DE, Himes JA, Comings BG. An epidemiologic study of Tourette's syndrome in a single school district. *J Clin Psychiatry* 1990; 51: 463-9.
67. Nomoto F, Machiyama Y. An epidemiological study of tics. *Jap J Psychiat Neurol* 1990; 44: 649-55.
68. Mason A, Banerjee S, Eapen V, Zeitlin H, Robertson MM. The prevalence of Tourette syndrome in a mainstream school population. *Dev Med Child Neurol* 1998; 40: 292-6.
69. Hornsey H, Banerjee S, Zeitlin H, Robertson M. The prevalence of Tourette syndrome in 13-14-years-olds in mainstream schools. *J Child Psychol Psychiat* 2001; 42: 1035-9.

# Transient movement disorders of infancy and childhood

**Mahendranath D. Moharir[1], Robert A. Ouvrier[1], Padraic Grattan-Smith[2]**

[1] T.Y. Nelson Department of Neurology and Neurosurgery, Royal Alexandra Hospital for Children, Westmead, Sydney, Australia
[2] Department of Neurology, Sydney Children's Hospital, Randwick, Australia

---

Movement disorders can be classified as transient, paroxysmal and chronic (Fernandez-Alvarez 1998) [1]. Transient movement disorders (TMDs) are simply defined as those that stop over time. In a review by Fernandez-Alvarez (1998), 19% of 356 children under the age of 18 with movement disorders had a TMD [1]. Most common in infancy, TMDs are readily recognised with experience. The generally benign and transient nature of these disorders has resulted in a lack of understanding (but no shortage of theories) as to the underlying cause in most cases. The following discussion approaches the TMDs on the basis of their age of presentation. The aim is to provide a practical approach to the recognition of the more common TMDs. There is insufficient space to discuss the possible theoretical basis of most of these conditions. The differentiation between a transient and a paroxysmal movement disorder is clearly somewhat artificial as many of the latter diminish or stop with time. Conditions such as transient tic disorder and paroxysmal kinesigenic dyskinesia (covered elsewhere in the book) will not be included in this chapter.

## ■ Benign Neonatal Sleep Myoclonus

Benign Neonatal Sleep Myoclonus (BNSM) was described by Coulter and Allen in 1982 [2]. Myoclonic jerks confined to sleep start in the neonatal period. They abruptly stop with arousal and are never seen in the awake state. The jerks are most frequent during NREM sleep but may appear during all stages. They may be unilateral or bilateral and often appear in short clusters and shift sides. The severity of individual jerks and duration of clusters may vary considerably [3]. The EEG is normal both during the jerks and inter-ictally. Detailed neurophysiological studies with back-averaging have not been performed. However, in *Figure 1* of the report of Daoust-Roy and Seshia, the EMG bursts appear to be at least 100 milliseconds, suggesting it is not a form of cortical myoclonus.

Rocking the bassinet or crib [4], touch and simple restraint [3] do not abolish the jerks and may actually induce them. Neurological examination and metabolic investigations are normal. BNSM is more common in pre-term newborns. Usually the jerks cease by 2-7 months of age. A recent report described completely normal follow-up in 5 siblings with BNSM seen 3-10 years after remission [5].

There have been case reports of BNSM being the presenting feature of neuroblastoma [6] and BNSM later followed by myoclonic-astatic epilepsy in childhood [7]. The association may, of course, have been coincidental. The relationship between BNSM and benign myoclonus of early infancy (BMEI) is not clear, although in one series 2/21 patients with BNSM were reported to have developed BMEI on follow-up [8].

## ■ Benign Myoclonus of Early Infancy

Benign myoclonus of early infancy (BMEI) was described by Lombroso and Fejerman in 1977 [9, 10, 11]. The usual age of presentation is between 3 and 15 months. The history is suggestive of infantile spasms with episodes of limb stiffening occurring in clusters. However, unlike infantile spasms the episodes usually occur in the awake state rather than in drowsiness and are often provoked by excitement or frustration. There are rarely more than 10 events in a cluster whereas with established infantile spasms many more episodes can be seen. There is no developmental delay or regression and the neurological examination is normal. Inter-ictal EEG is normal.

Pachatz *et al.* performed video-EEG and polygraphic studies on 5 infants [12]. They showed that the events varied in intensity from single subtle jerks to obvious spasms. Typically there were tonic spasms of the limbs with associated shuddering like movements of the trunk. EMG of the tonic limb spasms revealed durations as long as 2 seconds. The EEG was normal during the spasms. Therefore the term myoclonus is probably not appropriate for these events. Pachatz *et al.* suggested that there was a close similarity between BMEI and "non-epileptic reflex tonic seizures", a condition described by the same group where sustained tonic contractions occur only when the infant is held in someone's arms [12].

The jerking episodes become more prominent for a few weeks or months after onset but within an average of 3 months decrease considerably in most infants. They disappear spontaneously by 2 years of age [9]. Antiepileptic drugs do not stop the episodes. Most of the cases have been sporadic; however familial occurrence has been reported [13]. As well as infantile spasms, the differential diagnosis includes benign myoclonic epilepsy of infancy [11] where there are generalised ictal and inter-ictal EEG abnormalities.

## Shuddering Attacks

Shuddering or shivering attacks were described by Vanasse et al. in 1976 as "an early clinical manifestation of essential tremor" [14]. In a retrospective study of 666 children with paroxysmal non-epileptic events analysed by VEEG monitoring, 7% of the children had shuddering attacks [15]. Shuddering attacks may be mistaken for tonic, absence or myoclonic seizures. Onset of the episodes is as early as 3 to 6 months or after 3 years of age. They are often provoked or aggravated by excitement, fear, anger, frustration, the need to defecate/micturate or embarrassment [14]. The episodes last usually for a few seconds and appear to be a combination of body stiffening and trembling. There is adduction of the knees and arms, flexion of the head, elbows, trunk and knees and flexion or extension of the neck [14]. There may be hundreds of episodes per day. The parents describe the event as though water had been poured down the child's back or the child "had caught a chill" after going out into the cold. There is no alteration in consciousness and the inter-ictal EEG as well as the EEG during the event is normal.

In the study of Vanasse et al., 2 of the 6 children had a mild tremor and in 5, one of the parents had essential tremor [14]. However 3 of the children also had tics and tics were possibly present in 2 others. Subsequent studies by Holmes [16] and Kanazawa [17] did not find an association with a family history of essential tremor. An EMG recording during an attack in one of Kanazawa's patients showed a similar frequency to essential tremor.

In 2 of the children from the Vanasse study [14], the episodes stopped at 4 years and 7 years respectively. In most cases, no treatment is necessary. Treatment with antiepileptic medications has not been effective. Propranolol stopped the attacks in a child who was severely affected [18]. Reif-Lehrer and Stemmerman suggested the episodes might be provoked by ingested monosodium glutamate [19]. Vanasse et al. disagreed with this suggestion [14].

As in many of the TMDs, children with shuddering attacks can have developmental problems [17]. Kanazawa has suggested that shuddering attacks and benign myoclonus of early infancy are the same problem and the term *shuddering attacks of infancy* should be used for both conditions. However other authors disagree e.g. Pachatz et al. [12].

## Transient Idiopathic Dystonia of Infancy

This condition was first reported by Willemse in 1986 [20] and other reports followed [21, 22]. Onset is usually in the first 6 months. There is dystonic posturing of an upper limb and sometimes the trunk or a leg. The typical arm posture is forearm pronation with hyperflexion of the wrist. When prone, the affected arm often rests on the dorsum of the hand. Typically, the posture disappears with intentional movement, for example when reaching out to grab an object. Motor and mental development is usually normal. Deonna et al. [21] reported a slight delay in 2 infants. The posturing usually stops before the age of 2 years. Some cases seem to have more prominent dystonia and a more prolonged clinical course e.g. case 4 of Willemse had Achilles tendon surgery at 2 years and 8 months.

Two of Willemse's cases were siblings and in a personal case (PGS), the mother and a sibling had similar movements in infancy. Genetic factors may therefore have a role.

Symptomatic forms of dystonia are not uncommon in the first year of life and investigations are usually required but the normal development and the lack of functional abnormality suggest this diagnosis. Investigations have been reported to be normal, including imaging and tests for metabolic disorders. However, one report has documented a decreased perfusion of the basal ganglia and left temporomesial cortex using SPECT and decreased glucose metabolism in the basal ganglia and cerebellum in one patient [22]. Worsening of the dystonic posturing apparently induced by cisapride, a 5-HT receptor antagonist, has been described in 2 patients [22, 23].

Beltran and Coker described transient dystonia beginning in the newborn period to 3 months of age in 4 infants exposed to cocaine *in utero* [24]. Torticollis was a particular feature. Angelini [25] described 9 patients with paroxysmal episodes of dystonia involving limbs and trunk. The episodes lasted minutes to hours. It is not clear if this is the same condition.

## ■ Paroxysmal Tonic Upgaze

Ouvrier and Billson (1988) were apparently the first to describe this entity [26]. The clinical features are as follows: (1) onset usually under one year of age, (2) episodes of variably sustained conjugate upward deviation of the eyes, with neck flexion (chin down position) apparently compensating for the abnormal eye position, (3) downbeating saccades in attempted downgaze, (4) normal horizontal eye movements, (5) diurnal fluctuation of symptoms, (6) frequent relief by sleep, (7) exacerbation with febrile illnesses, (8) varying degrees of ataxia, (9) neurological examination usually otherwise normal, (10) absence of deterioration during long-term follow-up, (11) eventual improvement, (12) usually negative investigations, including EEG and CSF neurotransmitters.

Approximately forty-nine cases have been reported [27]. Aetiological factors have included autosomal dominant inheritance in four families and recessive inheritance in two others, foetal exposure to anticonvulsants (including sodium valproate and phenytoin) in several cases, and structural lesions in five (hypomyelination 2, periventricular leukomalacia, Vein of Galen malformation, pinealoma). The pathophysiology is still not understood.

The ocular movement disorder is the most obvious aspect of the condition. It has been reported to begin in the first week of life [28, 29], as late as seven years in an otherwise typical patient [30] or even at nine years in a patient with a pinealoma [31]. A video of the typical ocular findings is available [32].

In the large Melbourne series [28], age of onset was between one week and twenty-six months (mean 5.5 months) while resolution occurred from two days to seven years after onset (mean 2.6 years in ten cases). In the series of Verrotti and colleagues [30] in which six cases were followed for more than ten years, the age of onset varied between 2.6 and 7.4 years and the episodes stopped between one and four years later.

Onset sometimes occurs in the setting of a febrile illness or within twenty-four hours of immunization [28, 30, 31] but is usually insidious. The relationship to sleep may be paradoxical. On one hand, the ocular movement disorder may be absent on awakening and then begin several hours later to be subsequently relieved by sleep [26, 33]. On the other hand, relief by sleep may be variable or absent with the onset of the tonic upgaze occurring immediately after awakening [32; authors' observations]. With time, the duration and frequency of tonic upward gaze episodes decrease until complete cessation. Transient recurrences may occur for several years [28]. In the longer term, vertical or horizontal nystagmus, strabismus and hypometric saccades persist in about 20-25% of patients [27, 28].

Ataxia, occurring either intermittently at the time of attacks of tonic upgaze or as a chronic disability, is clearly an important accompaniment. It is difficult to obtain a clear picture of the frequency, nature and severity of the ataxia from many of the reports but at least twelve of the forty-nine reported cases had residual ataxia. In the video of a patient during an attack of ataxia [32] the patient does not appear to have tonic upgaze at the time suggesting that ataxia may occur independently from the ocular movement disorder. The ataxia appears to be mainly truncal in most cases. Vertigo has been described in a few patients [28; Echenne, – personal communication 2002].

Two of the original patients eventually showed cognitive impairment [26]. One had learning disabilities and the second had mild intellectual impairment and a behaviour disorder. In the Melbourne series of 17 cases [28], 69% had developmental delay, intellectual disability or language delay. Three of the eleven impaired Melbourne cases were siblings with rhizomelic short stature and congenital talipes or alternating exotropia. The cognitive disabilities in the latter family may have been related to the underlying syndrome rather than to the paroxysmal tonic upgaze. On the other hand, the six cases of Verrotti and colleagues were all normal on neurological and formal psychometric testing after a minimum follow-up of ten years [30].

Overall, about 50% of patients appear to have been intellectually normal. Some 40% have learning or mild intellectual deficits and about 10% have moderate to severe intellectual deficits. Verrotti et al. [30] suggested that cases with a later onset might have a better prognosis.

Several cases have had febrile convulsions as might be expected in a series of about fifty children [28, 30, 32]. One or two cases have had epilepsy [28] but repeated electro-encephalographic and videotelemetry studies have consistently excluded epileptic activity at the time of the tonic upgaze. Thus PTU does not appear to be epileptic in origin.

Treatment with the following agents has been unsuccessful: acetazolamide, ACTH and a variety of anticonvulsants. Several cases have had apparent improvement with low dosage L-dopa therapy [26, 33] and a short, carefully monitored treatment trial with the latter agent is probably worthwhile since, if the eye movement disorder is a manifestation of a focal deficit of dopamine, the other manifestations of the disorder such as ataxia and intellectual deficit might also be favourably affected.

## Benign Paroxysmal Torticollis

Snyder first reported this condition in 1969 [34]. Drigo et al. have recently reported a large series of 22 patients [35]. It is characterised by recurrent episodes of torticollis without persistent or obligatory head tilt, followed by subsequent spontaneous resolution. Onset is usually in the first year often between 2 and 8 months of age but sometimes as early as in the first week of life or as late as 30 months. Attacks tend to occur frequently at the onset (1-2 monthly) and sometimes with a striking regularity. Truncal posturing (retrocollis and tortipelvis) may also be seen [36]. A few cases have been familial [37].

The episodes last from 10 minutes to 14 days, may recur two or three times a month, and involve either side [34]. Drigo et al. have suggested the attacks can be subdivided into the more common "periodic torticollis" lasting hours or days and a "paroxysmal" form lasting only minutes and accompanied by ptosis and mydriasis. Many episodes appear in the morning [38] and may be precipitated by postural changes e.g. changing from the upright to the supine position [39]. There may be a prodrome of irritability, pallor, ataxia, distress or vomiting prior to the attack [40]. Ataxia may be a dominant feature [41]. Neurologic examination between attacks is normal. In most cases the attacks stop by 2 to 3 years of age without treatment.

EEG and neuroimaging are normal. Kimura and Nezu [42] performed surface EMG recordings of the left sternocleiodomastoid and right trapezius muscle in a child during an episode of left torticollis. Continuous electrical discharges were noted from both muscles when she was sitting. When lying on a bed, the sternocleiodomastoid activity continued but the trapezius muscle became silent. The authors concluded that the torticollis was a dystonic phenomenon.

The pathophysiology of benign paroxysmal torticollis is subject to speculation. The observation of eye rolling or deviation in some cases suggests labyrinthine involvement. Abnormal oculo-vestibular function has also been suggested [34]. Some believe that benign paroxysmal torticollis is related to benign paroxysmal vertigo & is a migraine-equivalent and may precede these conditions [34, 41, 43]. In a recent report 2 of 4 patients belonged to a kindred with familial hemiplegic migraine and linked to the CACNA1A mutation giving further support that BPT may be a "migraine-equivalent" or a channelopathy [44].

Children with apparent benign paroxysmal torticollis need to be carefully investigated. The differential diagnosis includes seizures, vertigo, gastroesophageal reflux, Sandifer's syndrome, dystonic reaction to drugs [45], posterior fossa, and craniocervical junction abnormalities (basilar impression, platybasia, atlantoaxial instability, Arnold-Chiari malformation, and Klippel-Feil syndrome). Vestibular testing may be difficult to perform and interpret in young children. EEG during the paroxysms is normal. Neuroimaging studies are necessary to exclude congenital and acquired lesions involving the craniocervical region.

Treatment with dimenhydrinate, meclizine, and chlorpromazine has not been successful [34]. The prognosis, however, is favourable and follow-up studies suggest spontaneous resolution in most cases.

## Stereotypies in Normal Children

A wide variety of repetitive movements is readily recognised by parents as part of normal development and these are not considered as TMDs. Body-rocking occurs in 6% to 19% of normal young children [46, 47], thumb-sucking in 21%-31% [48, 47], nail-biting in around 12% of pre-school children, and hair twisting in approximately 16% of normal children [48].

Stereotypic movements are well recognised among neurologically impaired children eg in autism and Rett syndrome. However, they are also commonly seen in children without major neurological impairment. In the authors' experience, they are the second most common movement disorder of childhood after tics. Despite this, there are surprisingly few reports of stereotypic movements in normal children. Tan et al. [49] defined stereotypies as "involuntary coordinated, patterned, repetitive, rhythmic, non-reflex non-goal directed motor activity *that is carried out in exactly the same way during each repetition*" (our italics). They described 10 normal children with stereotypies. Seven were boys. Only 2 of the 10 children seemed to be completely normal, the others had mild learning difficulties, speech problems and attention deficit disorder. The onset of the stereotypies was at 12 months or younger in 5 of the children. The oldest age of onset was 6 years. A large variety of movements were seen. The commonest were arm flapping and leg shaking. The movements appeared when the child was excited, stressed, bored or unoccupied. Follow-up was available to a maximum age of 11 years in 9 children and the stereotypies had completely stopped in only 2.

Stereotypies usually appear earlier than tics. Typically, the same basic movement persists over time although often with elaboration. In contrast with tics, there is usually a constant changing with one tic dominating for a while and then another taking over. The phenomenology of a stereotypic movement may be identical to that of a complex tic or a compulsion. The child's description of the event may help in the differentiation. There may be a sense of pleasure obtained from performing the stereotypy. This is in contrast to the feeling of physical discomfort and need to perform a tic to relieve the discomfort. Older children may report the association of obsessive thoughts with a compulsion.

Stereotypies may superficially resemble seizures but calling the child or interacting with them *e.g.* by tickling can immediately stop the movements. There is generally no need to attempt treatment. Even if the movements persist for a number of years, over time, the child tends to restrict the movements to times when they are not observed by others, for example when they are alone in their bedroom.

## Self-Stimulation (Infant Masturbation)

Infant masturbation was discussed in Still's textbook of 1915 [50]. It is usually only a diagnostic problem in young girls as it is readily recognised in boys. Infant masturbation can be mistaken for epileptic seizures, abdominal pain and paroxysmal dystonia [51-53]. Typically, the legs are tightly opposed and the feet crossed at the ankles. There may also be mechanical pressure over the supra-pubic or pubic area. Pelvic thrusting may be prominent. Irregular breathing, facial flushing sweating, irritable cries and grunting give an impression that the child is in pain. The episodes can last minutes to several hours. A fixed and glazed look may give the impression of altered consciousness but the episode can be usually stopped immediately by picking up the child. This may produce annoyance and resumption of the activity as soon as the child is put down again. Multiple observers have suggested that the infant experiences orgasm and this is often followed by exhaustion, or sleep giving the impression of a post-ictal state [54].

Still and many others since, postulated that the behaviour begins after an episode of local vulval irritation, which sensitises the child to pleasurable sensations arising from genital stimulation. Some young girls persist in the activity for many hours a day (so called "malignant masturbators"). Sexual abuse, family stress, deprivation of affectionate parental physical contact, parental feelings of guilt, anger, shame or perception of the child as vulnerable have all been suggested as underlying causes with very limited proof.

There are few follow-up studies. Bakwin described 3 girls [55]. One continued to perform the movements at 4 years of age. Another stopped at 6-7 months and there had been no recurrence up to age 8 years. The third child, at 12 months carried a large rag doll with her constantly and repeatedly threw it to the floor and would rhythmically press her body against it "as in the sexual act". By 4 years, she rarely exhibited the behaviour and when last seen was a medical student.

No treatment is necessary. It is important to explain to the parents that this is a normal behaviour, more pronounced in some children. Self-stimulation is a better term than masturbation, which carries with it thousands of years of both moral and medical prejudice. Judaic writers regarded it as a crime deserving death and St Thomas Aquinas condemned it as a "sin against nature" [56]. Strindberg vividly describes the supposed medical effects: "he was condemned to death or lunacy by the age of 25! His spinal marrow and brain would rot, his face would turn into a death's head, his hair would fall out, his hands would tremble" [57]. In this apparently enlightened age, a simmering anxiety continues beneath the surface of many parents. Considerable explanation may be required to prevent the use of unsuccessful coercive measures to try to stop this benign activity.

## ■ Movement Disorder of Cobalamin (Vitamin B12) Deficiency

Jadhav et al. described a movement disorder in Indian infants with nutritional cobalamin deficiency in 1962 [58] There have been many subsequent case reports from developed countries [59, 60, 61, 62]. Usually the infant is exclusively breast fed by a mother who is cobalamin deficient either because she has unrecognised pernicious anaemia or is a vegan. Developmental regression begins at around 4-8 months of age and by the time of diagnosis the infant may be profoundly obtunded. The movement disorder is variable in its timing and nature. It can appear before or after treatment. There may be mild choreoathetoid movements, an apparent tremor of one limb that mimics *epilepsia partialis continua* or what appears to be a mixture of tremor and myoclonus so severe as to shake the infant's cot [60]. When the tremor appears after treatment, it is often seen while the infant is less obtunded and otherwise shows neurological improvement. The movements gradually subside over a 1-2 month period. The cause of the movement disorder is not known. There may be a relatively rapid improvement in motor skills but long term intellectual problems often result from the cobalamin deficiency.

## ■ Midazolam Withdrawal Syndrome

Midazolam infusions have been increasingly used in intensive care units to provide sedation and analgesia for critically ill children. Sudden cessation of the midazolam can result in a withdrawal syndrome characterised by an altered state of consciousness, restlessness, irritability, vomiting, tremors and choreoathetoid and dystonic movements [63-66]. This may occur more frequently when the midazolam is combined with fentanyl [67]. In this setting, investigations are required to exclude metabolic disorders and non-convulsive status epilepticus but the possibility of a withdrawal syndrome should be kept in mind as it may be more common than is generally recognised.

## ■ Conclusion

The transient movement disorders of childhood are a distinctive group of disorders that are not rare. Over a number of years of practice, most general paediatric neurologists become familiar with them. They are usually seen in infants. Most require some investigation but recognition allows a limitation of what otherwise could be a very extensive diagnostic work-up. They are a satisfying group of disorders to deal with as most need no specific treatment and settle with time. The long-term neurological outcome is generally good, although some children subsequently are found to have learning and attentional problems.

## References

1. Fernández-Alvarez E. Transient movement disorders in children. *J Neurol* 1998; 245 (1): 1-5.
2. Coulter DL, Allen RJ. Benign neonatal sleep myoclonus. *Arch Neurol* 1982; 39: 191-2.
3. Daoust-Roy J, Seshia SS. Benign neonatal sleep myoclonus. *Am J Dis Child* 1992; 146: 1236-41.
4. Alfonso I, Papazian O, Aicardi J, Jeffries H. A simple manœuvre to provoke benign neonatal sleep myoclonus. *Pediatrics* 1995; 96 (6): 1161-3.
5. Vaccario ML, Valenti MA, Carullo A, Di Bartolomeo R, Mazza S. Benign neonatal sleep myoclonus: a case report and follow-up of four members of an affected family. *Clin Electroencephalogr* 2003; 34 (1): 15-7.
6. Kosaburo A, Watanabe K, Negoro T, *et al*. Neonatal myoclonus and neuroblastoma. *Lancet* 1993; 341: 1410-1.
7. Nolte R. Neonatal sleep myoclonus followed by myoclonic astatic epilepsy: a case report. *Epilepsia* 1989; 30 (6): 844-50.

8. Caraballo R, Yepez I, Cerosimo R, Fejerman N. Benign neonatal sleep myoclonus. *Revista de Neurologia* 1998; 26 (152): 540-4.
9. Lombroso CT, Fejerman N. Benign myoclonus of early infancy. *Ann Neurol* 1977; 1: 138-43.
10. Dravet C, Giraud N, Bureau M, et al. Benign myoclonus of early infancy or benign non-epileptic infantile spasms. *Neuropediatrics* 1986; 17: 33-8.
11. Maydell BV, Berenson F, Rothner D, Wyllie E, Kotagal P. Benign myoclonus of early infancy: an imitator of West's syndrome. *J Child Neurol* 2000; 16: 109-12.
12. Pachatz C, Fusco L, Vigevano F. Benign myoclonus of early infancy. *Epil Disord* 1999; 1: 57-61.
13. Galletti F, Brincotti M, Emanuelli O. Familial occurrence of benign myoclonus of early infancy. *Epilepsia* 1989; 30 (5): 579-81.
14. Vanasse M, Bedard P, Andermann F. Shuddering attacks in children: an early clinical manifestation of early tremor. *Neurology* 1976; 26: 1027-30.
15. Bye AME, Kok DJM, Ferenschild FTJ, Vles JSH. Paroxysmal non-epileptic events in children: a retrospective study over a period of 10 years. *J Ped Child Health* 2000; 36 (3): 244-8.
16. Holmes GL, Russman BS. Shuddering attacks. Evaluation using electroencephalographic frequency modulation radiotelemetry and videotape monitoring. *Am J Dis Child* 1986; 140: 72-3.
17. Kanazawa O. Shuddering attacks-report of four children. *Pediatr Neurol* 2000; 23 (5): 421-4.
18. Barron TF, Younkin DP. Propranolol therapy for shuddering attacks. *Neurology* 1992; 42: 258-9.
19. Reif-Lehrer L, Stemmermann G. Monosodium glutamate intolerance in children. *N Engl J Med* 1975; 293: 1204.
20. Willemse J. Benign idiopathic dystonia with onset in the first year of life. *Dev Med Child Neurol* 1986; 28: 355-63.
21. Deonna T-W, Zeigler A, Nielsen J. Transient idiopathic dystonia in infancy. *Neuropediatrics* 1990; 22: 220-4.
22. John B, Klemm E, Haverkamp F. Evidence for altered basal ganglia and cortical functions in transient idiopathic dystonia. *J Child Neurol* 2000; 15: 820-2.
23. Angelini L, Zorzi G, Rumi V, Nardocci N, Mennini T. Transient paroxysmal dystonia in an infant possibly induced by cisapride. *Ital J Neurol Sci* 1996; 17 (2): 157-9.
24. Beltran RS, Coker SB. Transient dystonia of infancy, a result of intrauterine cocaine exposure? *Pediatr Neurol* 1995; 12: 354-6.
25. Angelini L, Rumi V, Lamperti E, Nardoccci N. Transient paroxysmal dystonia in infancy. *Neuropediatrics* 1988; 19: 171-4.
26. Ouvrier RA, Billson F. Benign paroxysmal tonic upgaze of childhood. *J Child Neurol* 1988; 3: 177-80.
27. Ouvrier RA, Billson F. Paroxysmal tonic upgaze of childhood - A review. *Brain Dev* 2005. In press.
28. Hayman M, Harvey S, Hopkins IJ, Kornberg AJ, Coleman LT, Shield LK. Paroxysmal tonic upgaze: a reappraisal of outcome. *Ann Neurol* 1998; 43: 514-20.
29. Ahn JC, Hoyt WF, Hoyt CS. Tonic upgaze in infancy: a report of three cases. *Arch Ophthalmol* 1989: 107; 57-8.
30. Verrotti A, Trotta D, Blasetti A, Lobefalo L, Gallenga P, Chiarelli F. Paroxysmal tonic upgaze of childhood: effect of age-of-onset on prognosis. *Acta Paediatr* 2001; 90: 1343-5.
31. Spalice A, Parisi P, Iannetti P. Paroxysmal tonic upgaze: physiopathological considerations in three additional cases. *J Child Neurol* 2000; 15: 15-8.
32. Lispi ML, Vigevano F. Benign paroxysmal tonic upgaze of childhood with ataxia. *Epil Disord* 2001; 3: 203-6.
33. Campistol J, Prats JM, Garaizar C. Benign paroxysmal tonic upgaze in childhood with ataxia: a neuro-ophthalmological syndrome of familial origin? *Dev Med Child Neurol* 1993; 35: 436-9.

34. Snyder CH. Paroxysmal torticollis in infancy. A possible form of labyrinthitis. *Am J Dis Child* 1969; 117: 458-60.
35. Drigo P, Carli G, Laverda AM. Benign Paroxysmal Torticollis of infancy. *Brain Dev* 2000; 22 (3): 169-72.
36. Chutorian AM. Benign paroxysmal torticollis, tortipelvis and retrocollis in infancy. *Neurology* 1974; 24: 366-77.
37. Lipson EH, Robertson WC. Paroxysmal torticollis of infancy: familial occurrence. *Am J Dis Child* 1978; 132: 422-3.
38. Hanukoglu A, Somekh E, Fried D. Benign paroxysmal torticollis in infancy. *Clin Pediatr* 1984; 23: 272-4.
39. Cataltepe SE, Barron TF. Benign paroxysmal torticollis presenting as 'seizures' in infancy. *Clin Pediatr* 1993; 32: 564-5.
40. Chaves-Carballo E. Paroxysmal torticollis. *Sem Pediatr Neurol* 1996; 3: 255.
41. Deonna T, Martin D. Benign paroxysmal torticollis in infancy. *Arch Dis Child* 1981; 56: 956-9.
42. Kimura S, Nezu A. Electromyographic study in an infant with benign paroxysmal torticollis. *Pediatr Neurol* 1998; 19 (3): 236-8.
43. Eviatar L. Benign paroxysmal torticollis. *Pediatr Neurol* 1994; 11: 72.
44. Giffin NJ, Benton S, Goadsby PJ. Benign paroxysmal torticollis of infancy: 4 new cases and linkage to CACNA1A mutation. *Dev Med Child Neurol* 2002; 44 (7): 490-3.
45. Casteels Van Daele M. Paroxysmal torticollis in infancy. *Am J Dis Child* 1970; 120: 88.
46. Sallustro F, Atwell CW. Body rocking, head banging, and head rolling in normal children. *J Pediatr* 1978; 93 (4): 704-8.
47. Werry JS, Carlielle J, Fitzpatrick J. Rhythmic motor activities (stereotypies) in children under five: etiology and prevalence. *J Am Acad Child Psych* 1983; 22 (4): 329-36.
48. Troster H. Prevalence and functions of stereotyped behaviours in non-handicapped children in residential care. *J Abnormal Child Psychol* 1994; 22 (1): 79-97.
49. Tan A, Salgado M, Fahn S. The characterization and outcome of stereotypical movements in non-autistic children. *Mov Disord* 1997; 12 (1): 47-52.
50. Still GF. *Common Disorders and Diseases of Childhood, ed 3*. London: Oxford Medical Publications, 1915, 775 p.
51. Livingston S, Berman W, Pauli LL. Masturbation simulating epilepsy. *Clin Pediatr* 1975; 14 (3): 232-4.
52. Flesicher DR, Morrison A. Masturbation mimicking abdominal pain or seizure in young girls. *J Pediatr* 1990; 116: 810-4.
53. Mink JW, Neill JJ. Masturbation mimicking paroxysmal dystonia or dyskinesia in a young girl. *Mov Disord* 1995; 10: 518-20.
54. Bakwin H, Bakwin RM. *Clinical management of behaviour disorders in children, ed 2*. Philadelphia & London: WB Saunders Co, 1960: 394-6.
55. Bakwin H. Erotic feelings in infants and young children. *Am J Dis Child*; 126: 52-4.
56. The politics of masturbation. *Lancet Editorial* 1994; 344: 1714-5.
57. A Strindberg. *The son of a servant*. New York: Anchor Books Doubleday & Co., Inc. Garden City, 1966, 116 p.
58. Jadhav M, Webb JK, Vaishnava S, Baker SJ. Vitamin B12 deficiency in Indian infants: A clinical syndrome. *Lancet* 1962; 2: 903-7.
59. Sadowitz PD, Livingston A, Cavanaugh RM. Developmental regression as an early manifestation of Vitamin B12 deficiency. *Clin Pediatr* 1986; 25 (7): 369-71.
60. Grattan-Smith PJ, Wilcken B, Procopis PG, Wise GA. The neurological syndrome of cobalamin deficiency: developmental regression and involuntary movements. *Mov Disord* 1997; 12 (1): 39-46.

61. Emery ES, Homans AC, Colletti RB. Vitamin B12 deficiency: a cause of abnormal movements in infants. *Pediatrics* 1997; 99 (2): 255-6.
62. Ozer EA, Turker M, Bakiler AR, Yaprak I, Ozturk C. Involuntary movements in infantile cobalamin deficiency appearing after treatment. *Pediatr Neurol* 2001; 25 (1): 81-3.
63. Sury MR, Billingham I, Russell GN, Hopkins LS, Thornington R, Vivori E. Acute benzodiazepine withdrawal syndrome after midazolam infusion in children. *Crit Care Med* 1989; 17 (3): 301-2.
64. Bergman I, Steeves M, Burckart G, Thompson A. Reversible neurologic abnormalities associated with prolonged intravenous midazolam and fentanyl administration. *J Pediatr* 1991; 119 (4): 644-9.
65. van Engelen BG, Gimbrere JS, Booy LH. Benzodiazepine withdrawal reaction in two children following discontinuation of sedation with midazolam. *Ann Parmacother* 1993; 27 (5): 579-81.
66. Carnevale FA, Ducharme C. Adverse reactions to the withdrawal of opioids and benzodiazepines in paediatric intensive care. *Intensive & Critical Care Nursing* 1997; 13 (4): 181-8.
67. Fonsmark L, Rasmussen YH, Carl P. Occurrence of withdrawal in critically-ill sedated children. *Crit Care Med* 1999; 27 (1): 196-9.

# Early onset primary torsion dystonia

**Alfonso Fasano, Antonio E. Elia, Alberto Albanese**

*Istituto Nazionale Neurologico Carlo Besta,*
*Universita Cattolica del Sacro Cuore, Milano, Italy*

Dystonia is one of the several movement disorders that may arise in childhood. Primary torsion dystonia (PTD) is a syndrome of sustained muscle contractions usually producing twisting and repetitive movements or abnormal postures [1-3], which is not secondary to any known cause. Non-secondary forms of dystonia encompass primary torsion dystonia (PTD), in which dystonia is the one and only symptom of the observed condition (*e.g.* DYT1 dystonia), dystonia plus syndromes, in which dystonia is a prominent sign, yet associated with another movement disorder (*e.g.*, myoclonus-dystonia), and dystonia associated with heredodegenerative conditions (such as pantothenate kinase-associated neurodegeneration or Wilson's disease) *(Table I)*. All the non-secondary forms of dystonia can be observed in children and are considered to be of genetic origin. Advances in scientific knowledge have allowed to directly assess only a restricted number of dystonia types by genetic testing *(Table II)*.

**Table I. Classifications of dystonia.**

| |
|---|
| **By age at onset**<br>• *Early onset* (≤ 21 years): usually starts in a leg or arm and frequently progresses to involve other limbs and the trunk.<br>• *Late onset* (> 21 years): usually starts in the neck (including the vocal folds), the cranial muscles or one arm. Tends to remain localised with restricted progression to adjacent muscles. |
| **By distribution**<br>• *Focal:* single body region (*e.g.*, writer's cramp, blepharospasm).<br>• *Segmental:* contiguous body regions (*e.g.*, cranial and cervical, cervical and upper limb).<br>• *Multifocal:* non-contiguous body regions (*e.g.*, upper and lower limb, cranial and upper limb).<br>• *Generalised:* both legs and at least one other body region (usually one or both arms). |
| **By cause**<br>• *Primary (or idiopathic):* dystonia is the only clinical sign and there is no identifiable exogenous cause or other inherited or degenerative disease. Example: DYT1 dystonia.<br>• *Dystonia plus:* dystonia is a prominent sign, but is associated with another movement disorder. There is no evidence of neurodegeneration. Example: Myoclonus-dystonia (DYT11).<br>• *Heredo-degenerative dystonia* is a prominent sign, among other neurological features, of a heredo-degenerative disorders. Example: Wilson's disease.<br>• *Secondary dystonia* is a symptom of an identified neurological condition, such as a focal brain lesion, exposure to drugs or chemicals. Examples: dystonia due to a brain tumour, off-period dystonia in Parkinson's disease. |

**Table II. Genetic forms of childhood dystonia that can be diagnosed by direct testing.**

| Gene name (locus)[1] | Gene location | Disease | Trans-mission[2] |
|---|---|---|---|
| **Primary torsion dystonia** | | | |
| TOR1A (DYT1) | 9q34 | Early limb-onset or Oppenheim's dystonia | AD |
| **Dystonia plus syndromes** | | | |
| GCH1 (DYT5) | 14q22 | Dopa-responsive dystonia (DRD) or Segawa syndrome | AD |
| SGCE (DYT11) | 7q21.q31 | Myoclonus-dystonia | AD |
| TH | 11p15.5 | Dopa-responsive dystonia (DRD) | AR |
| **Heredodegenerative syndromes** | | | |
| PANK2 | 20p13 | Pantothenate kinase associated neurodegeneration (PKAN) or Hallervorden-Spatz disease | AR |
| PRKN (PARK2) | 6q25 | Autosomal recessive early-onset parkinsonism | AR |
| ATP7B | 13q14.3-q21.1 | Wilson's disease | AR |
| IT-15 | 4p16 | Huntington's disease | AD |
| FTL | 19q13.3 | Neuroferritinopathy | AD |
| Nuclear or mitochondrial DNA mutations | mDNA | Leigh's disease | M |
| DDP | Xq22 | Mohr-Tranebjaerg syndrome | XR |
| NPC1 | 18q11-q12 | Niemann-Pick disease, type C1 | AR |
| PLP1 | Xq22 | Pelizaeus-Merzbacher disease | XR |
| HEXA | 15q23-q24 | Tay-Sachs disease | AR |
| ATXN3 | 14q24.3-q31 | Machado-Joseph disease | AD |
| Mitochondrial DNA mutations | mDNA | Leber's disease | M |
| GCDH | 19p13.2 | Glutaricacidemia | AR |
| ARSA | 22q13.31-qter | Metachromatic leukodystrophy | AR |
| DJ1 (PARK7) | 1p36 | Autosomal recessive early-onset parkinsonism | AR |
| TBP (SCA17) | 6q27 | Spinocerebellar ataxia 17 | AD |
| HE1 (NPC2) | 14q24.3 | Niemann-Pick disease, type c2 | AR |
| MECP2 | Xq28 | Rett syndrome | XD |
| HPRT | Xq26-q27.2 | Lesch-Nyhan syndrome | XR |
| FUCA1 | 1p34 | Fucosidosis | AR |
| ATM | 11q22.3 | Ataxia-telangiectasia | AR |
| CLN3 | 16p12.1 | Ceroid-lipofuscinosis | AR |

[1] Abbreviations: ARSA, arylsulfatase A; ATM, ataxia-telangiectasia mutated gene; ATP7B, ATPase, $Cu^{++}$-transporting beta polypeptide; ATXN3, ataxin-3; CLN3, CLN3 gene; DDS, dystonia-deafness syndrome gene; DJ1, oncogene DJ1; FTL, ferritin light chain; FUCA1, alpha-L-fucosidase 1; GCDH, glutaryl-CoA dehydrogenase; GCH1, guanosine triphosphate cyclohydrolase I; HE1, epididymal secretory protein; HEXA, Hexosaminidase A alpha polypeptide; HPRT, hypoxanthine guanine phosphoribosyl-transferase 1; IT-15, important transcript 15 (huntingtin); MECP2, methyl-CpG-binding protein 2; NPC1, Niemann-Pick type C gene; PANK2, pantothenate kinase; PLP1, proteolipid protein 1; PRKN, parkin; SGCE, ε-sarcoglycan; TBP, TATA box-binding protein; TH, tyrosine hydroxylase; TOR1A, torsinA gene.
[2] Abbreviations: AD, autosomal dominant; AR, ausomal recessive; M, mitochondrial; XR, X-linked.

The diagnosis is based on clinical and laboratory work-out. Making a diagnosis of dystonia is not always straightforward, particularly among non-specialised neurologists or paediatricians, because the clinical spectrum is surprisingly broad, ranging from task-specific, to focal, segmental and generalised forms. *Figure 1* provides a flow chart to serve as a guide for the diagnosis. The clinical features of dystonia [3] must be distinguished from those of hypertonias (such as spasticity or rigidity) and from other movement disorders (*e.g.* tremor) that can be observed in childhood [4] *(Table III)*.

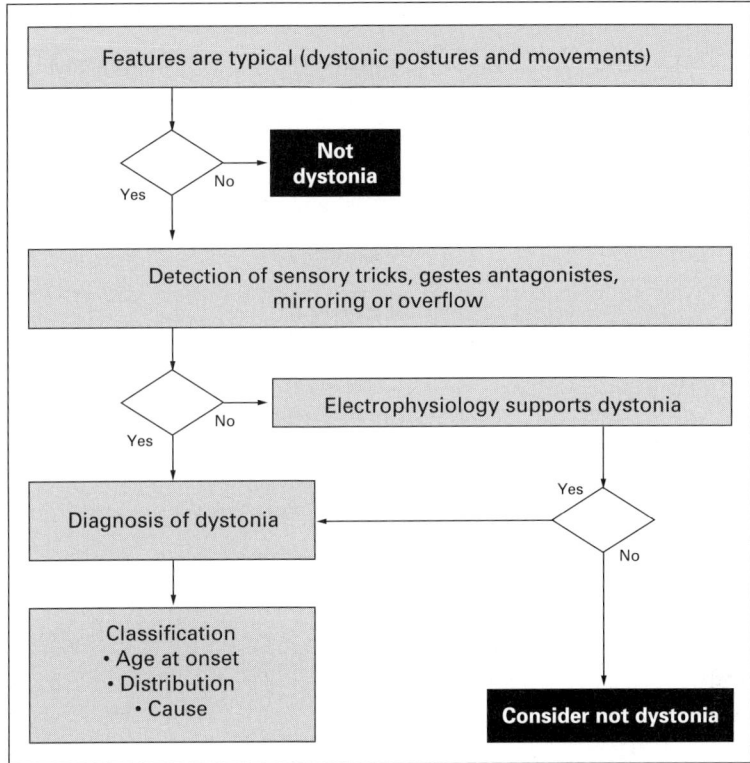

**Figure 1.** Flow chart for the clinical diagnosis of dystonia. Observation of characteristic clinical features [3] leads to the clinical diagnosis and to classification of dystonia, as reported in *Table I*.

The occurrence of dystonia in isolation (with or without dystonic tremor) points to PTD, whereas, when dystonia is combined to other forms of hypertonia or to other dyskinesias, the diagnosis is usually that of a dystonia plus syndrome or of dystonia associated with a neurodegenerative disease.

Aetiology is one of the three descriptors used to illustrate dystonia, the other two being age at disease onset and the topography of body regions affected (*Table I*). Age at onset is the single most important feature in determining outcome [5-7]; the earlier the age at onset the more likely symptoms will be severe, with dystonia spreading to multiple regions. Only a minority of PTD cases encountered in clinical practice are linked to known loci or genes; notwithstanding that, PTD is considered to be genetically determined in most cases, with a number of still unmapped genes remaining to be identified. The diagnosis of PTD requires ruling out of a non-primary form of dystonia, which may be an engaging task. The forms of non-primary dystonias that most commonly require a differential diagnosis will be briefly dealt with hereafter.

**Table III. Hypertonias observed in childhood have distinct features.**

|  | Spasticity | Dystonia | Rigidity |
|---|---|---|---|
| **Pathophysiology** | Increased short-latency stretch reflexes resulting from injury to the corticofugal projection originating from areas 4 and 6 ("upper motor neuron syndrome") | Simultaneous co-contraction of agonist and antagonist muscles and proximal "overflow" of muscle activation due to basal ganglia dysfunction | Enhanced long-latency stretch reflexes resulting from basal ganglia dysfunction |
| **Clinical features** | Velocity-dependent increase of resistance to externally imposed movement (varies with the direction of joint movement) | Sustained muscle contractions usually producing twisting and repetitive movements or abnormal postures. Dystonic postures and movements occur in variable combinations and are activated by voluntary motor tasks | Constantly increased resistance to passive motion with "plastic" quality |
| **Postural restructuring** | Flexion, adduction and intrarotation in the upper limbs; extension, abduction and extrarotation in the lower limbs | Torsion involves the main axis of the body part affected | Flexion of the body part affected |
| **Motor performance** | Muscle weakness (paralysis), loss of dexterity in distal movements | Muscle strength is unchanged, motor skilfulness is impaired | Muscle strength is unchanged, motor speed may be reduced (bradykinesia), repetitive movements may induce rapid fatiguing (akinesia) |
| **Deep tendon reflexes** | Increased | Unchanged | Unchanged |
| **Specific clinical signs** | Clasp-knife phenomenon, Babinski sign | *Gestes antagonistes*, sensory tricks, mirroring, overflow | Cog-wheeling |

## ■ Non-Primary Early Onset Dystonia

Non-primary dystonias encompass a host of disorders in which dystonia is a prominent sign, yet associated with another movement disorder (dystonia-plus syndromes), or it is a prominent symptom of a heredodegenerative disorder or, finally, it is secondary to exogenous factors (*e.g.* perinatal injury, neuroleptic medications, brain tumour, infections, etc.). Non-primary dystonias commonly start in paediatric age and require expert differential diagnostic work-out [8]. The most relevant forms of non-primary dystonias are the dystonia-plus syndromes.

*Dopa-responsive dystonia* (DRD) is characterized by childhood-onset dystonia, parkinsonism and sustained response to low doses of levodopa. The average age at onset is around 6 years. This syndrome has two main causes, namely: guanosine triphosphate cyclohydrolase I deficiency (DYT5: Segawa syndrome) [9], or tyrosine hydroxylase deficiency [10]. A new locus recently mapped to 14q13 (DYT14) [11] has been associated to a DRD phenotype; however, the direct observation, by one of us, of video tapes showing some of the affected family members, has not allowed to detect obvious DRD features.

The most common form of the disorder has long been called *Segawa syndrome*; it is transmitted by autosomal dominant trait with incomplete penetrance (about 30%) and a prevalence estimated around 0.5-1.0 per million [12]. The initial symptoms commonly consist of gait difficulties, due to action dystonia in a lower limb; the disease, however, can also start with upper limb or neck dystonia [13]. In addition to dystonia, increased tendon jerks and parkinsonian features (such as rigidity and rapidly induced fatiguing in repetitive motor tasks) are also common findings in the affected limb. By 10-15 years after onset, dystonia gradually spreads to all the limbs to become generalized. The resulting picture shows asymmetric involvement of the four limbs, with more severe features in the legs [13]. One of the most important features of DRD is the occurrence of diurnal fluctuations, with patients being less affected in the morning and more in the evening [14]. All DRD patients show complete and sustained response to low doses of levodopa (50-300 mg/day), however motor benefit can occur also within a few months after the beginning of treatment. This is the main reason why a short 3-month levodopa trial is justified to rule out DRD in patients with unclassified dystonia.

*Myoclonus dystonia* (MD) is a syndrome with onset in childhood; dystonia usually occurs in the first or second decade (average age being 5.4 years). Myoclonic jerks commonly affect the axial muscles [15]. MD has been associated with three different genetic defects: a deficiency of $\varepsilon$-sarcoglycan (DYT11) [16], a mutation in the D2 dopamine receptor [17] and a still unknown defect mapped to a new locus (DYT15) [18]. The most common form is $\varepsilon$-sarcoglycan deficiency, that is transmitted by autosomal dominant trait with incomplete penetrance and variable expressivity [15]. The initial symptoms usually consist of myoclonic jerks and dystonia mostly affecting the trunk and the upper limbs, with a prevalent proximal involvement. Jerky movements are very brief and are precipitated by voluntary action or by psychological stress, but they can also occur at rest. Progression is very slow and leg involvement is rare, although a dystonic gait disturbance can occasionally be observed in young patients [15]. A very typical feature of MD is the relief of both myoclonus and dystonia following the ingestion of alcohol; this clinical sign is not seen in all patients [19].

## ■ Early Onset primary torsion dystonia

The first observation of severe progression in patients with onset in childhood was made by Herz [20], who clearly recognized the rapid progression of the disease when it begins in childhood and classified dystonia into the three categories of early onset (shortly after birth), juvenile onset (between 5 and 15 years) and late onset (after 15 years). These observations were confirmed by Cooper [21], who differentiated dystonia patients into three age groups: childhood onset (between 4 and 6 years), adolescent onset (between 8 and 13 years) and adult forms; he also considered this classification to be of strict prognostic value. Marsden and colleagues [6] analyzed the natural history of 72 patients affected by PTD and identified age at onset as one of the most important features in determining outcome. They first observed that the frequency of age at onset presented a bimodal distribution and suggested that "one is dealing not with a single disease, but with two populations, one with onset in childhood, the other with onset in middle life". Nevertheless, they also noted an overlap between the two age groups and considered that the division into the two sets is based on a "gradual difference rather then on a clear distinction". A consensus meeting attended by the members of an *ad hoc* committee [1], who convened in 1984, identified three age groups: childhood onset (0-12), adolescent onset (13-20) and adult onset (> 20 years). Based on this, early onset (encompassing cases with onset in childhood and adolescence) was distinguished from adult onset by the threshold age of 21.

Later retrospective series have confirmed that the curve representing the frequency distribution of age at onset for PTD is bimodal, with a nadir separating two clusters of patients *(Table IV)*. These observations, however, have yielded inconsistent results on the most appropriate threshold age to distinguish the two clusters.

In a large series of 560 North American PTD patients followed at the Columbia University in New York, the frequency distribution of age at onset showed that dystonia cases clustered in two clearly distinct unimodal sets, a younger cluster with generalized dystonia and an older cluster with focal dystonia. In addition, the frequency distribution of segmental cases partially overlapped the two clusters of early- and adult-onset, giving rise to a bimodal plot with a nadir set at about 25 years [22] *(Figure 2)*. In a subsequent analysis of a series of 178 Ashkenazi Jews, the nadir separating the early and adult onset clusters was set at 27 years [23]. The authors observed that patients with onset before the age of 21 were more likely to have a generalized form than those with older age at onset.

In 1994 a similar bimodal frequency distribution of age at onset was observed in a series of 160 Ashkenazi Jewish patients, 90 of whom were carriers of a DYT1 mutation [24]. The majority of DYT1 positive patients in this series presented an earlier age at onset than DYT1 negative patients and were almost completely included into the early onset cluster. These observations led to conclude that DYT1 dystonia arises with particularly high frequency in the early onset group of patients, especially among North American Jews. Following up on this observation, the same group proposed that the threshold age of 26 years could serve as a ceiling in referring PTD patientsfor DYT1 genetic testing [25]. More recently, 26 years of age has also been considered the most appropriate threshold to distinguish early- from adult-onset PTD [26] *(Figure 3)*.

The afore-mentioned reports are useful criteria for defining a terminology used for classification of dystonia by age at onset; but they cannot be used to predict the outcome in individual cases. Indeed, the observation of a bimodal distribution of age at onset for PTD does not necessarily imply that the two age groups have a different disease progression or clinical prognosis. It is clear from the observations reported that, generally speaking, the earlier the age at disease onset the higher the likelihood of generalization. Nevertheless, these observations do not demonstrate that the

Table IV. Retrospective series reporting the frequency distribution of age at disease onset in dystonia.

| Recruiting centres | Patients | Age at onset (years) | Onset < 21 (% cases) | Age at onset (distribution) | Modes | Nadir | Reference |
|---|---|---|---|---|---|---|---|
| National Hospital (London) | 72 | 1-59 | 66 | Bimodal | 0-10 and 41-50 | 21-30 | (6) |
| St. Barnabas Hospital (New York) | 226 | NA | 82 | Bimodal | 9 and 16-20 | 15 | (82) |
| Columbia University (New York) | 560 | NA | 27 | Bimodal (for segmental dystonia) | 6-10 for generalized dystonia and 50-60 for focal and segmental | ~25 | (22) |
| Columbia University (New York) | 178 | NA | NA | Bimodal | 9 and 55 | 27 | (23) |
| Institute of Psychiatry, King's College Hospital, National Hospital, Hospital for sick children (London) | 107 | 2-70 | 65 | Bimodal | 5-10 and 45-50 | 30-35 | (83) |
| Columbia University (New York) | 160 | 4-74 | 58 | Bimodal | 0-10 and 31-40 | 21-30 | (24) |
| Gemelli Hospital (Rome) | 460 | 1-83 | 9.6 | Bimodal | 9 and 57 | 21 | (64) |

NA, not available.

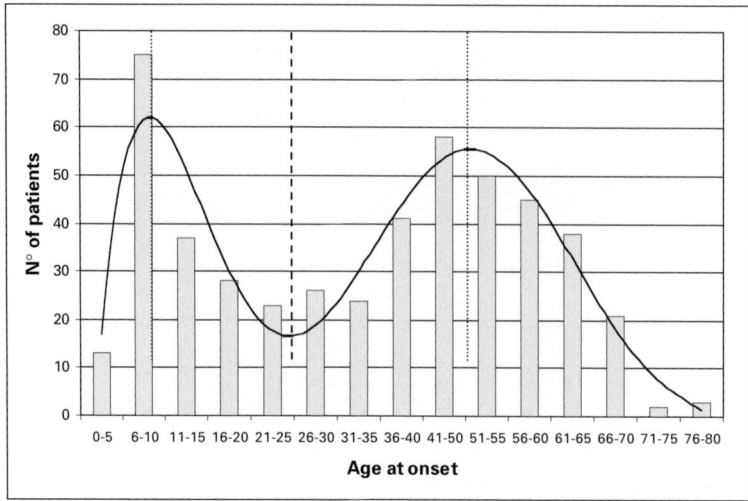

**Figure 2.** Frequency distribution of age at onset in 560 PTD cases seen at the Columbia University in New York. The bimodal distribution has a nadir at about 25 years (dashed line) and consists of two well-distinct clusters of patients with early and late disease onset. Dotted lines indicate modes at 6-10 years and 50-60 years, respectively (modified from [22]).

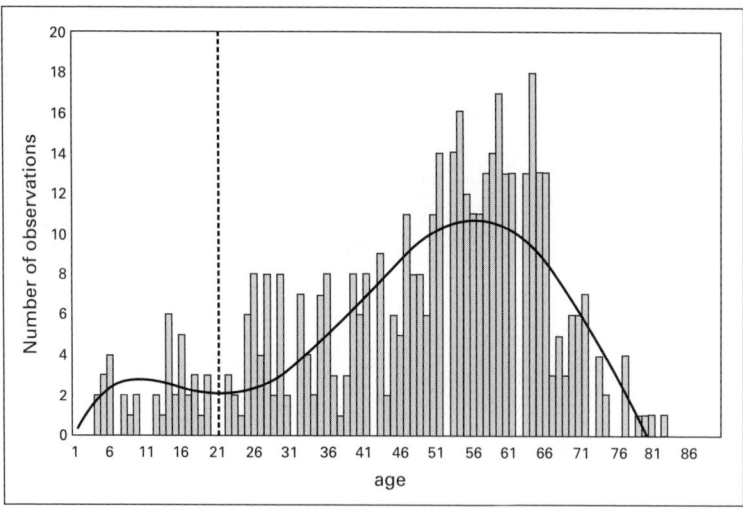

**Figure 3.** Frequency distribution of age at onset in 460 PTD cases seen at the Gemelli Hospital in Rome. This is a movement disorders clinic with a prevalence of adult referrals. The occurrence of a bimodal distribution is observed, with a nadir at 21 years (dashed line) that identifies two well-distinct clusters of patients with early and late disease onset.

retrospectively measured nadir of onset age distribution corresponds to a threshold predicting generalization. The issue of DYT1 testing further overlaps with this, because series of North American patients, which include a high proportion of Ashkenazi Jewish patients, do not necessarily apply to the European practice [27]. Ashkenazim or Sephardim are differently represented in North American and European patient series.

# DYT 1 Dystonia

## Typical and less typical phenotypes

The most known form of PTD is DYT1 dystonia, also called *Oppenheim dystonia* after the name of the German neurologist who first described generalized early-onset PTD as *"dystonia musculorum deformans"* [28]. The typical phenotype is characterized by early onset of dystonia, starting in one limb and rapidly progressing towards generalization. Selective or pronounced cranial-cervical involvement is considered unusual. The first symptom, especially in childhood, commonly is inversion of one foot, observed during walking. Later, the severity of dystonia increases; foot involvement occurs with less voluntary activity and later it is also observed at rest. When onset is in adolescence or in young adulthood the arms are often affected at first. DYT1 patients commonly develop generalized dystonia that can reach marked severity, and rarely have episodes of sudden worsening [29], which has been called dystonic storm (*see chapter by Nardocci et al.*). This classical phenotypic expression is particularly common in Ashkenazi Jewish patients. Indeed, it has been observed that the relatives of early-onset Ashkenazi probands have a very homogeneous phenotype, consisting of early limb involvement, onset before 40, and uncommon involvement of the cranial muscles [30]. Similar clinical features have been described in another North American series encompassing one non-Jewish and 12 Jewish families, whose phenotypes were characterized by early onset (on average at $14.4 \pm 3$ and $13.2 \pm 1$ years of age) in a limb [31]. In a series of 178 North American Ashkenazi Jewish patients it was found that age at onset of DYT1 dystonia carriers was 12.5 years (significantly earlier than that of non-carriers) [24]. In 94% of the DYT1 carriers, symptoms started in a limb, but only rarely in the neck and the larynx, whereas neck, larynx, or other cranial muscles were the site of onset in 79% of non-carriers. It was also reckoned that most cases of dystonia with early limb onset in Ashkenazi Jewish families carried the DYT1 gene. Thus, phenotypic expression of DYT1 dystonia in the Ashkenazim population seems to be constant, with preferential onset on the dominant side [32]. The clinical features of non-Jewish North American patients affected by DYT1 dystonia are more variable [33]: early onset in a limb is common, but the clinical expression in the affected relatives is milder and a significant proportion (10-15%) of affected family members have late onset (> 44 years). The clinical features of non-Jewish European patients are even less predictable, with variable phenotypic expression within a same family and a high prevalence of patients with cervical, laryngeal and cranial involvement [34].

After the identification of the DYT1 gene it has emerged that the phenotype associated with DYT1 mutations is broader than previously thought. So far, more than two hundred DYT1-positive patients have been reported (*Table V*) and unusual or uncommon phenotypes have emerged. The atypical DYT1 positive phenotypes can be summarized as follows.

Table V. Clinical features of DYT1 patients.

| Patients, n/total screened | Mean age at onset, yr (range) | Site of onset, n | Progression, n | Cranial involvement, n | Additional features | Reference |
|---|---|---|---|---|---|---|
| 5/7 | 14.9 (9-38) | Arm: 5 | Focal: 4<br>Unknown: 1 | No | Writer's cramp | (84) |
| 22/150 | 9.9 (2-21) | Arm: 3<br>Leg: 19 | Generalised: 19<br>Segmental: 2<br>Focal: 1 | Yes: 4 | | (34) |
| 4/57 | 9.8 (5-17) | Arm: 2<br>Leg: 2 | Generalised: 3<br>Multifocal: 1 | No | | (67) |
| 10/51 | 9 (5-20) | Arm: 9<br>Leg: 1 | Generalised: 7<br>Segmental: 2<br>Focal: 1 | Yes: 4 | Two patients with dysarthria, one with nystagmus | (50) |
| 3/49 | 12.7 (9-17) | Arm: 1<br>Leg: 2 | Generalised: 2<br>Focal: 1 | Yes: 1 | | (85) |
| 24/39 | NA | NA | Generalised: 22<br>Focal: 2 | NA | One patient with stuttering only and one with isolated hand tremor | (49) |
| 68/550 (40 clinical affected) | NA | NA | Generalised: 26<br>Segmental: 1<br>Focal: 2 | Yes: 1 | 19 patients with "unclassified movement disorder" A patient with tremor of the lips and jaw started at the age of 70 | (51) |
| 1/3 | 13 (NA) | Shoulder/trunk | Segmental: 1 | Yes | Axial dystonia | (39) |
| 5/100 | 8.6 (6-12) | Arm: 3<br>Leg: 2 | Generalised: 4<br>Segmental: 1 | Yes: 4 | | (35) |
| 97/267 | 14 (4-44) | Larynx: 1<br>Neck: 3<br>Arm: 47<br>Leg: 46 | Generalised: 55<br>Multifocal: 10<br>Segmental: 12<br>Focal: 20 | Yes: 9 | | (25) |
| 10 | 11.1 (0.3-18) | Arm: 8<br>Leg: 2 | Generalised: 5<br>Segmental: 1<br>Focal: 4 | Yes: 2 | One case with very early onset (4 months) | (86) |
| 3/50 | 13.3 (10-17) | Arm: 2<br>Leg: 1 | Generalised: 2<br>Segmental: 1 | Yes: 2 | A case of spontaneous remission after several months | (66) |
| 6/178 | 14 (9-35) | Arm: 4<br>Leg: 2 | Generalised: 3<br>Focal: 3 | NA | | (87) |
| 6/45 | 21 (7-64) | Arm: 4<br>Leg: 2 | Generalised: 3<br>Multifocal: 2 | Yes: 2 | All members of one family A case of dystonic storm with fatal outcome | (29) |

**Table V (continued).**

| Patients, n/total screened | Mean age at onset, yr (range) | Site of onset, n | Progression, n | Cranial involvement, n | Additional features | Reference |
|---|---|---|---|---|---|---|
| 5/30 | 8 (8-11) | Arm: 3<br>Leg: 2 | Generalised: 4<br>Segmental: 1 | Yes: 3 | | (27) |
| 1 | 9 | Leg | Generalised | No | Late progression and prominent tremor | (37) |
| 3/107 | NA | NA | Generalized: 3 | No | | (65) |
| 5 | 27 (5-50) | Neck: 1<br>Arm: 2<br>Leg: 2 | Generalised: 3<br>Multifocal: 1<br>Focal: 1 | No | 3 cases with dysarthria (one of them with severe dysphagia) 4 cases with late onset or progression (one triggered by injury and one by haloperidolo) | (38) |
| 6/256 | 14.5 (7-41) | Arm: 3<br>Leg: 3 | Generalised: 2<br>Multifocal: 2<br>Segmental: 2 | Yes: 2 | | (88) |
| 5/131 | 13 (3-31) | Neck: 1<br>Arm: 2<br>Leg: 2 | Generalised: 4<br>Multifocal: 1 | Yes: 1 | Neck involvement in 2 cases<br>Voice tremor in one case<br>One case with bulbar muscles involvement and mild tetraparesis | (89) |

NA, not available.

*Generalized dystonia with cranial-cervical involvement*

Early-onset dystonia usually starts in a limb, and takes a variable time to spread to the cranial, cervical or bulbar districts. This phenotype has been reported in several series and appears to be more frequent in Europe than in North America, reaching a frequency of 80% of DYT1 patients in a French series [35].

*Myoclonus-dystonia like phenotype*

Generalized DYT1 dystonia may be associated with rapid movements resembling myoclonic jerks; they are mostly proximal in the limbs and the trunk. This DYT1 variant appears to be more severe than DYT11 myoclonus-dystonia; jerks are not (or only partially) responsive to alcohol [36].

*Focal dystonia with slow progression*

Although DYT1 dystonia normally progresses to a generalized form during the first 5-10 years after onset, there are occasional reports of focal or segmental dystonia as the only clinical expression. Upper limb dystonia (writer's cramp) is the most frequent focal presentation in such cases. It has been observed that progression may occasionally occur several years after onset (even 50 [37] or 55 years [38]).

*Late onset dystonia*

Onset of dystonia may occur at a later age than 21 in some DYT1 patients. The oldest reported onset of dystonia was at 64 years [29]. Upper limb dystonia is the most frequent site of onset in these cases and the progression may be very slow, remaining limited to a focal form.

*Non-limb onset*

This is a very rare presentation of DYT1 dystonia: cervical onset has been reported in three cases, laryngeal onset has been described in one [25] and trunk onset also in one [39].

Despite the observed variable phenotypic expression of DYT1 dystonia, the majority of DYT1 patients shared similar phenotypic characteristics, namely limb onset in childhood, exclusion of the cranial district and progression of dystonia. The real incidence of atypical DYT1 presentations has not been established yet. Furthermore, it is unclear how broad it is phenotype heterogeneity associated with the DYT1 gene. The mere finding of a mutation in this gene is not sufficient to assess a diagnosis of DYT1 dystonia even in patients with a movement disorder [40]. Since the penetrance of DYT1 gene mutations does not exceed 40%, it is more likely for a DYT1 mutation carrier to be asymptomatic than symptomatic. Thus, it cannot be excluded that a patient with atypical features and a status of DYT1 carrier may express a coincident, yet undiscovered, gene defect.

## Clinical genetics

It was originally proposed that early-onset primary dystonia is inherited as autosomal recessive trait in Jews and as autosomal dominant trait in non-Jews [41]. Later, studies from Israel [42] and from the United States [30, 43], as well as the re-analysis of Eldridge's original data [44], showed that in Jews the disorder is not autosomal recessive, but rather autosomal dominant with reduced penetrance (around 30%). The first primary dystonia locus, named DYT1, was later mapped to the region 9q32-34 in a large North-American non-Jewish family of French Canadian ancestry [45]. Linkage of dystonia with markers in the same region was also found in 12 Ashkenazi families [31]. This suggested that the mutation causing the Ashkenazi Jewish disease was in the same gene as that causing dystonia in the non-Jewish kindred. It became later apparent that the Ashkenazi families shared a common haplotype. The area containing the DYT1 gene was delineated to a 6-cM region with a strong linkage disequilibrium suggesting a single mutation event or founder mutation [46].

It was later calculated that the mutation was introduced into the Ashkenazi population about 350 years ago and probably originated in Lithuania or Byelorussia [47]. It was also reckoned that the high prevalence of the disease in Ashkenazim (estimated to be about 1:3,000 to 1:9,000 with a gene frequency of about 1:2,000 to 1:6,000) was due to the tremendous growth of that population in the 18th century from a small reproducing founder population. A founder mutation and genetic drift, rather than a heterozygote advantage, is probably responsible for the high frequency of DYT1 dystonia in Ashkenazi Jews. Subsequently, the haplotype of 174 Ashkenazi Jewish individuals affected by PTD was calculated [24]. In this group, there were 90 carriers of the DYT1 haplotype and 70 non-carriers, showing relevant phenotypic differences. Discriminant analysis of limb onset, leg involvement, and age at onset distinguished haplotype carriers from non-carriers with 90% accuracy. In 23 of the 70 non-carriers, the disease was familial and included brachial, cervical, laryngeal, and facial dystonia. Later studies confirmed that DYT1 is a common cause of early onset PTD also in non-Jews from Europe; furthermore, the observed association between idiopathic torsion dystonia and the highly polymorphic loci argininosuccinate synthetase (ASS) and Abelson oncogene (ABL) was also found in some British Jewish families [48]. Evidence for linkage to the DYT1 locus was found in 5 of 7 non-Jewish families of Northern European or French-Canadian descent, with an estimated penetrance in non-Jews of 0.40 to 0.75, higher than that observed in Ashkenazi Jews [33]. None of these families carried the Ashkenazi Jewish haplotype.

In addition to Ashkenazims, the GAG deletion has also been found in non-Jewish individuals and in families of diverse ethnic background [34, 39, 49-51]. One proposed explanation for the genetic and clinical differences observed among these populations is that the disorder in Jews is genetically homogenous, whereas non-Jews show greater genetic heterogeneity of DYT1 dystonia. This means that in Jews the presence of a single founder mutation and a genetic drift are the most plausible reasons for the higher frequency of early onset dystonia [43]; thus most cases would be due to the same mutation event and clinical homogeneity would be expected. Non-Jews are a heterogeneous population with a lower disease prevalence; the disorder is likely to result from mutation/selection balance so that multiple mutations, including new mutations [52], are expected.

## Molecular genetics

The DYT1 gene is named TOR1A [53]. The mutation causing the disease has been identified as a deletion of one of a pair of GAG triplets from the carboxy terminal in torsin A, a previously unknown protein. De novo mutations causing this deletion are uncommon, but some have been encountered. The unique DYT1 haplotype found in North American and Russian Ashkenazi Jews has been observed in Europe as well [54]. With the notable exception of an 18 bp deletion found in families with PTD and myoclonus, that also harboured a mutation in ε-sarcoglycan [55-57], the original GAG deletion is the only disease mutation identified in TOR1A.

TorsinA is a heat-shock and ATP-binding protein and a member of the AAA+ family of proteins, that is believed to serve as a chaperon in the processing and repairing of damaged proteins. Six TorsinA proteins are thought to join together to form a ring, with each of these six proteins bound to its neighbour by ATP. This structure is believed to repair other proteins that have been damaged. If repairing is unsuccessful, the damaged proteins can aggregate or die by apoptosis. An impairment of TorsinA could explain why stress is capable to cause the onset or the worsening of dystonia. TorsinA mRNA has been mapped in normal human brain; it has an intense expression in dopamine neurons of the substantia nigra pars compacta, in the locus coeruleus, in the cerebellar dentate nucleus, in Purkinje cells, in several thalamic nuclei, and in the pedunculopontine nucleus, but it is also found in most cortical areas, in the basal ganglia and in other mid-brain nuclei [58, 59]. The normal protein is widely distributed in many species and is located in the endoplasmic reticulum [60, 61]. The immunohistochemical localization of TorsinA in a brain from a patient with DYT1 dystonia failed to reveal differences from control brains [62]. Finally, an intriguing, albeit unexpected, finding is the presence of torsinA in Lewy bodies [63].

## Guidelines for genetic testing

The availability of direct testing for the DYT1 mutation raises the issue of developing diagnostic guidelines for searching the GAG deletion in the appropriately selected patients. Based on the experience collected in North America, on Ashkenazi Jewish and non Jewish patients, an algorithm for selecting PTD patients for DYT1 testing has been proposed [25]. This algorithm suggests to perform testing in conjunction with genetic counselling in all PTD patients with onset before 26 years; this single criterion yielded a 100% detection of clinically ascertained carriers, with a specificity of 43% for non-Jewish patients and of 63% for Ashkenazi Jewish subjects. In addition, it is suggested to test patients with onset after 26 years if there is an affected relative with early onset PTD. A notable difference in the likelihood to identify DYT1 positive patients has been observed in the Jewish and non-Jewish populations. These guidelines on DYT1 testing, which are based on a North American population, cannot be directly applied to European patients. In Europe, the number of early-onset DYT1-negative cases of generalised dystonia is higher than in North America, possibly because of a lower representation of Ashkenazi Jews [27, 34, 64]. A revision of these recommendations has been proposed for the European population, where onset < 26 years as a single criterion does not appear to be an adequate factor to select non-Jewish individuals for DYT1 testing. It has been proposed that onset in a limb, in combination with onset < 26 years, is a better predictor of DYT1 carrier status [38].

As already mentioned, the penetrance of the DYT1 gene is not higher than 40%, meaning that the majority of those who carry a DYT1 gene mutation are not symptomatic. Therefore, it must be remembered that the identification of a DYT1 mutation is not sufficient to assert that the observed movement disorder is caused by the DYT1 gene. In keeping with this, a case of psychogenic movement disorder misdiagnosed as DYT1 dystonia, based on positive genetic testing, has been recently observed in the carrier of a DYT1 mutation [40]. A consistent clinical picture of dystonia must be observed in all cases undergoing genetic testing *(Figure 1)*. Due to its simplicity, genetic testing for the DYT1 mutation could be performed in every PTD patient. A negative test would rule out DYT1 dystonia, while a positive test would allow to confirm DYT1 PTD in the presence of a consistent clinical picture and a typical DYT1 phenotype.

## ■ Non DYT1 Early Onset Dystonia

DYT1 PTD is 3-5 times more common in Ashkenazi Jews compared to other ethnic groups [47], but is not the commonest cause of early onset generalized dystonia in the non-Jewish population. The frequency of the GAG deletion in non-Jewish

European patients has been estimated to be 2.8% in Danish patients [65], 6% in Serbian patients [66] and 7% in German patients [67]. Furthermore, in a large series of European PTD patients only 14% of patients were carriers of the DYT1 GAG deletion; such higher prevalence could be due to the high representation of familial cases in this series (66%) [34].

The DYT1 is the only mapped PTD gene. Available evidence shows that a large group of early-onset PTD cases are not associated with mutations of this gene. Some other loci have been linked to PTD in selected families; but the majority of early or late onset PTD cases remain genetically unmapped.

## Genetically classified early-onset PTD

Four forms of non-DYT1 dystonia have been observed to occur with early onset *(Table VI)*. They have been named DYT2, DYT4, DYT6 and DYT13. These forms of dystonia have been described in individual families and are considered to be rare; they possibly reflect the occurrence of private mutations in yet unmapped genes.

Table VI. Clinical features of DYT2, DYT4, DYT6, and DYT13 patients.

| Locus (patients, n) | Mean age at onset, yr (range) | Site of onset, n | Progression, n | Cranial involvement, n | Additional features | Ref. |
|---|---|---|---|---|---|---|
| DYT2 (3 affected) | 4.7 (1-8) | Leg: 2 Trunk: 1 | Generalised: 3 | Yes: 3 | Constant involvement of tongue and larynx AR inheritance | (70) |
| DYT4 (10 examined of 22 familial members affected) | NA (13-37) | Larynx: 7 Neck: 2 Leg: 1 | Generalised: 8 Segmental: 1 Focal: 1 | NA | Larynx involvement in 9 patients 2 relatives affected by Wilson's disease AD inheritance | (71) |
| DYT6 (15 affected) | 18 (5-38) | Cranial: 1 Tongue: 2 Larynx: 1 Neck: 3 Arm: 7 Leg: 1 | Generalised: 4 Segmental: 9 Focal: 2 | Yes: 8 | Frequent involvement of larynx (in 7 cases) and tongue (in 3 cases) AD inheritance | (72) |
| DYT13 (11 affected) | 16.6 (5-43) | Cranial: 2 Neck: 6 Arm: 3 | Generalised: 2 Segmental: 7 Focal: 2 | Yes: 9 | Possible anticipation between the first and the second generation AD inheritance | (75) |

AD: autosomal dominant; AR: autosomal recessive; NA: not available.

### DYT2

Autosomal recessive PTD has been described in three reports. The first observation [68] described three affected sibs whose parents were unaffected second-degree relatives. Another report described three consanguineous families of Spanish gypsies with early limb onset (average age at onset: 15 years) presenting generalized or segmental dystonia [69]. Cranial-cervical involvement was prominent. The supposed gene has been named DYT2, but linkage to a gene locus has not been demonstrated. Recently, a DYT2-like phenotype has been observed in a Sephardic Jewish family originating from Iran with 3 sibs affected by PTD [70]. The parents were first cousins, which suggest autosomal recessive inheritance. Age at onset was in childhood, with clinical features of dystonia becoming evident at 5, 7, and 8 years. Two patients first developed in-turning of the foot with gait abnormalities; all had cervical involvement, facial grimacing, blepharospasm, and dystonic posturing and jerking of the four limbs. Two patients had dysphagia.

## DYT4

A large Australian pedigree of PTD patients distributed along five generations had autosomal dominant transmission. Cranial dystonia was a prominent sign and impaired speech was common; few cases were affected by a generalized form. Age at onset varied from 13 to 37 years; the evident sign was speech dystonia in all patients but three, two of whom had cervical dystonia and later developed dysphonia. Wilson's disease was diagnosed in a brother and his sister belonging to a sibship of 11 subjects, three of whom had PTD. Linkage analysis using marker flanking the ATP7B gene yielded negative results, excluding the possibility that the disorder was due to an allele at the Wilson's disease locus on chromosome 13 [71].

## DYT6

This locus was identified in two Mennonite families [72]. The disease is transmitted as autosomal dominant trait with an estimated penetrance of 30%. The locus was mapped to 8p21-q22 and haplotypes across the candidate region were identical in the affected members of the 2 families, suggesting a founder effect and a common underlying mutation. Among 220 family members overall, a total of 15 definitely affected individuals were identified. The DYT6 phenotype has been described as "mixed type": early or young adult onset and prevalent segmental (cranial-cervical) distribution of features. The presentation at onset involves limb, cervical, and cranial muscles equally. Four patients developed a generalized dystonia. The authors reported that some affected individuals had a phenotype overlapping the classical early onset DYT1 PTD. Notwithstanding that, at variance with patients affected by DYT1 PTD, those with generalized DYT6 PTD had an older age at onset (range: 5-38; average: $18.9 \pm 11.9$ years); in addition, most of them presented with cranial or cervical involvement either at onset or later during the course of the disease. Furthermore, many patients were deeply disabled by the involvement of muscles in the cranial-cervical region [72].

## DYT13

This locus was mapped in a family with a phenotype described as "mixed type", consisting in prominent cervical-upper limb-cranial involvement. Onset was in infancy or adolescence in most cases [73]. Linkage with already known loci was excluded and a genome-wide search allowed mapping the DYT13 locus to chromosome 1p36 [74]. This family was followed up for several years and the affected individuals belonged to 3 consecutive generations. Anticipation of the age at onset and of the severity of symptoms was observed from the first to the second generation.

Two of 11 definitely affected individuals had generalized dystonia, with upper limb or cervical onset at 5 and 20 years, respectively. The first patient with generalized PTD was a woman, who presented a dystonic postural tremor of the upper limbs at the age of 5; dystonic movements progressively spread to the all body by the age of 26. At the age of 61 she had generalized dystonia of the larynx, the limbs, and the trunk; dystonic action tremor was prominent. Notwithstanding this widespread involvement, disability was mild. The second generalized patient was a man who reported onset at the age of 20, with mild cervical dystonia. The symptoms did not progress over the following 30 years, but started a mild progression in his fifties, with dystonic posturing of the right hand and involuntary jerks of both hands and the head. He was examined for the last time at the age of 56, and the clinical picture was that of a generalized dystonia, involving the neck, and the four limbs. Notwithstanding that, he could still work in a farm and was actually engaged in a full-time physical job. Two members of this family had early-onset cervical dystonia (at 5 and 15 years), that after several years progressed to a mild segmental form with cranial involvement. One patient exhibited cranial dystonia at 5 years of age; this progressed mostly in severity, but remained segmental with upper limb involvement [75].

## Genetically unclassified early onset PTD

It is not uncommon to observe PTD cases with early onset, which clinically resemble DYT1 dystonia, but turn out to be negative to DYT1 testing [64]. Most of such cases are sporadic. The Gemelli registry for movement disorders recorded 460 PTD cases of Caucasian origin. Forty-four of them (9.6%) had onset before age 21, there were 24 women and 20 men (male to female ratio of 0.83). All cases had focal dystonia at onset: in 22 patients (50%) PTD started in a limb (lower limb in 7 cases and upper limb in 15), in 12 subjects (27%) PTD made its appearance with cervical dystonia, in 5 (11%) with laryngeal involvement, in 4 (9%) with cranial dystonia and in one case (3%) the onset symptom was oro-mandibular dystonia. Progression of dystonia occurred in 34 cases (77%): after mean disease duration of $25.7 \pm 15.4$ years, 17 patients showed segmental dystonia and 17 generalized dystonia. Six of 10 focal cases had upper limb dystonia whereas other focal cases showed cranial or cervical dystonia (two in both cases).

The screening for GAG deletion in TorA gene was performed in 25 early onset cases: 7 patients (28%) carried the DYT1 mutation; all of them exhibited limb dystonia (lower limb in 5 cases and upper in two) and after a variable time (mean $3.1 \pm 2.5$ years) all reached generalization of symptoms; a positive family history for dystonia was found in 5 cases (71%). Eighteen early-onset patients (72%) did not carry the DYT1 mutation: 9 of them (50%) presented with cervical onset, 8 (44%) with limb involvement (upper limb in six cases, lower limb in two) and in one case (6%) dystonia started involving the larynx.

In all but two patients dystonia progressed to a second involved site: after several years of disease duration (mean $28.7 \pm 19.9$ years) two cases remained focal (both with cervical dystonia), 7 patients (38%) showed segmental dystonia and 9 (50%) cases had generalized dystonia (after a mean interval of $7.4 \pm 19.9$ years); a positive family history for dystonia was found in 12 cases (67%). The comparison of

DYT1-positive with DYT1-negative early-onset cases showed that, in carriers, progression to a generalized form was faster. Furthermore, the cranial and cervical muscles were involved in different proportion among DYT1+ and DYT1- patient: in the first group only one patient had cranial involvement (oro-mandibular dystonia) at the last visit, one patient had laryngeal dystonia and four had cervical dystonia. By contrast, 17 out of 18 non-carriers had cervical dystonia, 7 had cranial involvement and 6 had laryngeal dystonia. There was a comparable incidence of positive family history in DYT1 carriers and non-carriers. Analysis of disease progression showed that the number of new involved sites per year (starting at disease onset) increased with a time-dependent trend in DYT1 carriers and in non-carriers. In addition, DYT1 patients had a higher number of involved sites and reached generalization in a time interval significantly shorter than non-carriers *(Figure 4)*.

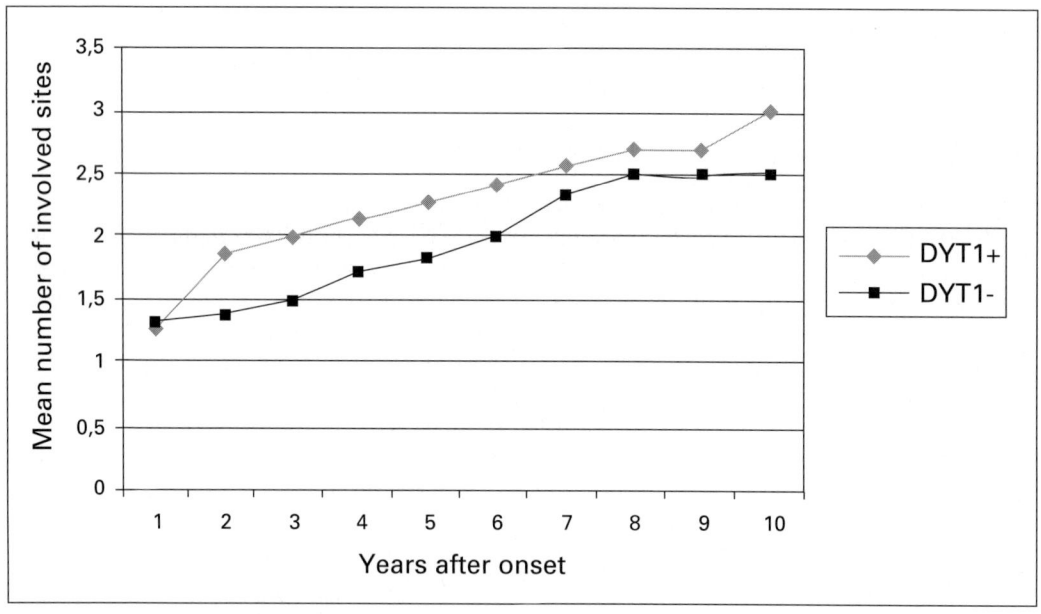

**Figure 4**. Mean number of involved body sites within 10 years from onset of dystonia in early onset PTD patients, of whom 18 were DYT1-negative and 7 were DYT1 carriers, followed at the Gemelli Hospital in Rome. Both groups show a progression after onset, but patients affected by DYT1 dystonia have a higher number of involved sites and reach generalization earlier than DYT1-negative PTD patients.
Abbreviations: DYT1+, DYT1-positive; DYT1-, DYT1-negative.

Several families with dystonia unlinked to known loci have also been described *(Table VII)*. The clinical features of these patients are heterogeneous and difficult to summarize into consistent phenotypes, although some remarkable differences with DYT1 dystonia can be drawn. As a rule, DYT1-negative families often show involvement of the cranial muscles and rarely have onset of dystonia in a limb. In addition, DYT1-negative cases have less tendency to generalize than DYT1-positive dystonia and frequently remain focal or segmental forms.

Table VII. Clinical features of unclassified early onset PTD cases.

| Patients, n | Mean age at onset, yr (range) | Site of onset, n | Progression, n | Cranial involvement, n | Additional features | Ref. |
|---|---|---|---|---|---|---|
| 1 | 7 | Leg: 1 | Generalization | Yes: 1 | Tongue involvement<br>Family with AD inheritance | (76) |
| 2 | 12,5 (12-13) | Neck: 1<br>Arm: 1 | Generalization: 2 | NA | Both familial cases<br>The only two cases generalised among 15 early onset cases | (90) |
| 4 | 18.3 (17-20) | Eye: 2<br>Larynx: 1<br>Arm: 1 | Generalised: 1<br>Multifocal: 2<br>Focal: 1 | Yes: 2 | Laryngeal involvement in 2 patients<br>Family with AD inheritance | (77) |
| 4 | 12.3 (8-17) | NA | Generalised: 1<br>Segmental: 2<br>Focal: 1 | NA | Cervical involvement in one case with onset at 8 | (85) |
| 2 | 6 (3-9) | Arm: 1<br>Leg: 1 | Segmental: 1<br>Focal: 1 | Yes: 1 | One case with anarthria | (51) |
| 7 | 13.6 (4-21) | Face: 1<br>Neck: 2<br>Arm: 3<br>Leg: 1 | Generalised: 3<br>Multifocal: 1<br>Segmental: 3 | Yes: 1 | 3 with familial history (none of the generalized cases)<br>One generalised case with cervical involvement | (67) |
| 2 | 17 (15-19) | Eye: 1<br>Neck: 1 | Segmental: 1<br>Focal: 1 | Yes: 1 | Members of 9 familial cases with AD inheritance | (78) |
| 6 | < 18 | Arm: 6 | Segmental: 3<br>Focal: 3 | No | All writer's cramp<br>Two familial cases | (81) |
| 2 | 2 both | Cervical: 2 | Focal: 2 | No | Identical twins (inheritance probably AD)<br>Alcohol-responder<br>Brief tics | (91) |
| 35 | 15.4 | NA | Generalised: 11<br>Segmental: 16<br>Focal: 8 | NA | | (66) |
| 25 | 7.7 (1.5-15) | Cranial: 1<br>Neck: 1<br>Arm: 12<br>Trunk: 2<br>Leg: 9 | Generalised: 22<br>Segmental: 3 | Yes: NA | Oromandibolar or laryngeal dystonia in 16 patients | (27) |
| 2 | 19 and 21 | Eye: 1<br>Neck: 1 | Focal: 2 | Yes: 1 | Family with AD inheritance | (92) |
| 7 | 15.9 | Eye: 2<br>Neck: 5 | Focal: 7 | Yes: 2 | All familial cases among 33 members affected belonged to 15 families | (80) |
| 2 | < 14 and < 18 | Eye: 2 | Focal: 2 | Yes: 2 | Members of 2 different families with blepharospasm AD inherited | (79) |
| 2 | 5.5 (2-9) | Leg: 1<br>Arm: 1 | Generalised: 1<br>Segmental: 1 | No | Myoclonus Dystonia-like phenotype<br>Familial occurrence AD | (93) |

AD: autosomal dominant; NA: not available.

A non-Jewish North-American family unlinked to DYT1 gene had seven members affected by cervical dystonia, and five of them also by dysarthria or dysphonia [76]. Onset was with cervical dystonia in five case; one patient had early onset with leg involvement and progression towards generalization. A Swedish family had autosomal dominant transmission and variable phenotypic expression, including involvement of the face and the larynx [77]. Onset in four of the ten patients occurred before the age of 21 (Figure 5).

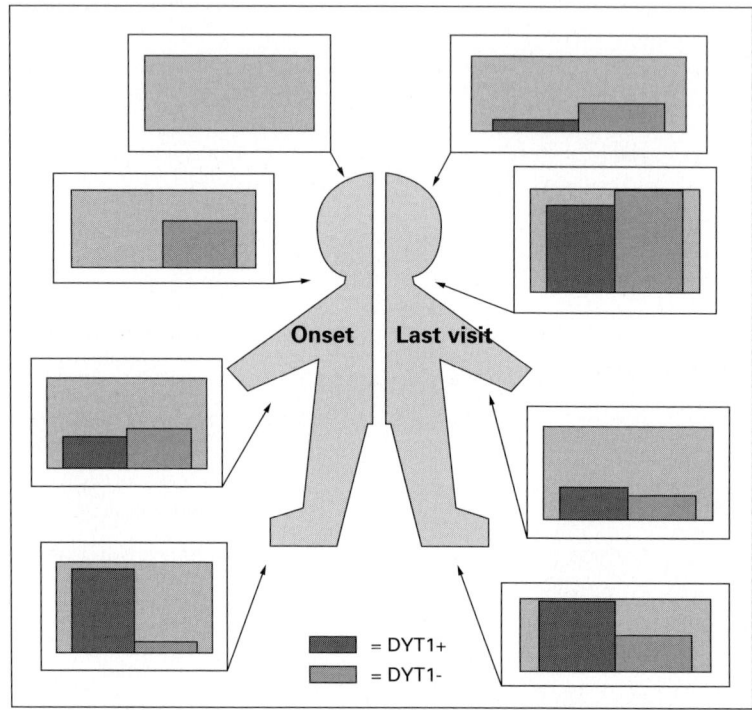

**Figure 5.** Body district affected at disease onset and at the last available visit in 25 early-onset PTD patients (18 DYT1-negative and 7 DYT1-positive, with a mean disease duration of 25.7 ± 15.4 years) seen at Gemelli Hospital in Rome. Histograms represent the percentage of patients who show involvement of cranial, cervical, upper limb or lower limb district at onset (left half of figure) or at the last visit (right half of figure). No DYT1-positive patient had cranial or cervical involvement at onset; at last visit all DYT1-negative patients had cervical or laryngeal dystonia whereas all DYT1-positive patients showed an involvement of lower limbs.

Young patients with DYT1-negative PTD with a severe involvement of the bulbar district leading to severe dysphagia or to anarthria have been described [51]. This is a rare observation in PTD patients, because bulbar involvement is commonly reported in secondary or heredodegenerative forms of dystonia. By contrast, cases with mild dystonia and focal forms without progression for long time have also been reported. A family from Yorkshire was characterized by cervical dystonia at onset with progression to the arms (78). Two of the 9 patients (5 definite and 4 probable cases) had early onset, one of them with blepharospasm. Blepharospam is very rarely observed in young PTD patients, because it is a focal dystonia of middle age. Two families with blepharospam in which two members had onset in childhood were recently reported [79]. Patients with blepharospasm at disease onset have been described also in another series from Germany [80]. Writer's cramp, a form of focal dystonia sometimes linked to DYT1 mutation, has been described in 6 DYT1-negative early-onset patients two of whom had a familial form [81]. In a series of 30 Italian patients (22 males and 8 females) affected by early-onset sporadic PTD, only 5 of them (23%) carried the DYT1 GAG mutation [27]. Their age at disease onset was on average 8 (range: 8-11). All carriers had onset in a limb (a leg in 2, one arm in 3). Four DYT1 carriers presented a generalised form; two of them had also oromandibular involvement. Twenty-five subjects (17 males and 7 females, M/F ratio: 2.4:1) were non carriers; their age at onset was 7.7 years (range: 1.5-15). Twenty-two of the DYT1-negative patients had generalized dystonia, 16 of whom with oromandibular or laryngeal involvement. Among the non-DYT1 carriers, onset was in a limb in 21 cases (the upper limb in 12, a lower limb in 9), in the trunk in 2 patients, in cranial muscles in one case, and in the neck in another one.

**Acknowledgement:** *The research reported in the present paper has been supported in part by Telethon grant E.1165.*

# References

1. Fahn S, Marsden CD, Calne DB. *Classification and investigation of dystonia*. In: Marsden CD, Fahn S, editors. Movement disorders 2. London: Butterworths, 1987: 332-58.
2. Fahn S, Bressman S, Marsden CD. Classification of dystonia. Adv Neurol 1998; 78: 1-10.
3. Albanese A. The clinical expression of primary dystonia. J Neurol 2003; 250: 1145-51.
4. Sanger TD, Delgado MR, Gaebler-Spira D, Hallett M, Mink JW. Classification and definition of disorders causing hypertonia in childhood. Pediatrics 2003; 111: e89-e97.
5. Marsden CD, Harrison MJ. Idiopathic torsion dystonia. Brain 1974; 97: 793-810.
6. Marsden CD, Harrison MJ, Bundey S. Natural history of idiopathic torsion dystonia. Adv Neurol 1976; 14: 177-87.
7. Fahn S. Concept and classification of dystonia. Adv Neurol 1988; 50: 1-8.
8. Jankovic J, Fahn S. *Dystonic disorders*. In: Jankovic J, Tolosa E, editors. *Parkinson's disease and movement disorders*. Baltimore: Williams and Wilkins, 1998: 513-51.
9. Ichinose H, Ohye T, Takahashi E, et al. Hereditary progressive dystonia with marked diurnal fluctuation caused by mutations in the GTP cyclohydrolase I gene. Nat Genet 1994; 8: 236-42.
10. Swaans RJ, Rondot P, Renier WO, van den Heuvel LP, Steenbergen-Spanjers GC, Wevers RA. Four novel mutations in the tyrosine hydroxylase gene in patients with infantile parkinsonism. Ann Hum Genet 2000; 64: 25-31.
11. Grotzsch H, Pizzolato GP, Ghika J, et al. Neuropathology of a case of dopa-responsive dystonia associated with a new genetic locus, DYT14. Neurology 2002; 58: 1839-42.
12. Nygaard TG. *Dopa-responsive dystonia: delineation of the clinical syndrome and clues to pathogenesis*. In: Narabayashi H, Nagatsu T, Yanagisawa N, Mizuno Y, editors. *Parkinson's disease: from basic research to treatment*. New York: Raven Press, 1993: 577-85.

13. Furukawa Y. Update on dopa-responsive dystonia: locus heterogeneity and biochemical features. *Adv Neurol* 2004; 94: 127-38.
14. Segawa M, Hosaka A, Miyagawa F, Nomura Y, Imai H. Hereditary progressive dystonia with marked diurnal fluctuation. *Adv Neurol* 1976; 14: 215-33.
15. Asmus F, Gasser T. Inherited myoclonus-dystonia. *Adv Neurol* 2004; 94: 113-9.
16. Zimprich A, Grabowski M, Asmus F, et al. Mutations in the gene encoding epsilon-sarcoglycan cause myoclonus-dystonia syndrome. *Nat Genet* 2001; 29: 66-9.
17. Klein C, Brin MF, Kramer P, et al. Association of a missense change in the D2 dopamine receptor with myoclonus dystonia. *Proc Natl Acad Sci USA* 1999; 96: 5173-6.
18. Grimes DA, Han F, Lang AE, George-Hyssop P, Racacho L, Bulman DE. A novel locus for inherited myoclonus-dystonia on 18p11. *Neurology* 2002; 59: 1183-6.
19. Vidailhet M, Tassin J, Durif F, et al. A major locus for several phenotypes of myoclonus-dystonia on chromosome 7q. *Neurology* 2001; 56: 1213-6.
20. Herz E. Dystonia I. Historical review: analysis of dystonic symptoms and physiologic mechanisms involved. *Arch Neurol Psychiat* (Chicago) 1944; 51: 305-18.
21. Cooper IS. *Involuntary movement disorders*. New York: Evanston, 1969.
22. Fahn S. Generalized dystonia: concept and treatment. *Clin Neuropharmacol* 1986; 9 (Suppl 2): S37-S48.
23. Bressman SB, de Leon D, Brin MF, et al. Inheritance of idiopathic torsion dystonia among Ashkenazi Jews. *Adv Neurol* 1988; 50: 45-56.
24. Bressman SB, de Leon D, Kramer PL, et al. Dystonia in Ashkenazi Jews: clinical characterization of a founder mutation. *Ann Neurol* 1994; 36: 771-7.
25. Bressman SB, Sabatti C, Raymond D, et al. The DYT1 phenotype and guidelines for diagnostic testing. *Neurology* 2000; 54: 1746-52.
26. Bressman SB. Dystonia genotypes, phenotypes, and classification. *Adv Neurol* 2004; 94: 101-7.
27. Zorzi G, Garavaglia B, Invernizzi F, et al. Frequency of DYT1 mutation in early onset primary dystonia in Italian patients. *Mov Disord* 2002; 17: 407-8.
28. Oppenheim H. Über eine eigenartige Krampfkrankheit des kindlichen und jugendlichen Alters (Dysbasia lordotica progressiva, Dystonia musculorum deformans). *Neurologische Centralblatt* 1911; 30: 1090-107.
29. Opal P, Tintner R, Jankovic J, et al. Intrafamilial phenotypic variability of the DYT1 dystonia: from asymptomatic TOR1A gene carrier status to dystonic storm. *Mov Disord* 2002; 17: 339-45.
30. Bressman SB, de Leon D, Brin MF, et al. Idiopathic dystonia among Ashkenazi Jews: evidence for autosomal dominant inheritance. *Ann Neurol* 1989; 26: 612-20.
31. Kramer PL, de Leon D, Ozelius L, et al. Dystonia gene in Ashkenazi Jewish population is located on chromosome 9q32-34. *Ann Neurol* 1990; 27: 114-20.
32. Inzelberg R, Zilber N, Kahana E, Korczyn AD. Laterality of onset in idiopathic torsion dystonia. *Mov Disord* 1993; 8: 327-30.
33. Kramer PL, Heiman GA, Gasser T, et al. The DYT1 gene on 9q34 is responsible far most cases of early limb-onset idiopathic torsion dystonia in non-Jews. *Am J Hum Genet* 1994; 55: 468-75.
34. Valente EM, Warner TT, Jarman PR, et al. The role of DYT1 in primary torsion dystonia in Europe. *Brain* 1998; 121: 2335-9.
35. Brassat D, Camuzat A, Vidailhet M, et al. Frequency of the DYT1 mutation in primary torsion dystonia without family history. *Arch Neurol* 2000; 57: 333-5.
36. Gatto EM, Pardal MM, Micheli FE. Unusual phenotypic expression of the DYT1 mutation. *Parkinsonism Relat Disord* 2003; 9: 277-9.
37. Chinnery PF, Reading PJ, McCarthy EL, Curtis A, Burn DJ. Late-onset axial jerky dystonia due to the DYT1 deletion. *Mov Disord* 2002; 17: 196-8.

38. Edwards M, Wood N, Bhatia K. Unusual phenotypes in DYT1 dystonia: a report of five cases and a review of the literature. *Mov Disord* 2003; 18: 706-11.
39. Ikeuchi T, Shimohata T, Nakano R, Koide R, Takano H, Tsuji S. A case of primary torsion dystonia in Japan with the 3-bp (GAG) deletion in the DYT1 gene with a unique clinical presentation. *Neurogenetics* 1999; 2: 189-90.
40. Bentivoglio AR, Loi M, Valente EM, Ialongo T, Tonali P, Albanese A. Phenotypic variability of DYT1-PTD: Does the clinical spectrum include psychogenic dystonia? *Mov Disord* 2002; 17: 1058-63.
41. Eldridge R. The torsion dystonias: literature review and genetic and clinical studies. *Neurology* 1970; 20: 1-78.
42. Zilber N, Korkzyn AD, Kahana E, Fried K, Alter M. Inheritance of idiopathic torsion dystonia among Jews. *J Med Genet* 1984; 21: 13-20.
43. Risch NJ, Bressman SB, de Leon D, et al. Segregation analysis of idiopathic torsion dystonia in Ashkenazi Jews suggests autosomal dominant inheritance. *Am J Hum Genet* 1990; 46: 533-8.
44. Pauls DL, Korczyn A. Complex segregation analysis of dystonia pedigrees suggests autosomal dominant inheritance. *Neurology* 1990; 40: 1107-10.
45. Ozelius L, Kramer PL, Moskowitz CB, et al. Human gene for torsion dystonia located on chromosome 9q32-q34. *Neuron* 1989; 2: 1427-34.
46. Ozelius LJ, Kramer PL, de Leon D, et al. Strong allelic association between the torsion dystonia gene (DYT1) and loci on chromosome 9q34 in Ashkenazi Jews. *Am J Hum Genet* 1992; 50: 619-28.
47. Risch N, de Leon D, Ozelius L, et al. Genetic analysis of idiopathic torsion dystonia in Ashkenazi Jews and their recent descent from a small founder population. *Nat Genet* 1995; 9: 152-9.
48. Warner TT, Fletcher NA, Davis MB, et al. Linkage analysis in British and French families with idiopathic torsion dystonia. *Brain* 1993; 116: 739-44.
49. Slominsky PA, Markova ED, Shadrina MI, et al. A common 3-bp deletion in the DYT1 gene in Russian families with early- onset torsion dystonia. *Hum Mutat* 1999; 14: 269.
50. Lebre AS, Durr A, Jedynak P, et al. DYT1 mutation in French families with idiopathic torsion dystonia. *Brain* 1999; 122: 41-5.
51. Klein C, Friedman J, Bressman S, et al. Genetic testing for early-onset torsion dystonia (DYT1): introduction of a simple screening method, experiences from testing of a large patient cohort, and ethical aspects. *Genet Test* 1999; 3: 323-8.
52. Klein C, Brin MF, de Leon D, et al. De novo mutations (GAG deletion) in the DYT1 gene in two non-Jewish patients with early-onset dystonia. *Hum Mol Genet* 1998; 7: 1133-6.
53. Ozelius LJ, Hewett JW, Page CE, et al. The early-onset torsion dystonia gene (DYT1) encodes an ATP-binding protein. *Nat Genet* 1997; 17:40-8.
54. Valente EM, Povey S, Warner TT, Wood NW, Davis MB. Detailed haplotype analysis in Ashkenazi Jewish and non-Jewish British dystonic patients carrying the GAG deletion in the DYT1 gene: evidence for a limited number of founder mutations. *Ann Hum Genet* 1999; 63: 1-8.
55. Leung JC, Klein C, Friedman J, et al. Novel mutation in the TOR1A (DYT1) gene in atypical early onset dystonia and polymorphisms in dystonia and early onset parkinsonism. *Neurogenetics* 2001; 3: 133-43.
56. Doheny D, Danisi F, Smith C, et al. Clinical findings of a myoclonus-dystonia family with two distinct mutations. *Neurology* 2002; 59: 1244-6.
57. Klein C, Liu L, Doheny D, et al. Epsilon-sarcoglycan mutations found in combination with other dystonia gene mutations. *Ann Neurol* 2002; 52: 675-9.
58. Augood SJ, Penney JBJ, Friberg IK, et al. Expression of the early-onset torsion dystonia gene (DYT1) in human brain. *Ann Neurol* 1998; 43 (5): 669-73.

59. Augood SJ, Martin DM, Ozelius LJ, Breakefield XO, Penney JB, Jr., Standaert DG. Distribution of the mRNAs encoding torsinA and torsinB in the normal adult human brain. *Ann Neurol* 1999; 46: 761-9.
60. Hewett J, Gonzalez-Agosti C, Slater D, *et al.* Mutant torsinA, responsible for early-onset torsion dystonia, forms membrane inclusions in cultured neural cells. *Hum Mol Genet* 2000; 9: 1403-13.
61. Kustedjo K, Bracey MH, Cravatt BF. Torsin A and its torsion dystonia-associated mutant forms are lumenal glycoproteins that exhibit distinct subcellular localizations. *J Biol Chem* 2000; 275: 27933-9.
62. Walker RH, Brin MF, Sandu D, Good PF, Shashidharan P. TorsinA immunoreactivity in brains of patients with DYT1 and non-DYT1 dystonia. *Neurology* 2002; 58: 120-4.
63. Shashidharan P, Good PF, Hsu A, Perl DP, Brin MF, Olanow CW. TorsinA accumulation in Lewy bodies in sporadic Parkinson's disease. *Brain Res* 2000; 877: 379-81.
64. Bentivoglio AR, Elia AE, Filippini G, Valente EM, Fasano A, Albanese A. Clinical presentation and progression of sporadic and familial primary torsion dystonia in Italy. *Adv Neurol* 2004; 94: 171-8.
65. Hjermind LE, Werdelin LM, Sorensen SA. Inherited and de novo mutations in sporadic cases of DYT1-dystonia. *Eur J Hum Genet* 2002; 10: 213-6.
66. Major T, Svetel M, Romac S, Kostic VS. DYT1 mutation in primary torsion dystonia in a Serbian population. *J Neurol* 2001; 248: 940-3.
67. Kamm C, Castelon-Konkiewitz E, Naumann M, *et al.* GAG deletion in the DYT1 gene in early limb-onset idiopathic torsion dystonia in Germany. *Mov Disord* 1999; 14: 681-3.
68. Santangelo G. Contributo clinico alla conoscenza delle forme familiari della dysbasia lordotica progressiva (spasmo di torsione). *Giornale di Psichiatria e Neuropatologia* 1934; 62: 52-77.
69. Gimenez-Roldan S, Delgado G, Marin M, Villanueva JA, Mateo D. Hereditary torsion dystonia in gypsies. *Adv Neurol* 1988; 50: 73-81.
70. Khan NL, Wood NW, Bhatia KP. Autosomal recessive, DYT2-like primary torsion dystonia: a new family. *Neurology* 2003; 61: 1801-3.
71. Ahmad F, Davis MB, Waddy HM, Oley CA, Marsden CD, Harding AE. Evidence for locus heterogeneity in autosomal dominant torsion dystonia. *Genomics* 1993; 15: 9-12.
72. Almasy L, Bressman SB, Raymond D, *et al.* Idiopathic torsion dystonia linked to chromosome 8 in two Mennonite families. *Ann Neurol* 1997; 42: 670-3.
73. Bentivoglio AR, Del Grosso N, Albanese A, Cassetta E, Tonali P, Frontali M. Non-DYT1 dystonia in a large Italian family. *J Neurol Neurosurg Psychiatry* 1997; 62: 357-60.
74. Valente EM, Bentivoglio AR, Cassetta E, *et al.* DYT13, a novel primary torsion dystonia locus, maps to chromosome 1p36.13-36.32 in an Italian family with cranial-cervical or upper limb onset. *Ann Neurol* 2001; 49: 362-6.
75. Bentivoglio AR, Ialongo T, Contarino MF, Valente EM, Albanese A. Phenotypic characterisation of DYT13 primary torsion distonia. *Mov Disord* 2003; DOI 10.1002/mds.10634.
76. Bressman SB, Heiman GA, Nygaard TG, *et al.* A study of idiopathic torsion dystonia in a non-Jewish family: evidence for genetic heterogeneity. *Neurology* 1994; 44: 283-7.
77. Holmgren G, Ozelius L, Forsgren L, *et al.* Adult onset idiopathic torsion dystonia is excluded from the DYT 1 region (9q34) in a Swedish family. *J Neurol Neurosurg Psychiatry* 1995; 59: 178-81.
78. Munchau A, Valente EM, Davis MB, *et al.* A Yorkshire family with adult-onset cranio-cervical primary torsion dystonia. *Mov Disord* 2000; 15: 954-9.
79. Defazio G, Brancati F, Valente EM, *et al.* Familial blepharospasm is inherited as an autosomal dominant trait and relates to a novel unassigned gene. *Mov Disord* 2003; 18: 207-12.
80. Maniak S, Sieberer M, Hagenah J, Klein C, Vieregge P. Focal and segmental primary dystonia in north-western Germany – a clinico-genetic study. *Acta Neurol Scand* 2003; 107: 228-32.

81. Kamm C, Naumann M, Mueller J, et al. The DYT1 GAG deletion is infrequent in sporadic and familial writer's cramp. *Mov Disord* 2000; 15: 1238-41.
82. Cooper IS, Cullinan T, Ricklan M. The natural history of dystonia. *Adv Neurol* 1976; 14: 157-69.
83. Fletcher NA, Harding AE, Marsden CD. A genetic study of idiopathic torsion dystonia in the United Kingdom. *Brain* 1990; 113: 379-95.
84. Gasser T, Windgassen K, Bereznai B, Kabus C, Ludolph AC. Phenotypic expression of the DYT1 mutation: a family with writer's cramp of juvenile onset [see comments]. *Ann Neurol* 1998; 44 (1): 126-8.
85. Leube B, Kessler KR, Ferbert A, et al. Phenotypic variability of the DYT1 mutation in German dystonia patients. *Acta Neurol Scand* 1999; 99: 248-51.
86. Nomura Y, Ikeuchi T, Tsuji S, Segawa M. Two phenotypes and anticipation observed in Japanese cases with early onset torsion dystonia (DYT1): pathophysiological consideration. *Brain Dev* 2000; 22 (Suppl. 1): S92-S101.
87. Matsumoto S, Nishimura M, Kaji R, et al. DYT1 mutation in Japanese patients with primary torsion dystonia. *Neuroreport* 2001; 12: 793-5.
88. Grundmann K, Laubis-Herrmann U, Bauer I, et al. Frequency and phenotypic variability of the GAG deletion of the DYT1 gene in an unselected group of patients with dystonia. *Arch Neurol* 2003; 60: 1266-70.
89. Kabakci K, Hedrich K, Leung JC, et al. Mutations in DYT1: extension of the phenotypic and mutational spectrum. *Neurology* 2004; 62: 395-400.
90. Bressman SB, Hunt AL, Heiman GA, et al. Exclusion of the DYT1 locus in a non-Jewish family with early-onset dystonia. *Mov Disord* 1994; 9: 626-32.
91. Wunderlich S, Reiners K, Gasser T, Naumann M. Cervical dystonia in monozygotic twins: case report and review of the literature. *Mov Disord* 2001; 16: 714-8.
92. Brancati F, Defazio G, Caputo V, et al. Novel Italian family supports clinical and genetic heterogeneity of primary adult-onset torsion dystonia. *Mov Disord* 2002; 17: 392-7.
93. Kock N, Kasten M, Schule B, et al. Clinical and genetic features of myoclonus-dystonia in 3 cases: a video presentation. *Mov Disord* 2004; 19: 231-4.

# Focal and segmental dystonia in children

**Teresa Temudo**

*Unidade de Neuropediatria, Serviço de Pediatria,*
*Hospital de Santo António SA, Porto, Portugal*

---

Dystonia is a neurological syndrome of sustained muscle contraction that frequently causes twisting and repetitive movements and abnormal postures [1].

These involuntary movements are often exacerbated during voluntary movements – so-called action dystonia – stress and fatigue and subside entirely during sleep. Many patients use "tricks" to reduce muscle contractions (*geste antagoniste*) such as touching the involved or adjacent body part.

We can classify dystonia according to temporal development, age at onset, topography (see p. 31) and aetiology (*Tables I-III*).

The current classification for aetiology [20] divides dystonias into two major categories: *idiopathic* and *symptomatic*. Adoption of the term primary is in fact preferred to idiopathic dystonia, because the later term may indicate an unknown aetiology, whereas for many forms of primary dystonia, abnormal genes have now been discovered as the possible cause. Symptomatic forms of dystonias may be subdivided into secondary, metabolic and heredodegenerative.

Secondary dystonia is defined as a dystonic disorder that develops mainly as the result of environmental factors that produce insult to the brain.

Heredodegenerative diseases are a category in which neurodegeneration produces dystonia as a prominent feature; usually other neurologic features, especially parkinsonism, also are present and can even predominate. In some patients with these disorders, dystonia may fail to appear, and other neurologic manifestations may be the presenting feature.

The distribution of dystonia is a partial indicator of its severity and is helpful in planning investigation and therapeutic strategy. The following features suggest that dystonia is secondary or metabolic/heredodegenerative: history of drug/toxin exposure, perinatal injury, central nervous system infection or head/neck trauma; atypical course with sudden onset and rapid progression; cranial onset with bulbar impairment

### Table I. Genetic Classification of the Dystonias [2].

| Name (ref) | Locus | Protein | Mode | Comments |
|---|---|---|---|---|
| DYT1 [3] | 9q34 | TorsinA | AD | Oppenheim dystonia |
| DYT2 [4] | ? | ? | AR | Spanish gypsies |
| DYT3 [5] | Xq13,1 | ? | X-R | Lubag (dystonia-parkinsonism), Filipino men |
| DYT4 [6] | ? | ? | ? | A whispering dysphonia family |
| DYT5 [7, 8] | 14q22,1 | GTPCH-I | AD | Dopa-responsive dystonia |
|  | 11p11,5 | TH | AR |  |
| DYT6 [9] | 8p21 | ? | AD | Mennonite/Amish, all ages & regions |
| DYT7 [10] | ?18p | ? | AD | Familial cervical dystonia |
| DYT8 [11, 12] | 2q33 | ? | AD | Paroxysmal non-kinesigenic dyskinesia |
| DYT9 [13] | 1p21 | ? | AD | Paroxysmal dyskinesia with spasticity |
| DYT10 [14-16] | 16p11 | ? | AD | Paroxysmal kinesigenic dyskinesia |
|  | 16q13 | ? | AD |  |
|  | 16p12 | ? | AD | PKD with infantile convulsions |
| DYT11 [17] | 7q21 | ε-sarcoglycan | AD | Myoclonus-dystonia |
| DYT12 [18] | 19q | ? | AD | Rapid-onset dystonia parkinsonism |
| DYT13 [19] | 1p36 | ? | AD | Cranial-cervical-brachial |

AD, autosomal dominant; AR, autosomal recessive; X-R, X-linked recessive;
GTPCH-I, GTP cyclohydrolase-I; TH, tyrosine hydroxylase.

### Table II. Secondary Dystonias.

**Drug-induced:**
Neuroleptic-induced (acute, tardive), anticonvulsants, levodopa

**Toxic:**
Manganese, carbon monoxide, carbon disulfide, cyanide, methanol, 3-nitroprorionic acid

**Infectious and postinfectious:**
Viral encephalitis, postinfectious, Reye's syndrome, subacute sclerosing leukoencephalopathy, wasp sting encephalopathy, HIV, Creutzfeld-Jacob disease

**Focal central nervous system lesions:**
Trauma, stroke, arteriovenous malformation, tumour

**Physical causes:**
Hypoxia, perinatal cerebral injury, electric shock, peripheral injury

**Autoimmune:**
Multiple sclerosis, antiphospholipid syndrome, Sjogren's syndrome

**Metabolic:**
Hypoparathyroidism

**Psychogenic**

**Table III. Metabolic and Heredodegenerative Dystonias.**

**Autosomal dominant:**
Rapid-onset dystonia-parkinsonism (RDP), Juvenile Parkinson's disease, Huntington's disease (Westfahl variant), Machado-Joseph disease (SCA3), Dentatorubro-pallidoluysian atrophy, other spinocerebellar degenerations

**Autosomal recessive:**
Wilson's disease, Niemann-Pick type C, juvenile neuronal ceroid-lipofuscinosis (Batten's disease), GM1 and GM2 gangliosidosis, metachromatic leukodystrophy, Lesch-Nyhan syndrome, homocystinuria, glutaric acidemia, methylmalonic aciduria, triose-phosphate isomerase deficiency, Hartnup's disease, ataxia telangiectasia, Hallervorden-Spatz syndrome, neuroacanthocytosis

**X-linked recessive:**
Lubag (dystonia-parkinsonism), deafness-dystonia syndrome (Mohr-Tranebjaerg syndrome)

**Others**
Rett syndrome
Familial basal ganglia calcifications
Progressive pallidal degeneration
Mitochondrial encephalopathies
Neurofibromatosis
Alternating hemiplegia of childhood

in childhood, and dystonia at rest at an early age; hemidystonia; presence of other neurologic abnormalities; systemic abnormalities; abnormal laboratory and neuroimaging studies. In this chapter we mainly discuss idiopathic or secondary focal dystonias.

Focal dystonia implies that a single body region is affected (eg, limb, spasmodic torticollis, blepharospasm, spasmodic dysphonia, writer's cramp).

Unlike adults, where focal dystonia is the most common type of dystonia, focal and segmental dystonias are rare forms of clinical presentation in childhood and usually represent only the initial phase of a generalized dystonia (idiopathic or symptomatic).

# ■ Primary Dystonias

## Idiopathic dystonia (torsion dystonia)

### *DYT1*

Early onset torsion dystonia, an autosomal dominant disease associated with the DYT1 locus on 9q34 [21], is the most frequent genetic dystonia.

This distinct genetic disorder was well characterized by Oppenheim in 1911, who coined the term *dystonia musculorum deformans* to describe it. The onset is early in life, usually in childhood, and in 80% of the cases before the age of 15 [22], but rare cases have been reported to present as late as 65 years [23].

One of the limbs is affected first in 90% of cases and the dystonia usually spreads to other body parts progressively; the cranial structures such as face, pharynx, and tongue tend to be spared [23].

In typical cases the onset is before the age of 10 and the first symptom is inversion of one foot during gait and initially this posture may appear only for some activities, especially when running [23]. Cases with limb onset usually generalize, especially if the disorder starts in a leg. Of the children evaluated by Green [24] in the young onset group (< 10 years) with presentation in the leg, 94% went on to develop dystonia in other body areas and 71% developed generalized dystonia. The spread from focal dystonia to generalized dystonia occurred approximately 5 years after disease onset.

Older children (> 10 years) had an increased frequency of symptom onset in the arm or neck region, and only 33% later developed generalized dystonia.

This dystonia is inherited in an autosomal dominant pattern with incomplete penetrance [25]. Even in the same family, the severity of the disease can vary considerably, with some family members manifesting generalized symptoms and others having only mild focal areas of involvement [26, 27].

## DYT6

Focal onset of dystonia in childhood (limb, cranial or cervical) may be the first sign of presentation of childhood and adult onset, familial cranial and limb dystonia (DYT6) [28]. The course of this disease may be limited or have a generalized spread.

This is an autosomal dominant primary dystonia with reduced penetrance and the abnormal gene has been mapped to 8p21-q22 [28].

## Dopa-responsive dystonia (DRD) or hereditary dystonia-parkinsonian syndrome of dopa-responsive dystonia (DYT5)

Doctor Masaya Segawa (Tokyo) was the first to delineate many of the particular characteristics of this disorder in a series of patients affected with hereditary progressive dystonia with marked diurnal fluctuation [29].

DRD is a rare autosomal dominant disorder with reduced but gender-influenced penetrance; it is more common in women. There is also a relatively high spontaneous mutation rate [30].

Many cases are caused by identified mutations of the gene for guanosine triphosphate cyclohydrolase I located at 14q 22.1 [30].

The important clinical features of DRD are onset of dystonia, usually affecting gait, in childhood; subsequent development of Parkinson signs; and a dramatic therapeutic response to DOPA [31]. A frequent but not invariable observation is the worsening of signs and symptoms later in the day (diurnal fluctuation). Approximately half of index cases with DRD report a family member affected with a similar disorder.

At onset dystonia affects one leg (foot inversion) in the majority of cases. A peculiar feature is a tendency to walk on the toes, instead of heel-striking. Writer's cramp [32] or cervical dystonia [33] are rare forms of presentation of the disease in childhood.

The disease is progressive but generally does not affect the trunk and the dystonia predominates in the lower limbs, even in the rare cases of the onset in the upper extremities. Some cases are wrongly diagnosed as spastic diplegia because of the presence of brisk deep tendon reflexes and, in long-lasting untreated cases, fixed dystonia and contractures. Administration of small doses (5-30 mg/kg/day) of L-dopa usually lead to a dramatic and rapid improvement of dystonia.

## Myoclonic dystonia (DYT11)

Myoclonic dystonia is an autosomal dominant disorder with variable expressivity and incomplete penetrance [34]. Mutations in the gene encoding epsilon-sarcoglycan were found to be responsible for this genetic dystonia [17].

Myoclonic dystonia is characterized by:
– Onset of myoclonus or dystonia in the first or second decade
– Both sexes are equally affected
– A benign course compatible with an active life with normal span
– Dominant mode of inheritance with variable severity (and variable character among family members)
– Absence of seizures, dementia, gross ataxia, and other neurological deficits
– Normal electroencephalogram.

Recognition of a familial occurrence and an essentially non-progressive character are of great importance for differential diagnosis.

In the largest family studied [34], myoclonus was the consistent abnormality, detected in almost everyone. Dystonia was present in three main forms: leg dystonia or hemidystonia in two cases (1-4 years old), writer's cramp in several teenagers and adults, and retrocollis and torticollis in two adult cases.

Leg dystonia resolved in both legs in one child and in one leg in another one. Transient dystonia has been described in babies born preterm with a good prognosis.

Dystonia symptoms and signs in infancy gradually improved during motor development, rather than progressing as in most other dystonic syndromes. Ambulation was possible at about the normal time, but the gait was abnormal since the action provoked inward leg rotation and tiptoe position. Writer's cramp in children of school age and adults did not increase with time but did worsen temporarily with stress and attempts to write quickly.

Neck dystonia only appeared in adults. Patients reported some benefit from benzodiazepines and alcohol.

## Cervical-cranial predominant dystonia (DYT 7)

Cervical-cranial predominant dystonia (DYT 7) may also begin in childhood [35].

The onset of this type of primary dystonia is usually in the neck, but dystonia often spreads to involve the cranial structures as well, and occasionally the arm [36].

# Secondary Dystonias

## Tardive dystonia

Tardive dystonia is seen equally in children and adults. There is a tendency for younger patients to demonstrate more generalized involvement, while older patients usually have a focal or segmental distribution.

Prerequisites for diagnosis of tardive dyskinesia are [37]:
– History of at least three months total cumulative (continuous or discontinuous) neuroleptic exposure
– Presence of at least "moderate" abnormal involuntary movements (using an accepted rating scale) in one or more body areas or at least "mild" movements in two or more body areas
– Absence of other conditions that might produce abnormal involuntary movements.

In a study of 300 patients with cervical dystonia [38] tardive dystonia was found as a cause of secondary CD in 6% of the patients.

In another study of 42 patients with tardive dystonia [39] the symptoms began 3 to 11 days after antipsychotic therapy. In a few patients spontaneous remission occurred, but dystonia persisted in most. The most frequent helpful medications were tetrabenazine and anticholinergics.

## Trauma

Progressive hemidystonia due to focal basal ganglia lesion after mild head trauma was reported by Brett [40]. Focal dystonia appeared days after the incident and progressed during a two-year period. A CT Scan revealed a discrete area of low attenuation in the basal ganglia of the contralateral hemisphere with the appearance of an old infarct.

In a large study of 300 patients (including children) with cervical dystonia [38] 15% of the patients had secondary forms of cervical dystonia and in 11% of all patients CD developed within one year after trauma of the neck. Although acute neck extension-flexion (whiplash) injuries are common, only a few are followed by CD [41].

These sequelae, however, may develop in genetically or otherwise predisposed individuals [42].

## Cerebral vascular abnormalities

Cerebral vascular injury caused by ischemia may also be a cause of secondary focal dystonia in children and adults.

A case of an infarct in the lentiform nucleus followed by focal dystonia of the contralateral hand was described in a 43-year-old patient [43]. Giraud and Dumas [44] described three cases of focal dystonia in children secondary to an infarct of the territory of the lenticular striate arteries.

A 12-year-old girl with a 3-year history of writer's cramp in association with arteriovenous malformation was reported by Kurita *et al.* [45]. The lesion was localized to the left globus pallidus and putamen, extending to the adjacent white matter of the frontal lobe.

## Ketogenic diet

Focal dystonia was also a complication of ketogenic diet in a five-year-old girl with a cryptogenic epileptic encephalopathy. Cranial magnetic resonance imaging (MRI) demonstrated bilateral putaminal lesions that were not present before starting the diet. These radiographic abnormalities resolved after stopping the diet, although movement disorder persisted [46].

## Delayed onset dystonia

This term refers to the cases in which the appearance of dystonia follows a period (usually several years) of an apparent static motor disorder. In one study by Saint Hilaire et al., of ten patients with perinatal asphyxia [47] the mean age of onset of dystonia was 12.9 years, and the arm or hand was the most frequent site of onset. Progression occurred over a mean period of 7.1 years.

Delayed onset dystonia may also appear following an acquired insult, such as a cerebral infarct [48].

## Infections and parainfectious diseases of CNS

Infections and parainfectious diseases of the CNS may also be responsible for the appearance of focal dystonia in children.

Basal ganglia involvement is not unusual in postinfectious encephalomyelitis [49, 50] and focal dystonia may be one of the neurologic manifestations of this disease [51]. Movement disorders may also appear during tuberculous meningitis (TbM). In a large study of 180 patients with TbM, 30 patients had movement disorders and among these three had dystonia [52].

## Tumours of CNS

Tumours of the CNS can be responsible for focal dystonia in children.

Narbona et al. [53] reported one case of an 8-year-old boy who developed focal dystonia of the left hand secondary to an astrocytoma originating in the right putamen.

A case of acute onset focal dystonia of the left upper limb was also observed in a patient with a homolateral cerebellar hemisphere mass (tuberculoma). Both the limb dystonia and the tuberculoma resolved with the continuation of antituberculous treatment [54].

## Dystonia in Rasmussen's encephalitis

Rasmussen's encephalitis is a rare autoimmune disorder characterized by intractable epilepsy and progressive hemispheric dysfunction [55]. More recently, attention has been focused on athetosis, dystonia or choreic movements, correlating with atrophy of the caudate nucleus in addition to the focal cortical atrophy which characteristically involves mainly the frontal and perisylvian areas [56, 57].

Frucht [58] reported a 19-year-old woman with Rasmussen's encephalitis whose clinical presentation was dominated by foot dystonia, athetosis and *epilepsia partialis continua*.

## Environmental toxins

Environmental toxins such as manganese, carbon monoxide, methanol and 3-nitroproprionic acid may cause symptomatic dystonia [59, 60].

The mycotoxin 3NPA is responsible for a toxic encephalopathy followed by delayed dystonia. The dystonia syndrome that follows acute encephalopathy induced by 3-NPA poisoning occurs in severely affected patients who are in a coma for more then 3 days during the acute stage, and usually appears 7-40 days after consciousness is regained.

The involuntary movements are diverse, showing a wide range of speed, amplitude, rhythmicity, torsion, forcefulness, and distribution in the body. In most instances, the movements are somewhat unpatterned but usually repetitive, either segmental or generalized.

Parkinsonism has not been observed in any of the dystonic patients; therefore, 3-NPA-induced dystonia differs clinically from the extrapyramidal sequelae of acute carbon monoxide poisoning and chronic manganese poisoning, which manifest mainly as muscular hypertonia and bradykinesia and seldom show choreoathetosis.

The CTs and MRIs of all the dystonic patients showed striking hypodensity in the bilateral lenticular nuclei. Both the putamen and globus pallidus were consistently involved [61].

## Electrical injury

Electrical trauma may produce central or peripheral nervous system complications acutely or delayed for up to several weeks or months following injury [62-65].

In recent years, dystonia has been recognized following peripheral electrical injury [66-69].

Dystonia has been reported affecting one of the upper limbs (that received the electric shocks) or a hemidystonia, cervical dystonia or lingual dystonia.

The pathophysiology of electrically induced dystonia remains highly speculative but is considered to be a type of trauma-induced movement disorder. Post-traumatic dystonia occurs after both central and peripheral lesions. Some authors have postulated an underlying genetic predisposition, previous neural damage or prior drug exposures. Pathophysiologic theories advocate direct damage to the nervous system as well as a variety of delayed indirect effects, including aberrant neuronal sprouting, denervation, supersensivity, ephaptic transmission and oxidative reactions [70].

The majority of the cases reported in the literature did not respond to botulinum toxin.

## ■ Other Rare Causes

### Chromosome abnormalities

Gorgon FM et al. [71] described the first case of dystonia in a patient with deletion of 18q, a 36-year-old woman who developed a movement disorder with mixed features of dystonia and tremor in the cranial-brachial regions.

Awaad Y. et al. [72] reported a case of dystonia with partial deletion of the short arm of chromosome 8. Neurological findings in the 18p syndrome include mental retardation, seizures, incoordination, tremor, and chorea. These authors described progressive asymmetric dystonia in a 15-year-old girl with a denovo 18p deletion. She only responded to intrathecal baclofen therapy.

## Neurofibromatosis

Hyperintense areas in the left thalamic and sub-thalamic regions on MRI were responsible for right hand dystonia in a 13-year-old girl with neurofibromatosis type I. Over a two-year follow-up, the lesions showed a reduction in size, apparently correlated with a reduction in symptoms [73].

## Alternating hemiplegia of childhood (AHC)

In a typical attack the infants have a prodrome of screaming and restlessness and appear to be in pain. Oculomotor abnormalities appear early. Surprisingly, there may be unilateral nystagmus, but this may also be bilateral and episodes of dystonic stiffening frequently occur. Subsequently, multiple attacks of flaccid hemiplegia develop lasting from minutes to days. Paralysis is often accompanied by autonomic symptoms such as alterations in skin color, temperature, and sweating.

In some patients, bilateral hemiplegic attacks occur, characterized by generalized flaccidity, often associated with pseudo bulbar features such as dysphagia, dysarthria, and respiratory difficulties.

In the bilateral attacks, the level of consciousness may be reduced. The episodes are dramatically relieved by sleep but may recur after the child wakes. Focal dystonia or other symptoms may precede by months the appearance of hemiplegic attacks or occur in isolation [74]. The cause of AHC is unknown. It has often been regarded as a subtype of complicated migraine and some of the first reports included patients with familial hemiplegic migraine [75].

In a series of 44 patients with alternating hemiplegia, 95% had dystonia [76]. Dystonic and tonic events of the limbs, neck and trunk were usually short and lasted from a few seconds to several hours. In many of the patients the dystonic episodes did not exceed a few minutes. Dystonic or tonic posturing often appeared intermittently during the hemiplegic events. Not all hemiplegic events, however, were accompanied by dystonia, and dystonic episodes often occurred independently. Posturing could appear ipsilateral or contralateral to the hemiplegia. Two patients had dystonic events almost exclusively, with only rare hemiplegic attacks [76].

## Rett syndrome

Rett syndrome is a neurodegenerative disorder described in 1966 by Andreas Rett [77] and clinically delineated by Bent Hagberg et al. in 1983 [78]. A mutation in the gene $MECP_2$ was recognized in 1999 [79]. Extrapyramidal disturbances are prominent in this syndrome from the beginning of the disease or at the final stages [80]. Dystonia is a very common sign in Rett syndrome, particularly focal dystonia involving upper or lower extremities.

In one series of 32 patients, dystonia was present in 59% [81] and in another study of 37 girls with MECP$_2$ mutation 54% had focal dystonia [80].

## ■ Treatment

The prognosis for childhood dystonia remains guarded. There is no therapy that can halt the spread of symptoms or cure dystonia with the exception of the dramatic response of DRD to low doses of levodopa. However, pharmacological interventions can provide some relief in many children and improve their quality of life. Therapies for dystonia are divided into 3 categories: oral medications, intramuscular botulinum toxin injections, and surgical procedures. We will discuss only medical treatment.

Standard oral pharmacological therapies include anticholinergic agents, baclofen, clonazepan and levodopa. Tetrabenazine, a catecholamine depleting agent, has also been shown to improve symptoms but often causes serious side effects. A variety of other medications have been tried and found to be of some benefit in an occasional patient. Overall, approximately 40% of the patients will improve on oral therapy. The limitation of many oral agents is the occurrence of side effects: sedation, dry mouth, dysphoria, anxiety, depression, blurred vision, nausea and others. With the exception of levodopa, these agents must all be initiated at low doses with a gradual increase in dose as tolerated until benefit occurs or side effects intervene.

Levodopa is the first drug recommended for all children with primary dystonia. It is a safe drug with minimal side effects that can be administered for an indefinite time. Pediatric doses of levodopa range from 5 to 30 mg/kg divided in two or three doses a day (medium 10 mg/kg/day). The dose may be increased every 3-7 days until improvement occurs or a dose of 600 mg/day is reached. There are no withdrawal effects from the sudden discontinuation of levodopa.

If levodopa is ineffective, anticholinergics are the second line. Trihexyphenidyl is the most frequent preparation used. The initial dose is 1 mg twice a day. Trihexyphenidyl is increased slowly, usually 1 mg/day every week until the patient benefits or side effects occur – dryness of mouth, constipation, blurred vision, urinary hesitancy, anorexia, chorea, confusion and psychosis – to reach doses as high as 80 mg/day in children.

When trihexyphenidyl fails, a combination of trihexyphenidyl, tetrabenazine (75 mg/day) and pimozide (6-12 mg/day) can be used. Tetrabenazine is a difficult drug to use. Starting at low doses of 12.5 mg one to two times a day, it is often necessary to increase on a monthly schedule in order to determine whether the dose is effective or side effects occur (depression, dysphoria, parkinsonism) [82] or a combination of trihexyphenidyl and progressively increasing doses of clonazepan or diazepam [83].

Baclofen, clonazepan or diazepam are usually considered if anticholinergic therapy is unsuccessful. Baclofen is initiated at a dose of 10 mg, two to three times daily, until a maximal dose of 120 mg/day, unless side effects intervene (lethargy, dry mouth and dizziness). A rapid decrease in the dose of baclofen may produce seizures or psychosis [84]. Clonazepan is started at low doses of 0.5 mg/day at bedtime, and then slowly increased to include daytime doses.

# References

1. Fahn S. Concept and classification of dystonia. *Adv Neurol* 1988; 50: 1-8.
2. Nemeth AH. The genetics of primary dystonias and related disorders. *Brain* 2002; 125: 695-721.
3. Ozelius LJ, Hewett JW, Page CE, et al. The early-onset torsion dystonia gene (DYT1) encodes an ATP-binding protein. *Nat Genet* 1999; 71: 40-8.
4. Gimenez-Roldan S, Delgado G, Marin M, et al. Hereditary torsion dystonia in gypsies. *Adv Neurol* 1998; 50: 73-81.
5. Muller U, Haberhausen G, Wagner T, et al. DXS106 and DXS559 flank the X-linked dystonia-parkinsonism syndrome locus (DYT3). *Genomics* 1994; 23: 114-7.
6. Parker N. Hereditary whispering dysphonia. *J Neurol Neurosurg Psychiatry* 1985; 48: 218-24.
7. Ichinose H, Ohye T, Takahashi E, et al. Hereditary progressive dystonia with marked diurnal fluctuation caused by mutations in the GTP cyclohydrolase I gene. *Nat Genet* 1994; 8: 236-42.
8. Knappskog PM, Flatmark T, Mallet J, et al. Recessively inherited L-DOPA-responsive dystonia caused by a point mutation (Q381K) in the tyrosine hydroxylase gene. *Hum Mol Genet* 1995; 4: 1209-12.
9. Almasy L, Bressman SB, Raymond D, et al. Idiopathic torsion dystonia linked to chromosome 8 in two Mennonite families. *Ann Neurol* 1997; 42: 670-3.
10. Leube B, Rudnicki D, Ratzlaff T, et al. Idiopathic torsion dystonia: Assignment of a gene to chromosome 18p in a German family with adult onset, autosomal dominant inheritance and purely focal distribution. *Hum Mol Genet* 1996; 5: 1673-67.
11. Fouad GT, Servidei S, Durcan S, et al. A gene for familial paroxysmal dyskinesia (FPD1) maps to chromosome 2q. *Am J Hum Genet* 1996; 59: 135-9.
12. Fink JK, Rainer S. Wilkowski J, et al. Paroxysmal dystonic choreoathetosis: Tight linkage to chromosome 2q. *Am J Hum Genet* 1996; 59: 140-5.
13. Auburger G, Ratzlaff T, Lunkes A, et al. A gene for autosomal dominant paroxysmal choreoathetosis/spasticity (CSE) maps to the vicinity of a potassium channel gene cluster on chromosome 1p probably within 2 cM between DIS443 and DIS197. *Genomics* 1996; 31: 90-4.
14. Tomita H, Nagamitsu S, Wakui K, et al. Paroxysmal Kinesigenic choreoathetosis locus maps to chromosome 16p11.2-2q12.1. *Am J Hum Genet* 1999; 65: 1688-97.
15. Valente EM, Spacey SD, Wali GM, et al. A second paroxysmal kinesigenic choreoathetosis locus (EKD2) mapping on 16q13-q22.1 indicates a family of genes wich give rise to paroxysmal disorders on human chromosome 16. *Brain* 2000; 123; 2040-5.
16. Szepetowski P, Rochette J, Berquin P, et al. Familial infantile convulsions and paroxysmal choreoathetosis: A new neurological syndrome linked to the pericentromeric region of human chromosome 16. *Am J Hum Genet* 1997; 61: 889-98.
17. Zimprich A. Grabowski M. Asmus F, et al. Mutations in the gene encoding epsilon-sarcoglycan cause myoclonus-dystonia syndrome. *Nat Genet* 2001; 29: 866-9.
18. Kramer PL, Mineta M. Klein C, et al. Rapid-onset dystonia-parkinsonism: Linkage to chromosome 19q13. *Ann Neurol* 1999; 46: 176-82.
19. Valente EM, Bentivoglio AR, Cassetta E, et al. DYT13, a novel primary torsion dystonia locus, maps to chromosome 1p36.13-36.32 in an Italian family with cranial-cervical or upper limb onset. *Ann Neurol* 2001; 49: 362-6.
20. Fahn S, Bressman SB, Marsden CD: *Classification of dystonia*. In: *Dystonia 3: Advances in Neurology*, vol 78, edited by Fahn S, C.D. Marsden and M. DeLong. Philadelphia: Lippincott-Raven Publishers, 1998: 1-10.
21. Marsden CD, Harrison MJG. Idiopathic torsion dystonia (dystonia musculorum deformans). A review of forty-two patients. *Brain* 1974; 97: 793-810.

22. Bressman SB, de Leon D, Kramer PL, et al. Dystonia in Ashkenazi Jews: clinical characterization of a founder mutation. *Ann Neurol* 1994; 36: 771-7.
23. Fernández-Alvarez E, Peña J, Lorente I. *Distonia muscular deformante.* In: Fernández-Alvarez E, Fejerman N, Campos J (eds). *Actualidades en Neuropediatria.* Barcelona: Edición Medicina y Técnica, 1980; 179-203.
24. Green P, Kang UJ, Fahn S. Spread of symptoms in idiopathic dystonia. *Movement Disorders* 1995; 10: 143-52.
25. Kramer PL, Heinman GA, Gasser T, et al. The DYT1 gene on 9q34 is responsible for most cases of early limb-onset idiopathic torsion dystonia in non-Jews. *Am J Hum Genet* 1994; 55: 468-75.
26. Bressman SB, Sabatti C, Raymond D, et al. The DYT1 phenotype and guidelines for diagnostic testing. *Neurology* 2000; 54: 1747-52.
27. Marsden CD, Harrison MJ, Bundey S. Natural history of idiopathic torsion dystonia. *Ad Neurol* 1976; 14: 177-87.
28. Almasy L, Bressman SB, Raymond D, et al. Idiopathic torsion dystonia linked to chromosome 8 in two Mennonite families. *Ann Neurol* 1997; 42: 670-3.
29. Segawa M, Mosaka A, Miyagawa F, Namura Y, Imai H. Hereditary progressive dystonia with marked diurnal fluctuations. *Adv Neurol* 1976; 14: 215-33.
30. Furukawa Y, Lang AE, Trugman JM, et al. Gender-related penetrance and the novo GTP-cyclohydrolase I gene mutations in dopa-responsive dystonia. *Neurology* 1998; 50: 1015-20.
31. Nygaard TG, Marsden CD, Duvoisin RC. Dopa-responsive dystonia. *Adv Neurol* 1988; 50: 377-84.
32. Deonna T, Roulet E, Ghika J, Zegiger P. Dopa-responsive childhood dystonia: a forme fruste with writer's cramp, triggered by exercise. *Dev Med Child Neurol* 1997; 39: 49-53.
33. Nygaard TG, Trugman JM, Yebanes JG, Fahn S. Dopa-responsive dystonia: the spectrum of clinical manifestations in a large North American family. *Neurology* 1990; 40: 66-9.
34. Kyllerman M, Forsgren L, Sanner G, Holmgren G, Wahlstrom J, Drugge U. Alcohol-responsive myoclonic dystonia in a large family: Dominant inheritance and phenotypic variation. *Mov Disord* 1990; 5: 270-9.
35. Bentivoglio AR, Delgrosso N, Albanese A, Cassetta E, Tonali P, Frontali M. Non-DYT1 dystonia in a large Italian family. *J Neurol Neurosurg Psychiatry* 1997; 62: 357-60.
36. Bressman SB, Heiman GA, Nygaard TG, et al. A study of idiopathic torsion dystonia in a non-Jewish family: evidence for genetic heterogeneity. *Neurology* 1994; 44: 283-7.
37. Weiner WJ, Lang AE. *"Tardive Dyskinesia" in movement disorders: A comprehensive survey.* New York: Futuro Publishing company, Inc 295 Main Street, PO. Box 330. Mount Kisco, 1989; 10549.
38. Jankovic J, Leder S, Warner D, Schwartz K: Cervical dystonia: clinical findings and associated movement disorders. *Neurology* 1991; 41: 1088-91.
39. Burke RE, Fahn S, Jankovic J, Marsden CD, Lang Gollomp S, Ilson J. Tardive dystonia: late-onset and persistent dystonia caused by antipsychotic drugs. *Neurology* 1982; 32: 1335-46.
40. Brett EM, Hoore RD, Sheehy MP, Marsden CD. Progressive hemidystonia due to focal basal ganglia lesion after mild head trauma. *J Neurol Neurosurg Psychiatry* 1981; 44: 460-1.
41. Pearce JM. Whiplash injury: a reappraisal. *J Neurol Neurosurg Psychiatry* 1989; 52: 1329-31.
42. Jankovic J, Van der Linden C. Dystonia and tremor induced by peripheral trauma: predisposing factors. *J Neurol Neurosurg Psychiatry* 1988; 51: 1512-9.
43. Troub M, Ridley A. Focal dystonia in association with cerebral infarction. *J Neur Neurosurg Psychiatry* 1982; 45: 1073-4.
44. Giraud M, Dumas R. Dystonie secondaire à un infarctus putamino-capsulo-caudé chez l'enfant. *Rev Neurol* 1988; 144; 5: 375-7.
45. Kurita H, Sasaki T, Susuki I, Kirino T: Basal ganglia arteriovenous malformation presenting as "writer's cramp": *Childs Nerv Syst* 1998; H (6): 285-7.

46. Erickson JC, Jabbari B, Difazio MP. Basal ganglia injury as a complication of the Ketogenic diet. *Mov Disord* 2003; 18 (4): 448-51.
47. Saint Hilaire M-H, Burke RE, Bressman SB, Brin MF, Fahn S. Delayed-onset dystonia due to perinatal or early childhood asphyxia. *Neurology* 1991; 41: 216-22.
48. Factor SA, Sanchez-Ramos J, Weiner WJ. Delayed-onset dystonia associated with cortico-spinal tract dysfunction. *Mov Disord* 1988; 3: 201-10.
49. Danovan MK, Lenn NJ. Postinfectious encephalomyelitis with localized basal ganglia involvement. *Pediat Neurol* 1989; 5 (5): 311-3.
50. Dale RC, Church AJ, Cardose F, et al. Poststreptococcal acute disseminated encephalomyelitis with basal ganglia involvement and auto-reactive antibasal ganglia antibodies. *Ann Neurol* 2001; 50 (5): 588-95.
51. Leite BAL, Costa A, Cunha J, Silva NF, Teixeira J, Temudo T. Acute disseminated encephalomyelitis in children: clinical and magnetic resonance imaging features. *Rev Neurol* 2003; 36: 490 (Abst).
52. Alarcon F, Duenas G, Cevallos N, Lees AJ. Movement disorders in 30 patients with tuberculous meningitis. *Movement Disord* 2000; 15: 561-9.
53. Narbona J, Obeso JA, Tunon T, Lage MJM, Marsden CD. Hemi-dystonia secondary to focalised basal ganglia tumour. *J Neurol Nerosurg Psychiatry* 1984; 47: 704-9.
54. Alarcón F, Tolosa E, Muñoz E. Focal limb dystonia in a patient with a cerebellar mass. *Arch Neurol* 2001; 58: 1125-7.
55. Rasmussen TB, Olszewski J, Lloyd-Smith D. Focal seizures due to chronic localized encephalitis. *Neurology* 1958; 8: 435-45.
56. Bhatjiwale MG, Polkey C, Cox TC, Dean A, Deasy N. Rasmussen's encephalitis: neuroimaging findings in 21 patients with a closer look at the basal ganglia. *Pediatr Neurosurg* 1998; 129: 142-8.
57. Ben Zeev B, Nass D, Polack S, et al. Progressive unilateral basal ganglia atrophy and hemidystonia: A new form of chronic focal viral encephalitis. *Neurology* 1999; 51 (suppl. 1).
58. Frucht S. Dystonia, athetosis, and epilepsia partialis continua in a patient with late-onset Rasmussen's encephalitis. *Mov disord* 2002; 17: 610-2.
59. Marsden CD. *The investigation of dystonia*. In: Fahn S, Marsden CD, Calne DB, eds. *Advances in neurology*. New York: Raven Press 1988; 53: 35-44.
60. Calne DB, Lange AE. *Secondary dystonia*. In: Fahn S, Marsden CD, Calne DB, eds: *Advances in neurology*. New York: Raven Press 1988; 50: 9-34.
61. He F, Zhang S, Qian F, Zhang C. Delayed dystonia with striatal CT lucences induced by a mycotoxin (3-nitroproprionic acid). *Neurology* 1995; 45: 2178-83.
62. Critchley M. Neurological effects of lightening and of electricity. *Lancet* 1934; 1: 68-72.
63. Silversides J. The neurological sequelae of electrical injury. *Can Med Assoc J* 1964; 91: 195-204.
64. Fannell DF, Starr A. Delayed neurological sequelae of electrical injuries. *Neurology* 1968; 18: 601-6.
65. Grube BJ, Heimbach DM, Engrav LH, et al. Neurologic consequences of electrical burns. *J Trauma* 1990; 30: 254-8.
66. Colosino C, Kocen RS, Powell M, et al. Torticollis after electrocution. *Mov disord* 1993; 8: 117.
67. Tarsy D, Sudarsky L, Charness ME. Limb dystonia following electrical injury. *Mov Disord* 1994; 9: 230-2.
68. Boonkogchuen P, Lees A. Case of torticollis occurring following electrical injury. *Mov Disord* 1996; 11: 109-10.
69. Ondo W. Lingual dystonia following electrical injury. *Mov Disord* 1997; 12: 253.
70. Jankovik J. Pos-traumatic movement disorders: central and peripheral mechanisms. *Neurology* 1994; 44: 2006-14.

71. Gordon FM, Bressman S, Brin FM, et al. Dystonia in a patient with deletion of 18 q. *Mov Disord* 1995; 10 (4): 496-9.
72. Awaad Y, Munoz S, Nigro M. Progressive dystonia in a child with chromosome 18p deletion, treated with in intrathecal baclofen. *J Chid Neurol* 1999; 14: 75-7.
73. Di Capua M, Lispi ML, Giannotti A, Longo D, Faniello G. Neurofibromatosis type I presenting with hand dystonia. *J Child Neurol* 2001; 16: 606-8.
74. Silver K, Anderman F. Alternating hemiplegia of childhood: A study of 10 patients and result of flunarizine treatment. *Neurology* 1993; 43: 36-41.
75. Verret S, Steel JC. Alternating hemiplegia in childhood: a report of eight patients with complicated migraine in infancy. *Pediatrics* 1971; 47: 675-80.
76. Mikati MA, Kramer U, Lupank ML, Shanahan RJ. Alternating hemiplegia in childhood: clinical manifestations and long-term outcome. *Ped Neurol* 2000; 23: 134-41.
77. Rett A. Über ein eigarties hinartrophisches Syndrom bei Hyperammoniamie in Kindesalter. *Wien Med Wochenschr* 1966; 116: 723.
78. Hagberg B, Aicardi J, Dias K, Ramos O. Progressive syndrome of autism, dementia, ataxia and loss of purposeful hand use in girls: Rett's syndrome: report of 35 cases. *Annals of Neurol* 1983; 14: 471-9.
79. Amir RE, Veyver IB, Wan M, Tran CQ, Francke U, Zoghbi HY. Rett syndrome is caused by mutations in X-linked MECP2, encoding methyl. CpG-binding protein 2. *Nature Genetics* 1999; 23: 185-8.
80. Temudo T, Santos MJ, Dias K, et al. Rett syndrome in Portugal: mutation analysis and tentative of clinical correlations. *Rev Neurol* 2004; 38: 32-3 (Abst).
81. Fitzgerald PM, Jankovic J, Glase DG, Schultz R, Percy AK. Extrapyramidal involvement in Rett's syndrome. *Neurology* 1990; 40: 243-5.
82. Marsden CD, Marion MH, Quinn N. The treatment of severe dystonia in children and adults. *J Neurol Neurosurg Psyquiatry* 1984; 47: 1116-73.
83. Fernández-Alvarez E, Aicardi J. *Disorders with dystonia or athetosis*. In: Fernández-Alvarez E, Aicardi J, eds. *Movement disorders in children*. Mac Keith Press for the INCA 2001; 77-129.
84. Green P. *Medical and surgical therapy of idiopathic torsion dystonia*. In: Kurlan R (ed). *Treatment of movement disorders*. Philadelphia: JB Lippincott 1995: 153-81.

# Status dystonicus in children

**Nardo Nardocci\*, Terasa Temudo\*\*, Bernard Echenne\*\*\*, Agathe Roubertie\*\*\* for the European Study Group on Movement Disorders in Children**

\* Division of Child Neurology, Istituto Nazionale Neurologico "C. Besta", Milano, Italy
\*\* Serviço de Pediatria, Hospital de Santo António, Porto, Portugal
\*\*\* Service de Neuropédiatrie, Hôpital Saint-Éloi, Montpellier, France

---

Status dystonicus is a rare clinical syndrome characterized by a severe, life-threatening dystonia occurring in patients with dystonic syndromes of different aetiologies. Patients should be managed on intensive care unit for sedation and ventilation since they may develop respiratory and metabolic complications. Pharmacological treatment is very difficult, drugs such as anticholinergics, pimozide, haloperidol, and tetrabenazine may be beneficial in some cases. In drug resistant patients surgical procedures can be considered. We report 10 children affected by a broad spectrum of dystonic syndromes who developed during the course of the disease a status dystonicus, describing the clinical features and the therapeutical strategies of this rare condition.

## ■ Introduction

Patients with primary and secondary dystonia may develop during the course of the disease severe episodes of generalized dystonia and rigidity which may be refractory to standard drug therapy. The most severe cases may develop bulbar and ventilatory complications. As a consequence of the intense muscle activity, metabolic complications such as rhabdomyolysis, leading to acute renal failure, may occur. Such condition has been described in isolated reports under different terms such as devastating dystonia, dystonic storm, life threatening dystonia or malignant dystonia [1-9]. In 1998 Manji et al. [9] reported under the term of Status Dystonicus (SD) a series of twelve patients which included five children describing the main clinical features of the syndrome and suggesting some therapeutical guidelines. However, the syndrome is rare and the management of these patients remains difficult. We therefore report 10 children, with a broad spectrum of dystonic syndromes, who developed severe dystonia culminating in status dystonicus necessitating management on an intensive care unit.

## ■ Patients and Methods

Eight out of the ten patients (eight males and two females) were followed at National Neurological Institute of Milan; one patient was treated at the Service de Neuropédiatrie-Hôpital Saint-Éloi, Montpellier (Prof. B. Echenne and Dr. A. Roubertie) and one case at the Servico de Pediatria-Hospital Geral de Santo Antonio, Porto (Dr. T. Temudo).

According to Manji et al. [9], patients were defined as having status dystonicus when they developed increasingly frequent and severe episodes of generalized dystonia necessitating hospital admission. All suffered one or more of the following life-threatening complications: bulbar weakness with risk of pulmonary aspiration; progressive impairment of respiratory function leading to respiratory failure; severe exhaustion and pain and metabolic derangements. All patients were investigated for secondary causes of dystonia. Investigations included some or all of the following: routine haematology and biochemistry; uric acid; copper and caeruloplasmin; CSF examination; plasma and CSF lactate and pyruvate; plasma and urinary amino acids; white cell enzymes; urinary amino acids, oligosaccharides, mucopolysaccharides and organic acids; muscle biopsy for evidence of a mitochondrial cytopathy; slit lamp examination; cranial CT and/or MRI; evoked responses; nerve conduction tests and electromyography; electroencephalography.

### Clinical features

The age at onset of SD ranged between 5 and 14 years with latency between the onset of dystonia and the status ranging between 1 and 9 years. The underlying diagnoses were variable: primary DYT1-positive dystonia (1 patient), primary DYT1-negative dystonia (2 patients), athetoid cerebral palsy (2 patients), Huntington's disease (1 patient), mitochondrial encephalopathy (1 patient) and unknown symptomatic dystonia (3 patients).

The onset of SD was acute in seven patients and slowly progressive during weeks in three. In four out of the ten patients the development of SD coincided with an intercurrent infection. In three out of the five patients who remained on intensive treatment unit for a period longer than 30 days an exacerbation of their severe dystonic spasms with episodes of pneumonia or urinary tract infection was noted. Pure dystonia characterized by generalized dystonic movements and spasms involving neck, trunk and cranial muscles was present in two patients. In the remaining children, the status dystonicus was characterized by the association of dystonia with more rapid hyperkinesias such ballism, chorea and myoclonus.

### Management on intensive care unit

Seven of the ten patients underwent tracheal intubation and mechanical ventilation due to bulbar and respiratory compromise, severe discomfort and exhaustion or metabolic derangement. The mean duration of ventilation was 39 days (range 3-120 days). Tracheotomy was performed in one patient. As a result of the severe dystonic spasms, five patients developed rhabdomyolysis leading to renal failure Pneumonia and deep vein thrombosis occurred in three and one patient respectively.

Patients who were not ventilated were admitted to the intensive care unit because the levels of sedation required to control dystonia necessitated a close monitoring of cardiovascular and respiratory indices.

## Pharmacological treatment

A series of antidystonic agents were tried in various combination and dosages. They included: trihexyphenidyl, pimozide, tetrabenazine, haloperidol, clozapine, risperidon, olanzapine, clotiapine, oral and intrathecal baclofen, levodopa, carbamazepine and valproate.

Oral baclofen was tried in six patients without benefit. In two cases an intrathecal infusion of baclofen was also unhelpful. Two patients seemed to improve with adding pimozide to tetrabenazine and trihexyphenidyl. An improvement in the status dystonicus was related to the starting of tetrabenazine in one case; in another, the adding of olanzapine coincided with the onset of improvement of the SD Finally, sedation and treatment with intravenous antibiotics correlated with a clinical improvement which led to the resolution of the SD in one patient.

## Surgical treatment

Bilateral globus pallidus stimulation was performed in four patients after having verified the ineffectiveness of the pharmacological treatment. Surgery was performed at the National Neurological Institute "C. Besta" of Milano (Prof. G. Broggi) in three patients and at the School of Medicine University of Montpellier (Prof. P. Coubes) in one case. Three patients showed a clear improvement in the first days from starting stimulation which led to a complete resolution of the status within one week. In the remaining case, the improvement was slower and after progressively reduction, sedation and ventilation were totally discontinued at 3 months.

## Outcome

One patient died due to pneumonia after 29 days on intensive treatment. After the resolution of SD, six patients returned to their pre-status neurological conditions and three were worse. One patient suffered a relapse after 3 months.

## ■ Discussion

Status dystonicus is a rare clinical condition. Jankovic and Penn [1] reported an 8-year-old boy with autosomal dominant primary torsion dystonia who deteriorated over 6 months and required mechanical ventilation. His crisis seemed to respond to treatment with levodopa. Marsden et al. [2] described two children with primary generalized dystonia who at 12 and 15 years of age showed a "life-threatening" worsening of dystonia with generalized dystonic movements and painful dystonic spasms. A combined treatment with trihexyphenidyl, pimozide and tetrabenazine was effective in one patient. The same triad of drugs was not effective in the other patient who showed an acute dystonic reaction to pimozide. Narayan et al. [3] described an 18-year-old man with dystonia, due to cerebral palsy who deteriorated markedly after spinal surgery. Treatment with anticholinergics, tetrabenazine and oral baclofen were ineffective, while intrathecal infusion of baclofen led to the resolution of the status. Vaamonde et al. [4] used the term 'dystonic storm' to describe two patients affected by primary dystonia and a probable Hallervorden-Spatz disease. The first patient deteriorated over a period of 2 months following a febrile illness. Treatment with benzhexol, tetrabenazine, pimozide and diazepam was ineffective and he received general anaesthesia because of severe discomfort and respiratory distress. Treatment with baclofen and haloperidol, in addition to the four drugs above, was of little benefit; with the introduction of carbamazepine, primidone and valproic acid his dystonic storm seemed to abate. The second patient presented with a rapid deterioration of general condition due to a generalized dystonic spasms which depressed his respiration. General thiopentone anaesthesia combined with chlorpromazine, haloperidol, pimozide, diazepam and benzhexol was ineffective and his condition improved with the introduction of baclofen. Manji et al. [9] under the term status dystonicus described twelve cases which included five children. Four out of the five children required mechanical ventilation. Two died during the course of the status; a combined treatment with trihexyphenidyl, pimozide tetrabenazine, high doses of baclofen and the association of haloperidol and acetazolamide correlated with the resolution of the status in the remaining patients. Bilateral thalamotomy performed in one case did not show benefit. Considering the clinical features and the response to treatment observed in the whole series, the authors concluded that patients with SD should be managed on intensive care unit due to the frequent occurrence of respiratory and metabolic complications and that drug therapy with trihexyphenidyl, tetrabenazine, pimozide or haloperidol may be beneficial in some patients.

Angelini et al. [5] reported a 13-year-old boy who developed severe refractory dystonia-dyskinesias as an abrupt worsening of a previously non progressive movement disorder. The patient required mechanical ventilation and continuous sedation in the intensive care unit. Various drugs and drugs combination (trihexyphenidyl, tetrabenazine, pimozide) failed to achieve control. Bilateral pallidal stimulation led to the resolution of the status within one week from starting the stimulation. Opal et al. [6] described a large family affected by DYT1 dystonia with a broad variability of the clinical spectrum, including a patient who succumbed in his second decade to malignant dystonia. Various drugs (Levodopa, ethopropazine, tetrabenazine, baclofen) caused only transient improvement and a ventrolateral thalamotomy was ineffective.

In the present series an underlying infection was an important precipitating factor leading to staus dystonicus and in one case sedation and treatment with intravenous antibiotics correlated with the resolution of the SD. A possible infection must therefore sought and treated as a first therapeutical step. In most cases of this series it was necessary to institute paralysis, ventilation and sedation in order to avert the bulbar and respiratory complications or to relieve the severe exhaustion and the pain resulting from the incessant dystonic spasms.

The present series indicates that tetrabenazine which depletes all three monoamine neurotransmitters may be helpful and that, as suggested by Marsden et al. [2] and Manji et al. [9], a combined treatment with tetrabenazine, trihexyphenidyl and pimozide should be tried. It is worth to note that such drugs may have significant side effects that may require their withdrawal. The poor understanding of the pathopharmacological mechanisms of dystonia makes it difficult to explain the reports suggesting the efficacy of drugs such as baclofen, levodopa and anticonvulsants [4]. It may reflect the fact that different pathophysiological mechanisms underlie the clinical syndrome.

Surgical intervention may be indicated in drug-resistant cases. Stereotactic thalamotomy has been tried with equivocal results [9] and bilateral pallidotomy associated with temporary intrathecal baclofen infusion seemed to be effective in a 9-year-old boy affected by Hallervorden-Spatz disease [7]. Four patients of the present series underwent pallidal stimulation after having verified the inefficacy of various drugs. Two of them have been already reported [5, 10]. In three patients the SD resolved within few days from starting stimulation. In the remaining patient the condition subsided slowly over 3 months casting doubt on the role of stimulation; however turning off stimulation on separate occasions always provoked the appearance, within a few hours, of dystonic spasms requiring higher doses of sedation and resolving with the turning on of the stimulation.

In conclusion, the present series and the literature indicate that children with status dystonicus should be managed in an intensive care unit due to the risk of respiratory and metabolic complications. Sedation itself and the cure of possible underlying infection may lead to a resolution of SD. The pharmacological approach remains empirical; however trihexyphenidyl, tetrabenazine and pimozide should be tried since they may have a beneficial effect. If such treatment fails, baclofen, anticonvulsant drugs and levodopa should be used. Intrathecal baclofen may prove a further useful option. Finally, pallidal stimulation should be considered when conventional treatments are ineffective.

# References

1. Jankovic J, Penn AS. Severe dystonia and myoglobinuria. *Neurology* 1982; 32: 1195-7.
2. Marsden CD, Marion MH, Quinn N. The treatment of severe dystonia in children and adults. *J Neurol Neurosurg Psychiatry* 1984; 47: 1166-73.
3. Narayan RK, Loubser PG, Jankovic J, Donovan WH, Bontke CF. Intrathecal baclofen for intractable axial dystonia [see comments]. *Neurology* 1991; 41: 1141-2. Comment in: *Neurology* 1992; 42: 1639-40.
4. Vaamonde J, Narbona J, Weiser R, Garcia MA, Brannan T, Obeso JA. Dystonic storms: a practical management problem. *Clin Neuropharmacol* 1994; 17: 344-7.
5. Angelini L, Nardocci N, Estienne M, Conti C, Dones I, Broggi G. Life-threatening distonia-dyskinesias in a child: successful treatment with bilateral pallidal stimulation. *Mov Disord* 2000; 15: 1010-2.
6. Opal P, Tintner R, Jankovic J, *et al*. Intrafamilial phenotypic variability of the DYT1 dystonia: from asymptomatic TOR1A gene carrier status to dystonic storm. *Mov Disord* 2002; 17: 339-45.
7. Kyriagis M, Grattan-Smith P, Scheinberg A, Teo C, Nakaji N, Waugh M. Status dystonicus and Hallervorden-Spatz disease: treatment with intrathecal baclofen and pallidotomy. *J Paediatr Child Health* 2004; 40: 322-5.

8. Giménez-Roldàn S, Mateo D, Martìn M. ¹Life-threatening cranial dystonia following trihexyphenidyl withdrawal. *Mov Disord* 1989; 4: 349-53.
9. Manji H, Howard RS, Miller DH, *et al*. Status dystonicus: the syndrome and its management. *Brain* 1998; 121: 243-52 *et al*.
10. Coubes P, Echenne B, Roubertie A, *et al*. Traitement de la dystonie généralisée à début précoce par stimulation chronique bilatérale des globus pallidus internes. À propos d'un cas. *Neurochirurgie* 1999; 45: 139-44.

# Deep brain stimulation in paediatric dystonia

Laura Cif, Hassan El Fertit, Nathalie Vayssière, Simone Hemm, Daniel Gaudin, Stéphanie Serrat, Philippe Coubes

*Research Group on Movement Disorders in Children, Department of Pediatric Neurosurgery, School of Medicine, University of Montpellier, Centre Gui de Chauliac, Montpellier, France*

Generalized dystonia, especially with onset in childhood is a severe medical condition with poor response to pharmaceutical treatment.

In November 1996 we proposed Deep Brain Stimulation (DBS) in a patient with very severe, life threatening generalized dystonia.

Since then, more than 100 patients have been treated for bilateral stimulation of the Internal Globus Pallidus (Gpi) in the department of Neurosurgery in Montpellier.

Our method is well adapted to paediatric population. Its originality consists of the use of stereotactic MR imaging for the target determination, without microelectrode recordings. This considerably reduces the duration of the procedure, which is important especially in children, as well as the risk of hemorrhage. Furthermore, the surgery, performed under general anesthesia is more adapted to patients with permanent involuntary movements.

We will present the management of the paediatric population and the results obtained by DBS in this subgroup.

In order to discuss the criteria for selecting the patients with dystonia, we will briefly discuss the features of this medical condition.

Dystonia has been defined as a neurological syndrome characterized by involuntary, sustained muscle contractions, causing twisting and repetitive movements or abnormal postures [1].

It can be classified according to the distribution of the symptoms to different body parts, to the age of onset or by etiology.

According to distribution, dystonia is classified into one of the following categories: focal, segmental, multifocal, hemidystonia and generalized dystonia.

The age of onset is another important way of characterization because an early disease is more likely to generalize and to more severely worsen than adult-onset dystonias.

Dystonia can also be classified by etiology. In primary dystonia, dystonia is the only symptom and can be sporadic or inherited (DYT1 dystonia [2]). Dystonia-plus is a group of syndromes where dystonia is usually associated to other neurological condition such as parkinsonism or myoclonus (Dopa responsive dystonia, myoclonus-dystonia syndrome). The group of heredodegenerative dystonias includes a big number of diseases and in this group, dystonia is typically not pure. Amino acid disorders, lipid disorders, Lesch-Nyhan disease, pantothenate kinase-associated neurodegeneration (PKAN), mitochondrial disesases, Wilson's disease, Huntington's disease, Juvenile parkinsonism-dystonia [3, 4] and many others are heredodegenerative dystonias. Secondary dystonias are generated by insults such as drugs, strokes, tumors, infections [1] and this subgroup also includes dystonia-dyskinesia secondary to cerebral palsy (CP).

In 40% of the patients with early-onset dystonia a specific cause might be found. The etiologic diagnosis is established by clinical evaluation, neuroimaging and molecular analysis in primary dystonias. When the clinical examination and the brain MRI suggests a heredogenerative dystonia, further investigations will be performed such as blood work-up, urine sample analysis, CSF testing, electrophysiologic studies, muscle, skin, liver biopsies, eye slit-lamp examination, PET.

The identification of the etiology is very important for the prognosis of the dystonia and because of the existence of very few diseases having a specific treatment such as Dopa-Responsive dystonia, creatine deficiency or Wilson's disease.

Several drugs are available to treat dystonic symptoms but their efficacy is often limited, transient and difficult to assess. The most important drugs to be used are Levodopa (also as a diagnosis trial in Dopa responsive dystonia), anticholonergics, benzodiazepines, baclofen [5], Botulinum toxin injection especially for the treatment of focal dystonias [6, 7].

Because of the poor efficacy of the pharmaceutical treatment in front of the very severe forms of generalized dystonia encountered in children, we were led to find another therapeutic strategy in order to control the symptoms generating life-threatening complications.

Based on the experience with brain lesioning surgery (pallidotomy) in a young patient with idiopathic generalized dystonia [8] and deep brain stimulation in Parkinson's disease [9, 10], a very important improvement was obtained in patients presenting with primary generalized dystonia after chronic bilateral stimulation of the Gpi.

## Patients (population)

Between November 1996 and July 2003, we treated 45 children with generalized dystonia using bilateral chronic electrical stimulation of the GPi. Population was separated in two groups: the first group included 27 patients with primary dystonia and the second group 18 children with secondary dystonia and heredodegenerative diseases. In order to check for the influence of the DYT1 mutation on the outcome, we divided primary dystonia into two subgroups: primary DYT1 dystonia and primary dystonia without the DYT1 mutation *(Table I)*. For the patients included in this study, the follow-up was at least of 6 months.

Table I. Patients.

|  | Etiologies | Number of Patients | Gender |
|---|---|---|---|
| **Primary Dystonia** 27 children Mean age (months): 11,5 +/- 3,3 | DYT1+ | 15 | 6 male/9 female |
|  | DYT1- | 12 | 4 male/8 female |
| **Secondary Dystonia and Heredodegenerative Diseases** 18 children Mean age (months): 9,9 +/- 2,6 | PKAN | 4 | 1 male/3 female |
|  | Cerebral Palsy | 5 | 1 male/4 female |
|  | Mitochondrial Cytopathy | 4 | 3 male/1 female |
|  | Lesch-Nyhan C | 1 | 1 male |
|  | Others | 4 | 1 male/3 female |

## Clinical Evaluation

Dystonic movements and abnormal postures were evaluated using the Burke-Marsden-Fahn-Dystonia-Rating scale (BMFDRS, motor and disability part) [11] before the surgical procedure, several times during the post-operative hospital stay, every month during the first year and every three months afterwards.

## Surgical Procedure

Bilateral electrode implantation was performed in a single session under general anesthesia [12, 13]. The MR-compatible Leksell stereotactic frame was applied and a 3D-SPGR (spoiled gradient recall) acquisition was performed. The postero-ventral part of the GPi was located through axial, sagittal and coronal MRI studies *(Figure 1)*. The target coordinates (x, y, z) and the trajectory angles ($\alpha$, $\beta$) were calculated using a dedicated software.

Two four contact electrodes (DBS 3389, Medtronic, Minneapolis) were implanted under strict profile radioscopic control. Immediate postoperative control MRI was obtained with the stereotactic frame on. Electrodes were connected to pulse generators five days later (Itrell II or III, Kinetra and Soletra Medtronic, Minneapolis, USA) which were subcutaneously introduced in the abdominal area.

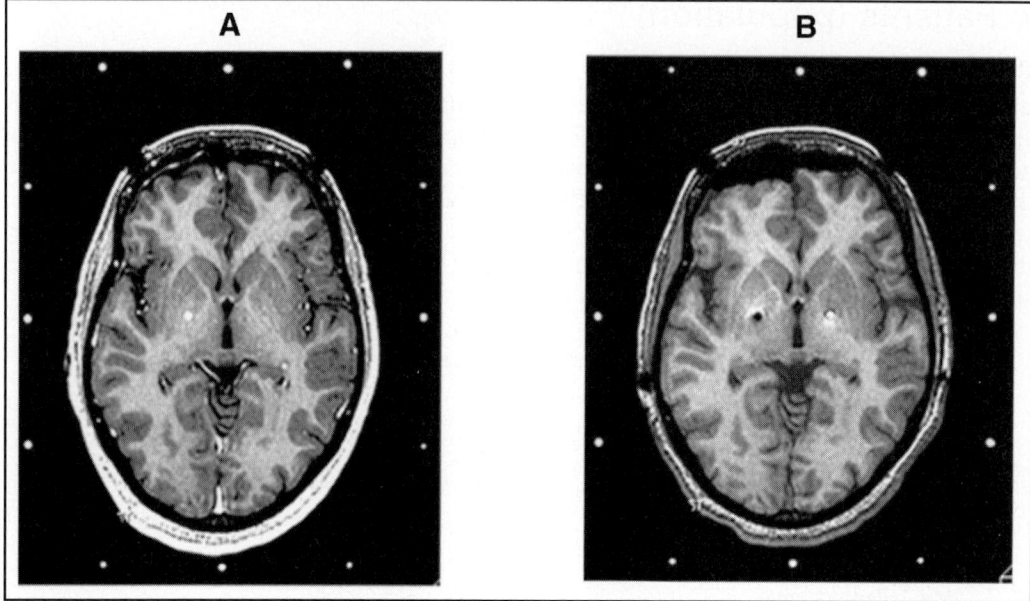

**Figure 1.** Pre- (A) and postoperative (B) stereotactic MRI.

## ■ Electric Parameter Settings

After implantation, stimulators were switched on. Electrical variables were set at high frequency (130 Hz), 450 μsec for the pulse width, with one contact negatively activated. Intensity was progressively increased according to the needs of each patient and the clinical evolution. Usually the first levels for the voltage were between 0.5 V-0.8 V. Over time, we modified the electric parameters in several patients, by activating a second contact or increasing the voltage. The mean steady state value of the voltage was 1.6 ± 0.3 V [14].

## ■ Clinical Results

Clinical and functional scores' evolution (BMFDRS) for primary and secondary dystonia is presented in *Table II and III*. Within each group, the improvement was progressive over the time. With more than 3 years of follow-up, the clinical improvement was comparable for the two groups of primary dystonia (82% of improvement on the motor scale). The results obtained in the group of secondary dystonia and heredodegenerative diseases are less important but yet around 40% with 3 years of follow-up. After three years, the functional improvement was superior in the group of primary DYT1 dystonia (80%) compared to non-DYT1 primary dystonia (56%) and to secondary dytonia (19%). Even if the group of secondary dystonia and heredodegenerative diseases is a very heterogeneous group, because of the few number of patients by etiology, we present the results for all etiologies together.

Table II. Clinical scores (BMFDRS) of dystonic children treated by DBS.

| Motor score | Mean follow-up (months) | Before surgery /120 | 6 months after surgery /120 (%)[1] | 1 year after surgery /120 (%)[1] | 2 years after surgery /120 (%)[1] | > 3 years after surgery /120 (%)[1] |
|---|---|---|---|---|---|---|
| PGD[2] DYT1+[3] | 46.6 ± 16.6 | 53.4 ± 18.1 $n^4 = 15$ | 11.1 ± 10.7 (79) $n^4 = 13$ | 10.9 ± 13.5 (77) $n^4 = 13$ | 10.6 ± 10.7 (76) $n^4 = 12$ | 8.3 ± 8.2 (82) $n^4 = 10$ |
| PGD[2] DYT1- | 52.3 ± 17.5 | 58 ± 27 $n^4 = 12$ | 17.7 ± 12.8 (72) $n^4 = 12$ | 14.8 ± 11.5 (74) $n^4 = 12$ | 18.4 ± 12 (68) $n^4 = 10$ | 11.5 ± 4.2 (82) $n^4 = 8$ |
| Secondary dystonia | 29.5 ± 20.2 | 69.2 ± 15.9 $n^4 = 18$ | 47.1 ± 21.9 (33) $n^4 = 14$ | 39.8 ± 21.9 (39) $n^4 = 11$ | 38.1 ± 11.2 (36) $n^4 = 9$ | 45.7 ± 0.7 (40) $n^4 = 5$ |

Mean values ± SD. The values in brackets represent the mean improvement in percent. A reduction in the score indicates an improvement in function. BMFDRS denotes Burke-Marsden Fahn's Dystonia Rating Scale.
[1] The improvement in percent is calculated based on the maximal possible gain $(Score_{preop} - Score_{postop})/(Score_{preop})$.
[2] Primary generalized dystonia.
[3] DYT1 mutation.
[4] Number of patients.

Table III. Functional scores (BMFDRS) of dystonic children treated by DBS.

| Disability score | Mean follow-up (months) | Before surgery | 6 months after surgery /120 (%)[1] | 1 year after surgery /120 (%)[1] | 2 years after surgery /120 (%)[1] | > 3 years after surgery /120 (%)[1] |
|---|---|---|---|---|---|---|
| PGD[2] DYT1+[3] | 46.6 ± 16.6 | 14.1 ± 4.7 $n^4 = 15$ | 5.8 ± 6.1 (55) $n^4 = 13$ | 4.2 ± 5.2 (62) $n^4 = 13$ | 3.6 ± 3.4 (63) $n^4 = 12$ | 1.7 ± 2.1 (80) $n^4 = 10$ |
| PGD[2] DYT1- | 52.3 ± 17.5 | 18.3 ± 7.8 $n^4 = 12$ | 11 ± 7.5 (42) $n^4 = 12$ | 9.3 ± 6.8 (52) $n^4 = 12$ | 8.7 ± 5.9 (56) $n^4 = 10$ | 10.4 ± 7.6 (56) $n^4 = 8$ |
| Secondary dystonia | 29.5 ± 20.2 | 23.4 ± 4.7 $n^4 = 18$ | 20.1 ± 6.6 (16) $n^4 = 14$ | 19.7 ± 6.9 (19) $n^4 = 11$ | 21.5 ± 1.5 (18) $n^4 = 9$ | 19.5 ± 7 (19) $n^4 = 5$ |

Mean values ± SD. The values in brackets represent the mean improvement in percent. A reduction in the score indicates an improvement in function. BMFDRS denotes Burke-Marsden Fahn's Dystonia Rating Scale.
[1] The improvement in percent is calculated based on the maximal possible gain $(Score_{preop} - Score_{postop})/(Score_{preop})$.
[2] Primary generalized dystonia.
[3] DYT1 mutation.
[4] Number of patients.

# Discussion

We report here our experience on efficiency of bilateral chronic electrical stimulation of the internal globus pallidus in the treatment of generalized dystonia [15-17].

Since the first child has been operated, 44 other children underwent surgery for deep brain stimulation in our department.

While at the beginning deep brain stimulation was proposed in children with primary generalized dystonia (with or without DYT1 mutation), criteria for selection were revisited and enlarged to now include other types of dystonia. Several patients with generalized dystonia associating myoclonus underwent surgery for chronic electrical stimulation of the GPi and we could see an early and complete control of myoclonus. These findings led us to propose this treatment in a child with genetically proven myoclonus-dystonia syndrome (MDS, DYT11, mutation in the epsilon-amino sarcoglycan gene [18, 19]) and we obtained a very satisfactory improvement of his symptoms.

Being confronted with very severe clinical conditions in patients with secondary dystonia and heredodegenerative diseases, in which the efficacy of the medical treatment was poor and dystonic movements and postures comparable with those met in primary dystonia, we proposed deep brain stimulation in several selected patients of these groups.

The criteria for patient's selection in this group were clinical, electrophysiological and based on brain imaging.

We performed surgery for DBS in patients in whom dystonia and dyskinesia were prominent compared to spasticity, the motor pattern was preserved and in patients presenting with severe or life threatening symptoms due to dystonia (swallowing difficulties, permanent opisthotonus, painful muscle spasms).

Electroencephalogram, electroretinogram, visual, brainstem and somatosensory evoked responses were obtained. Motor evoked potentials were performed in elder children to identify pyramidal tract impairment. In order to exclude brain abnormalities contraindicating surgery (major cortical atrophy, severe periventicular leucomalacia especially met in cerebral palsy, basal ganglia and thalamic lesions), brain MR under general anesthesia was performed in all patients.

As shown in *Tables II and III*, best results were obtained within the group of patients with DYT1 mutation [15, 20, 21]. The surgery of abnormal movements should intervene before the occurrence of skeletal deformities. Within the population of non-DYT1 dystonia and especially in secondary and heredodegenerative dystonias, results are not so predictable. The improvement of dysarthria is variable.

Stimulation switch-off systematically causes the recurrence of symptoms within some hours or days.

In the secondary dystonia group, the efficacy of stimulation is far more limited. We were led to propose it for very handicapped patients for whom other therapeutical strategies failed to improve dystonia, as already mentioned. The clinical and etiological heterogeneity among this group almost prevents any global interpretation of these results. In this group, a frequently associated hypertonia of pyramidal origin influences the dystonic component.

An important prognostic factor under stimulation is the existence of a permanent hypertonia at rest, whatever may be its origin. Although we are not yet able to predict the long-term prognosis, we observed an interesting improvement with dyskinesia-dystonia secondary to a perinatal anoxia (dyskinetic forms of cerebral palsy account for less than 10% of all forms CP) [22], PKAN and mitochondrial diseases treated by GPi stimulation. A constant control of pain associated with muscle spasms was obtained in patients suffering from secondary dystonia.

The progression of the causal disease is of critical importance for patient's prognosis.

Using this surgical method based on MRI [12, 13], the associated morbidity is low. We didn't observe hemorrhage due to the intracerebral tracts as reported before in other series (our experience reaches 236 electrodes if adult patients are included) [23]. Secondary infection of the stimulation system remains the major complication of this technique and was observed in three children. We summarize the complications observed in this paediatric population in Table IV.

Table IV. Complications.

| Complications | Number |
|---|---|
| Hemorrage | 0 |
| Infection | 3 |
| Lead fracture | 2 |
| Extension fracture | 2 |

The remarkable tolerance of the internal pulse generator in children must be emphasized. We never observed any complication due to displacement with growth. As shown in Figure 2 and 3, a residual length was enrolled around the battery and the electrode in order to compensate for growth in children and to provide some flexibility with movements in the system. Furthermore, it appears that growth does not interfere with stimulation, and the implantation of a single 90-cm extension compensates adequately for the growth of the child.

The children's physical development (height, body weight) was followed as well as hormonal levels (Insuline-like Growth Factor-IGF1, Insuline-like Growth Factor Binding Protein 3-IGF-BP3, Estradiol, Testosterone, Folliculine Stimulating Hormone-FSH and Luteinizing Hormone-LH) in order to check puberty development.

# ■ Conclusion

Despite its cost, bilateral chronic electrical stimulation can be proposed as first line treatment for early onset primary generalized dystonia when pharmacologically intractable. It is conservative, adaptable, reversible and well tolerated by the pediatric population. It must be applied soon, especially in primary dystonia before complications occur. The complication rate remains low.

For secondary dystonia, pallidal stimulation can partially improve dystonic syndrome, with important control of pain and swallowing difficulties.

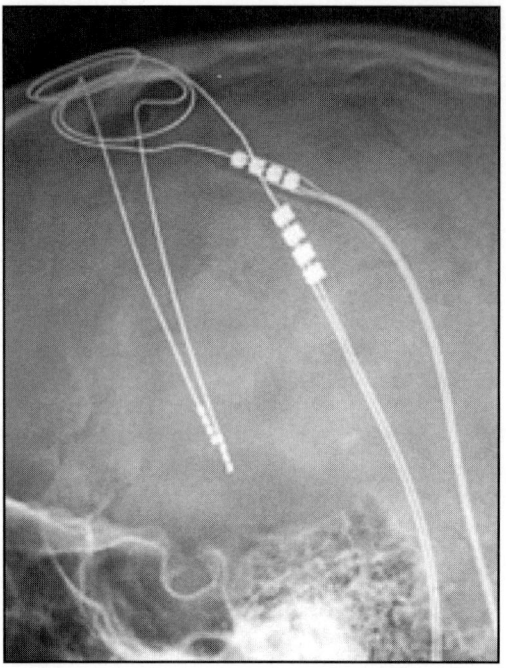

**Figure 2.** X-Ray of implanted leads with a length reserve to compensate growth.

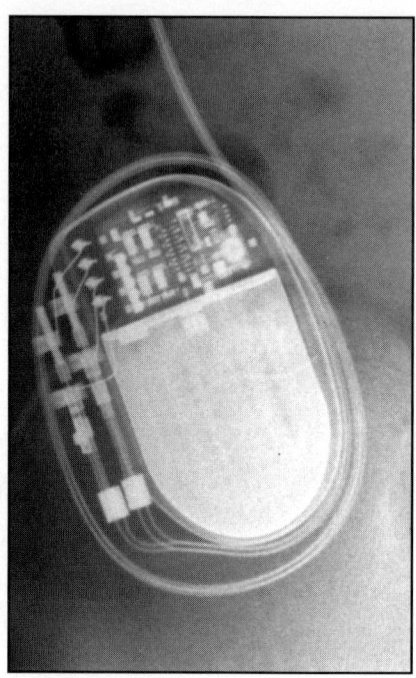

**Figure 3.** X-Ray of the implanted stimulator with a length reserve.

# References

1. Fahn S. Concept and classification of dystonia. *Adv Neurol* 1988; 50: 1-8.
2. Ozelius LJ, Hewett J, Kramer P, et al. Fine localization of the torsion dystonia gene (DYT1) on human chromosome 9q34: YAC map and linkage disequilibrium. *Genome Res* 1997; 7: 483-94.
3. Dwork AJ, Balmaceda C, Fazzini EA, MacCollin M, Cote L, Fahn S. Dominantly inherited, early-onset parkinsonism: neuropathology of a new form. *Neurology* 1993; 43: 69-74.
4. Ishikawa A, Takahashi H. Clinical and neuropathological aspects of autosomal recessive juvenile parkinsonism. *J Neurol* 1998; 245: 4-9.
5. Ford B, Greene PE, Louis ED, Bressman SB, Goodman RR, Brin MF, Sadiq S, Fahn S. Intrathecal baclofen in the treatment of dystonia. *Adv Neurol* 1998; 78: 199-210.
6. Tsui JK, Fross RD, Calne S, Calne DB. Local treatment of spasmodic torticollis with botulinum toxin. *Can J Neurol Sci* 1987; 14: 533-5.
7. Marion MH. Treatment of dystonias. *Presse Med* 1999; 28: 312-5.
8. Iacono RP, Kuniyoshi SM, Lonser RR, Maeda G, Inae AM, Ashwal S. Simultaneous bilateral pallidoansotomy for idiopathic dystonia musculorum deformans. *Pediatr Neurol* 1996; 14: 145-8.
9. Benabid AL, Pollak P, Seigneuret E, Hoffmann D, Gay E, Perret J. Chronic VIM thalamic stimulation in Parkinson's disease, essential tremor and extra-pyramidal dyskinesias. *Acta Neurochir Suppl (Wien)* 1993; 58: 39-44.
10. Benabid AL, Pollak P, Louveau A, Henry S, de Rougemont J. Combined (thalamotomy and stimulation) stereotactic surgery of the VIM thalamic nucleus for bilateral Parkinson disease. *Appl Neurophysiol* 1987; 50: 344-6.

11. Burke R, Fahn S, Marsden C. Validity and reliability of a rating scale for the primary torsion dystonia. *Neurology* 1985; 35: 73-7.
12. Vayssière N, Hemm S, Zanca M, *et al.* Magnetic resonance imaging stereotactic target localization for deep brain stimulation in dystonic children. *J Neurosurg* 2000; 93: 784-90.
13. Vayssière N, Hemm S, Cif L, *et al.* Comparison of atlas- and magnetic resonance imaging-based stereotactic targeting of the globus pallidus internus in the performance of deep brain stimulation for treatment of dystonia. *J Neurosurg* 2002; 96: 673-9.
14. Hemm S, Diakonova N, Mennessier G, Vayssière N, Cif L, Coubes P. Stimulated volume and energy consumption in improved dystonic patients treated by high frequency GPi stimulation. *Mov Disord* 2002; 17: S302.
15. Coubes P, Roubertie A, Vayssière N, Hemm S, Echenne B. Treatment of DYT1-generalised dystonia by stimulation of the internal globus pallidus. *Lancet* 2000; 355: 2220-1.
16. Coubes P, Cif L, Azais M, *et al.* Traitement des syndromes dystoniques par stimulation électrique chronique du globus pallidus interne. *Arch Pediatr* 2002; 9 (suppl 2): 84s-86s.
17. Cif L, El Fertit H, Vayssière N, *et al.* Treatment of dystonic syndromes by chronic electrical stimulation of the internal globus pallidus. *J Neurosurg Sci* 2003; 47: 52-5.
18. Zimprich A, Grabowski M, Asmus F, *et al.* Mutations in the gene encoding epsilon-sarcoglycan cause myoclonus-dystonia syndrome. *Nat Genet* 2001; 29: 66-9.
19. Gasser T. Inherited myoclonus-dystonia syndrome. *Adv Neurol* 1998; 78: 325-34.
20. Coubes P, Echenne B, Roubertie A, *et al.* Treatment of early-onset generalized dystonia by chronic bilateral stimulation of the internal globus pallidus. A propos of a case. *Neurochirurgie* 1999; 45: 139-44.
21. Roubertie A, Echenne B, Cif L, Vayssière N, Hemm S, Coubes P. Treatment of early-onset dystonia: update and a new perspective. *Childs Nerv Syst* 2000; 16: 334-40.
22. Lin JP. The cerebral palsies: a physiological approach. *J Neurol Neurosurg Psychiatry* 2003; 74 (suppl 1): 23-9.
23. Starr P, Feiwell R, Marks W, Jr. Placement of deep brain stimulators into the subthalamic nucleus: technical approach. *Stereotact Funct Neurosurg* 1999; 72: 247.

# Essential tremor in children

Elan D. Louis

GH Sergievsky Center, Department of Neurology, and the Taub Institute for Research on Alzheimer's Disease and the Aging Brain, College of Physicians and Surgeons, Columbia University, New York, NY, USA

Although it is often viewed as a disease exclusively of the elderly, essential tremor (ET) may also affect children, with estimates that approximately 5% of ET cases arising during childhood [1]. Given the propensity for this disease to be both functionally disabling and progressive over time [2, 3], it is important to understand ET in children. In addition, the study of ET in children may enhance our insights about the disease in general, as the disease in children might differ from the disease as it is expressed in adults. The purpose of this chapter is to review the literature on ET in children and to relate this literature to the broader context of ET in all ages.

## Basic Clinical Characteristics and Anatomical Basis

ET is a neurological disease that is characterized by a kinetic tremor of the arms that is mild at the outset and often worsens gradually with age [2, 4]. Being a kinetic tremor, the tremor is present with movement (*e.g.*, performing the finger-to-nose maneuver during the neurological examination or while performing everyday activities like writing or holding a cup). A characteristic feature of the development of ET over time is the somatotopic spread of tremor; the tremor almost always begins in the arms and later spreads to involve cranial structures (head, voice). This spread to involve cranial structures occurs in 30-50% of ET cases [5] and the spread may occur years or decades after the onset of arm tremor. In adults with ET, rest tremor (*i.e.*, tremor that is visible when the arms are resting in the patient's lap or while the arms are hanging at the side while lying, standing, or walking) can occur and is seen in nearly 20% of adults with ET who are attending a specialty clinic for movement disorders [6].

The precise neuro-anatomical basis for ET is not well-understood, although evidence from imaging studies, including positron emission tomography, functional magnetic resonance imaging and magnetic resonance spectroscopic imaging suggests that the cerebellum or cerebellar outflow pathways may be involved [7-9]. The underlying pathology may eventually spread to involve more widespread regions of the cerebellum (thereby resulting in head tremor) and the basal ganglia (resulting in rest tremor), although this has yet to be demonstrated on pathological studies, which are for the most part lacking in ET. ET is very common; indeed, it is one of the most common movement disorders. In epidemiological studies, the prevalence is as high as 4% in individuals age 40 and older [10, 11]. Although the prevalence and incidence of the disorder peak later in life, an epidemiological study in Rochester, MN, indicated that 5% of incident ET cases arise during childhood [1], indicating that the problem of ET in childhood is not a minor one.

## ■ Essential Tremor in childhood

The study of ET cases in childhood cases can yield important insights into the mechanisms of this progressive disease. Four series of childhood ET cases have been published, including that of Paulson (5 cases in 1976) [12], Fernández-Alvarez and Lopez-Casas (28 cases in 1996) [13], Louis et al. (19 cases in 2001) [14], and Fusco et al. (9 cases in 2003) [15]. The series of Fernández-Alvarez and Lopez-Casas [13] and Fusco [15] overlap to some extent, so the total number of published cases from these four studies is 52. The following paragraphs summarize some of the consistent results that may be found across these case series.

ET in children is characterized by action tremor that is often mild but functionally disabling. In most series, the age of onset is below ten years of age for the majority of cases [12-15], although some cases begin in the second decade of life as well. Not all cases have a family history of ET so that sporadic cases are thought to occur. In the series of Louis et al. [14], major complaints at the time of onset of tremor included difficulty with the following activities of daily living: using a spoon, drinking from a cup, writing, drawing on a blackboard, and playing the piano. Fernández-Alvarez and Lopez-Casas [13] noted that the most common handicap was in writing, which created difficulties at school, followed by eating (e.g., drinking from a glass or eating with a fork or spoon). In some instances, this tremor was aggravated by stress and created social embarrassment and avoidance of situations in which the tremor was most apparent or most embarrassing (e.g., going to restaurants). The clinical evaluation of patients in most series included thyroid function tests and ceruloplasmin. Despite being bothersome, most series have indicated that a minority of pediatric ET patients are undergoing treatment. In the series of Paulson [12], two of five cases were under treatment whereas in the series of Louis et al. [14], five (26%) of nineteen had been prescribed medication for the tremor. In the series of Fernández-Alvarez and Lopez-Casas [13], 7 (25%) of 28 cases were tried on medication. In most series, propranolol and primidone were the most commonly used agents. The benefit of these medications has been difficult to judge although may be slight to moderate. A concern about cognitive side effects of medications in school age children is a major issue.

A consistent finding across studies has been the male predominance of childhood ET cases. Four of five of Paulson's cases were male [12], and thirteen of the nineteen cases reported by Louis et al. were male [14]. In the series of Fernández-Alvarez and Lopez-Casas [13], 21 of 28 were male. In summary, 38 (73.1%) of 52 published cases have been male. This male-predominance, across all series, is in contrast to what is seen in adults, in which the prevalence of ET seems to be similar in the two genders. The explanation for this gender predominance in children is not clear. It could represent a difference in health seeking behavior between the genders (*i.e.*, because there may be more motor challenges for boys, tremor might be perceived as more of a problem for them). An alternative explanation is that it could be a result of a modification of disease expression (*i.e.*, age of onset) by gender such that males manifest the disease at an earlier age than do females. Supporting the latter explanation are the following data. First, in a community-based epidemiological study of ET in Sweden in which subjects were not ascertained through doctors' offices [16], 3% of males with ET had manifested the disease by age 18 years versus 0% of females. The respective proportions of male *vs* female ET cases who had manifested the disease at later ages were as follows: 8% *vs* 4% (28 years), 26% *vs* 19% (43 years), 80% *vs* 76% (58 years), 100% *vs* 100% (73 years). In an epidemiological study from Rochester Minnesota [1], the overall incidence of ET in males and females was reported to be similar. However, examination of their results reveals that the incidence of ET in children (individuals 1-19 years of age) was 42% higher in males than in females (2.7 *vs* 1.9 cases per 100,000).

While head tremor occurs in 30-50% of ET cases who are adults [5], in the series published to date, head tremor seems to be uncommon in children. In the series of Louis *et al.* [14], only one of nineteen ET cases had head tremor while in the series of Fernández-Alvarez and Lopez-Casas [13], head tremor seemed to have been observed in only one case. There is a sense in the ET literature that in adults, tremor begins in the hands and only later on spreads to the head and other body regions. This pattern of spread suggests that the neuropathological changes also develop somatotopically. Head (*i.e.*, axial) tremor might be the result of midline or more extensive bilateral pathological changes, which may occur later in the temporal evolution of the illness. Jager and King [17] examined a large five-generation ET kindred with multiple affected members. None of those in the youngest generation (ages 12-28 years) exhibited head or voice tremor, compared with approximately 50% of affected individuals in older generations. These data support the notion that there is somatotopic organization to the temporal development of ET, and that childhood cases of ET may not have had ET for long enough for the tremor to have spread to the head.

Finally, rest tremor was not observed in any children. This contrasts with the situation observed in adults with ET in whom rest tremor may be present [6]. Adults with ET and rest tremor tend to have severe disease of longer duration [6]. As is the case with head tremor, it might be that childhood cases have not had ET for long enough for the tremor-causing pathology to have spread to the basal ganglia.

## ■ Conclusions

In summary, while a small number of children with ET have been noted in the literature, epidemiological studies suggest that as many as 5% of the cases of this highly prevalent disease may arise during childhood. The published literature suggests that childhood and adult forms of ET may differ in several important respects.

Differences in the gender distribution and anatomical location of tremor could provide clues about the biology of this common neurological disorder, which is still poorly understood. The clinical characteristics of ET in children indicate that several of the features of adults with ET may have not had time to develop in children. This supports the view of ET as a clinically and perhaps pathologically progressive disorder.

## References

1. Rajput AH, Offord KP, Beard CM, Kurland LT. Essential tremor in Rochester, Minnesota: a 45-year study. *J Neurol Neurosurg Psychiatry* 1984; 47: 466-70.
2. Louis ED. Clinical Practice: Essential tremor. *N Engl J Med* 2001; 345: 887-91.
3. Louis ED, Barnes LF, Albert SM, et al. Correlates of functional disability in essential tremor. *Mov Disord* 2001; 16: 914-20.
4. Brennan KC, Jurewicz E, Ford B, Pullman SL, Louis ED. Is essential tremor predominantly a kinetic or a postural tremor? A clinical and electrophysiological study. *Mov Disord* 2002; 17: 313-6.
5. Hardesty DE, Maraganore DM, Matsumoto JY, Louis ED. Increased risk of head tremor in women with essential tremor: Longitudinal data from the Rochester Epidemiology Project. *Mov Disord* 2004; 19: 529-33.
6. Cohen O, Pullman S, Jurewicz E, Watner D, Louis ED. Rest tremor in essential tremor patients: Prevalence, clinical correlates, and electrophysiological characteristics. *Arch Neurol* 2003; 60: 405-10.
7. Wills AJ, Jenkins IH, Thompson PD, Findley LJ, Brooks DJ. Red nuclear and cerebellar but no olivary activation associated with essential tremor: A positron emission tomographic study. *Ann Neurol* 1994; 36: 636-42.
8. Bucher SF, Seelos KC, Dodel RC, Reiser M, Oertel WH. Activation mapping in essential tremor with functional magnetic resonance imaging. *Ann Neurol* 1997; 41: 32-40.
9. Louis ED, Shungu D, Chan S, Mao X, Jurewicz EC, Watner D. Metabolic abnormality in patients with essential tremor: A proton magnetic resonance spectroscopic imaging study. *Neurosci Lett* 2002; 333: 17-20.
10. Dogu O, Sevim S, Camdeviren H, et al. Prevalence of essential tremor. Door-to-door neurologic exams in Mersin Province, Turkey. *Neurology* 2003; 61: 1804-6.
11. Louis ED, Ottman R, Hauser WA. How common is the most common adult movement disorder? Estimates of the prevalence of essential tremor throughout the world. *Mov Disord* 1998; 13: 5-10.
12. Paulson GW. Benign essential tremor in childhood. *Clin Ped* 1976; 15: 67-70.
13. Fernández-Alvarez E, Lopez-Casas J. *Essential tremor in childhood.* In: Arzimanoglou A, Goutieres F, eds. *Trends in Child Neurology.* Paris: John Libbey Eurotext, 1996: 147-55.
14. Louis ED, Dure L, Pullman S. Essential tremor in childhood. *Mov Disord* 2001; 16: 921-3.
15. Fusco C, Vals-Sole J, Iturriaga C, Colomer J, Fernandez-Alvarez E. Electrophysiological approach to the study of essential tremor in children and adolescents. *Develop Med Child Neurol* 2003; 45: 24-627.
16. Larsson T, Sjogren T. Essential tremor: a clinical and genetic population study. *Acta Pychiatr Neurol Scand* 1960; 36 (suppl 144): 1-176.
17. Jager BV, King T. Hereditary tremor. *Arch Intern Med* 1955; 95: 788-93.

# Diagnostic considerations in juvenile parkinsonism

**Dominic C. Paviour, Andrew J. Lees**

*National Hospital for Neurology and Neurosurgery, Queen Square, London, United Kingdom*

---

Parkinsonism refers to the collection of signs that make up the core clinical features of Parkinson's disease (PD), namely bradykinesia, and at least one other of rigidity, a resting tremor and postural instability. PD is a common neurodegenerative disorder, with a prevalence of between one and two percent among those over 65 years of age [1].

When parkinsonism is present between the ages of 21 and 40 years, it is described as young onset Parkinson's disease (YOPD) and when the clinical features are apparent before the age of 21, the term juvenile parkinsonism (JP) [2] has been proposed. Parkinsonian syndromes with onset in the first year of life are also recognised. These have been termed infantile parkinsonism-dystonia, and most are caused by autosomal recessive inborn errors of dopamine metabolism [3].

YOPD is generally considered to represent the lower end of the age spectrum for idiopathic Parkinson's disease and typical Lewy body pathology has been found in most pathologically studied cases [4]. Genetic causes are, however, more frequently identified in this group than when the malady presents in the second half of life. In contrast, Lewy bodies have only been identified in one case of JP and even here, different pathological interpretations of the case have been published [5, 6]. This suggests that JP may be pathologically distinct from PD.

Whilst parkinsonism in juveniles is rare, even in specialist neuropaediatric services [7], it has been described in the early medical literature, including a case with onset aged 15 and a disease duration of 25 years [8] with *post mortem* revealing atrophy of the *globus pallidus*.

Quinn et al. described four patients with an age of onset below 21 years [2]. All four had at least one first degree relative with Parkinson's disease in whom the condition began before the age of 40. In a follow up to this study [9], 10 patients are described with JP, of whom half had a family history. Two of these familial cases have subsequently been found to carry parkin mutations. If the Queen Square brain bank criteria [10] are applied strictly then none of the familial cases would fit a diagnosis of Parkinson's disease.

Juvenile parkinsonism, therefore would seem to be a better term than juvenile Parkinson's disease.

## Genes and Juvenile Parkinsonism

Most Parkinson's disease cases in adults are sporadic and of uncertain aetiology. In contrast, in one genetic study, mutations in the parkin gene on chromosome 6 are implicated in approximately 50% of cases of early onset, autosomal recessive parkinsonism and 18% of sporadic early onset cases. In cases of onset of parkinsonism before 21 years of age, 77% (10 of 13) of sporadic cases had mutations in the parkin gene. In contrast, in those over the age of 30, only 3% had parkin mutations [11].

Whilst there are now ten different genetic linkages associated with Parkinson's disease, only PARK2 (parkin mutations on chromosome 6q) causing autosomal recessive juvenile parkinsonism (ARJP) [11-13] and the Contursi kindred of alpha-synuclein mutations on chromosome 4q [14] (PARK 1) associated with autosomal dominant (AD) parkinsonism, have so far been associated with onset before the age of 21 years.

### Parkin mutations

Parkin mutations are the most common cause in juveniles of a clinical picture resembling Parkinson's disease. *Table I* lists the clinical cases in the literature, documenting ages at onset and age ranges. From this information it appears that up to 20% of parkin mutations may result in parkinsonism with onset before the age of 21. The parkin mutation was originally described in a Japanese kindred [15] and has subsequently been described in many families and individuals worldwide (*Table I*). These families are either homozygotes or compound heterozygotes for point mutations and deletions. These different mutations may impart different susceptibility to parkinsonism and result in subtly different phenotypes. In those with a younger age of onset and a parkin mutation, the mutation probably plays a greater role in the aetiopathogenesis.

In the families reported in the literature, the initial manifestations are usually bradykinesia and dystonia and tremor of the leg. Progression is very slow and behavioural problems are said to be common but dementia absent. The response to l-dopa is uniformly good at low doses but dyskinesias and motor fluctuations occur early. Brisk reflexes are common and mild cerebellar and pyramidal signs as well as early autonomic dysfunction have been rarely reported [16, 17]. PET studies in patients with parkin mutations and young onset or juvenile parkinsonism show reductions in the uptake of fluorodopa in the caudate nucleus comparable to that found in the putamen [18], a finding not typically seen in PD [19]. In a larger study of patients with YOPD with and without parkin mutations, the putamen was more affected than the caudate, with no significant difference between the two cohorts [20]. Serial PET studies in patients with parkin mutations and clinical disease have also confirmed a slower rate

**Table I. Onset age of symptoms in clinical reports of parkin mutations.**

| Author | Date | n | n < 21 years | Onset age range (years) |
|---|---|---|---|---|
| Kitada [15] et al. | 1998 | 7 | 1 (+ others NR) | 18-27 |
| Leroy [133] et al. | 1998 | 5 | 2 | 13-41 |
| Tassin [134] et al. | 1998 | 23 | At least 1 (+ others NR) | 7-58 mean 35 (+/- 11) |
| Hayashi [25] et al. | 2000 | 1 | 0 | 32 |
| Maruyama [135] et al. (including cases from Ishikawa et al. originally described as familial juvenile dystonia-parkinsonism) | 2000 | 17 | 5 | 8-40 |
| Klein [136] et al. | 2000 | 11 | 0 | 31-76 |
| Lucking [11] et al. | 2000 | 18[a] 83[b] | 10 NR | 7-58 mean 21 (+/- 9) mean 32 (+/- 9) |
| Van de Warrenberg [22] et al. | 2001 | 3 | 1* | 18-40 |
| Jeon [12] et al. | 2001 | 1 | 1 | 12 |
| Nisipeanu [137] et al. | 2001 | 4 | 0 | 30-37 |
| Farrer [24] et al. | 2001 | 7* | 0 | 24-64 |
| Khan [21] et al. | 2002 | 4 | 0 | 27-32 |
| Hedrich [138] et al. | 2002 | 6[a] 17[b] | 2 8 | 14-41 10-50 |
| Munoz [139] et al. | 2002 | 7 | 1 | 20-46 |
| West [140] et al. (only 5 newly reported, other prev reported in Lucking et al.) | 2002 | 5 | 1 4 | 18 29-45 |
| Hoenicka [141] et al. | 2002 | NR | NR | NR |
| Khan [23] et al. (excluding 4 already reported) | 2003 | 20 | 9 | 13-54 |
| Periquet [16] et al. | 2003 | 20 | 3 | 7-45 |
| Illarioshkin [142] et al. | 2003 | 8 | 4 | 12-40 |
| Lohmann [143] et al. (new reports only) | 2003 | 18 | NR | NR |
| Rawal [144] et al. (9 new reports) | 2003 | 9 | 3 | 11-47 |
| **TOTAL** | | 294 | 56 (+ others NR) | |

NR: not recorded.
a: number with sporadic parkinsonism.
b: number with apparent AR parkinsonism.
*: post mortem tissue available.

of change in fluorodopa uptake compared to PD [21]. Interestingly, subjects in this kindred, heterozygous for the parkin mutation and without clinical disease, also had reduced fluorodopa uptake at baseline with no deterioration over a mean of 7 years, despite developing mild extrapyramidal signs. $I^{123}$-IBZM-SPECT and β-CIT-SPECT in parkinsonism with parkin mutations [22] suggest that the dopaminergic dysfunction is located in the pre-synaptic part of the nigro-striatal pathway. Another interesting difference between parkin disease and PD is that olfaction seems to be normal in the former [23].

*Post mortem* neuropathological analysis has been done in only a few parkin cases. The most consistent finding is marked depigmentation of the *substantia nigra pars compacta* (SNpc) with neuronal loss, gliosis and an absence of Lewy bodies [22, 24-26]. Other findings have included the presence of tau positive neurofibrilliary tangles and neuropil threads.

In a single case, a compound heterozygote with a 40bp deletion of exon 3 in the parkin gene and an exon 7 substitution, with onset aged 41 and accidental death aged 52 [24], Lewy bodies were seen in the SN and *locus ceruleus*. Interestingly, another family in this report contained a member who died aged 93 with no clinical features of parkinsonism and no features suggestive of Parkinson's disease at autopsy, despite having the same exon 3 parkin mutation. The pathology in the 52 year old did not differ in any respect from that seen in mild to moderate Parkinson's disease. These findings suggest that the parkin protein may have a more direct role in typical LB parkinsonism than previously thought and that heterozygous mutations might confer increased susceptibility to PD.

## Other important, potentially treatable causes of juvenile parkinsonism

*Dopa responsive dystonia*

Dopa-responsive dystonia (DRD) is characterised by limb dystonia with diurnal worsening of symptoms in some cases [27]. Most patients have an excellent and sustained response to both low doses of l-dopa (300 mg/day) and anticholinergics without the emergence of a long-term l-dopa syndrome. The clinical spectrum of the disease is broad, encompassing a minor focal dystonia, a cerebral palsy like picture with some associated pyramidal signs, a severe generalised dystonia and a predominantly parkinsonian picture. The prevalence of DRD is thought to be around 0.5-1.0 per million [28], but this is likely to be an underestimate as many cases are still missed. Despite its rarity, it is recommended that all children with dystonia, parkinsonism or cerebral palsy (athetoid form) should be given a 6-week trial of l-dopa (125 mg t.i.d).

DRD is inherited as an autosomal dominant trait, with variable penetrance and the disease locus has been assigned to 14q11-q24.3, coding for GTPCH 1. This is the rate-limiting enzyme in the biosynthesis of tetrahydrobiopterin (BH4), an essential cofactor for the amino acid monooxygenases, necessary for the production of dopamine. Tyrosine hydroxylase (TH) is a monooxygenase and this explains why a very similar clinical picture to that of DRD can arise with mutations in the TH gene [29] or in rare examples of TH deficiency [30] effectively causing autosomal recessive DRD. In these rare inborn errors of metabolism, infantile bradykinesia, rigidity and dystonia which responds to l-dopa is the usual presentation (infantile parkinsonism) [31].

In an analysis of 22 families with a DRD phenotype, multiple mutations were identified resulting in differing clinical presentations [32]. A patient with lower limb spasticity previously diagnosed as spastic paraplegia was found to have a GTPCH 1 mutation and to be l-dopa responsive. Additional atypical features in some of these cases included postural tremor, oromandibular dystonia, delayed speech onset and oculogyric crises, all of which respond to l-dopa.

The absence of l-dopa induced dyskinesias following sustained treatment helps to distinguish DRD from dystonia due to parkin mutations. This is thought to be due to a lack of dopaminergic cell loss in the SN in DRD. The recent discovery of l-dopa-induced dyskinesias in a few cases with GTPCH 1 mutations has however partly blurred this distinction [32]. In three of the families in this study, no GTPCH 1 mutation was detected, but screening for the parkin mutation revealed abnormalities. All these cases had predominant dystonia at onset with subsequent progressive parkinsonism and l-dopa induced dyskinesias. More recently, in a GTPCH 1 mutation confirmed case of DRD with onset of an asymmetric leg tremor at 15 years of age, polymorphisms in the parkin gene were present on each allele, raising the possibility that these polymorphisms may have altered the clinical presentation.

At present, as for parkin mutations, GTPCH 1 mutations can only be screened for in a research context and there is no routinely available genetic test. FP-CIT is a SPECT ligand that binds to the pre-synaptic dopamine transporter. A patient with atypical DRD underwent FP-CIT SPECT scanning which was found to be normal compared to a case of parkin associated JP where uptake ratios were reduced in the putamen [33]. In addition, in PET studies in DRD, striatal 18F-dopa uptake is either normal or only mildly reduced compared to age matched controls [34]. DRD as a cause for JP would be suggested by an excellent response to low doses of l-dopa without early emergence of dyskinesias, a normal dopamine transporter ligand SPECT (DAT scan) or F-Dopa PET and an abnormal phenylalanine loading test [35]. The phenylalanine loading test involves oral administration of 100 mg/kg body weight of phenylalanine at least 2 hours after the last meal. Blood should be drawn just prior to administration and subsequently at one, two, four and six hours after administration. Recently, a simpler method of carrying out the test, with a single sampling point, has been suggested [36]. The plasma from the heparinised tubes should be separated and stored immediately at $-70°$ C until analysed. Plasma phenylalanine is elevated in patients post loading and plasma tyrosine and biopterin is reduced. The abnormality in plasma measurements does not seem to correlate with disease severity suggesting that this test may detect asymptomatic disease carriers. Other factors such as absorption, the oral contraceptive pill, diurnal variation, age and obesity can affect phenylalanine levels and heterozygotes for phenyl-ketonuria (PKU) may have a similar plasma profile after phenylalanine load.

*Wilson's disease*

Early treatment of Wilson's disease (WD) may prevent potentially permanent neurological and psychiatric disabilities. It is a rare autosomal recessive condition with a prevalence of one in 30,000, with approximately 10 new cases presenting neurologically, annually in the UK[37]. More than 190 mutations in the ATP7B gene on chromosome 13 have been identified. Mutations in the protein product probably compromise oxidative phosphorylation in mitochondria [38]. Genetic screening for WD is not routinely available although some genetic laboratories offer screening for the commoner regional mutations.

A large series of 136 cases presenting with neurological features [37] suggested that in both juveniles and adults, the commonest manifestation was with parkinsonism. However, most of the cases also had other signs, which would exclude them from a clinical diagnosis of PD. Most of these cases also failed to respond to l-dopa.

Other common neurological presentations include dystonia and a pseudo-sclerotic phenotype with a "wing beating" tremor similar to that seen in MS. Neurobehavioural disturbances, a dystonic face (risus sardonicus) with drooling and a distinctive marked "mixed" dysarthria are frequent findings. Delay in diagnosis is common with the mean delay from symptom onset being 13 months. Neurological presentation of Wilson's disease before puberty is very rare and abnormalities of gait are never the presenting symptom. Wilson's disease should be excluded with a serum copper and caeruloplasmin measurement, slit lamp examination looking for Kayser-Fleischer (K-F) rings, 24 hour urinary free copper estimation and if necessary a liver biopsy to estimate liver copper concentration. A diagnosis of neurological Wilson's disease in the absence of K-F rings is likely to be incorrect. Diagnosis can be hampered by problems with standardisation of serum copper and caeruloplasmin levels in many laboratories [39] and unfamiliarity with the appearance of the K-F ring. The treatment of choice is with the chelating agent penicillamine but about 20% of cases with neurological Wilson's get worse after treatment initiation. Other valuable treatments include trientene HCL, tetrathiomolybdate, oral zinc and British-anti-Lewisite (BAL) injections. Controlled trials are urgently needed to determine if any of these are superior to penicillamine as initial treatment.

## Other genetic causes of juvenile parkinsonism

### Huntington's disease (HD)

HD is an autosomal dominant CAG repeat disorder. It usually presents in the fourth or fifth decade of life, most commonly with behavioural disturbances and chorea. Anticipation results in more severe disease earlier in life and juvenile onset is characterised by a bradykinetic rigid syndrome (Westphal variant). The presentation with atypical movement disorders in HD was recently studied in a cohort of 376 affected subjects in Italy [40]. A younger age at onset, with atypical symptoms, was associated with a larger number of CAG repeats. Two cases in this series presented before the age of 21 with isolated bradykinesia and rigidity and a number of juveniles with parkinsonism were also described in the Lake Maracaibo family from which huntingtin was first isolated [41]. The parkinsonian features in these juvenile cases, may respond to l-dopa [42].

### The spino-cerebellar ataxias (SCA)

In the past decade, the genetic cause for most cases of adult-onset dominant cerebellar ataxia have been identified.

SCA2 and SCA3 (Machado-Joseph disease) have recently been associated with a presentation with parkinsonism, especially in Afro-Americans and Afro-Caribbeans (SCA3) [43] and Orientals (SCA2) [44]. SCA6 has also been associated with parkinsonism but not in juveniles [45]. Extrapyramidal signs are most common in SCA3. Bradykinesia, rigidity, reduced arm swing and slowed alternating movements may be seen at presentation [46]. An Antiguan kindred [43] had an almost pure parkinsonian syndrome, which responded to l-dopa, although none of these cases had juvenile onset. Numerous cases with juvenile onset and parkinsonism have been described [47], but features that would exclude a diagnosis of Parkinson's disease such as an ataxic gait and slowing of saccadic eye movements were present. There was no correlation between the length of repeats and the clinical phenotype.

In a study of 28 Japanese patients with SCA2, 2 patients were documented with predominant parkinsonism but neither was under the age of 21 [48]. Ataxia in association with slow eye movements and hyporeflexia is usual. Pseudobulbar dysphagia and pyramidal signs are also commonly present. A 12 year old case with parkinsonism and SCA2 has been described in another series [49] raising the possibility that in other SCA2 families, as the age of onset gets younger with anticipation, the parkinsonian phenotype at presentation may be more common. In one Chinese SCA2 family, there was parkinsonism and subsequent ataxia as the repeat length increased [44]. The response of the parkinsonian features to l-dopa in these SCA2 cases was variable. More recently, analysis of 136 probands with a family history of parkinsonism (fitting the Queen Square Brain Bank clinical criteria, excepting the family history) revealed borderline SCA2 mutations (32-35 repeats) in 2 cases [50]. These patients had l-dopa responsive parkinsonism suggesting that it is not simply the length of the expansion that confers the clinical phenotype.

*Neuroacanthocytosis*

Chorea acanthocytosis may present before 21 years of age. A combination of prominent stereotyped orofacial dyskinesias with lip and cheek biting together with mild limb chorea and dystonia is most characteristic. Parkinsonism has been reported amongst the spectrum of clinical manifestations [51] and even as a presenting feature [52]. Five cases in this series, presented before the age of 21, but only one had clear parkinsonian features, and these occurred as part of a constellation of other clinical signs including chorea, dystonia and developmental delay. The gene for chorea-acanthocytosis (CHAC) maps to chromosome 9q21 and many different "private" mutations have already been found [53]. Diagnosis hinges on the presence of more than 3% acanthocytes on fresh wet blood films and it is recommended that if the condition is suspected, a minimum of six separate wet blood films should be taken before excluding the condition. A number of cases also have an elevated creatine kinase level in the serum.

Acanthocytes can also occur in association with neurological disease in abetalipoproteinaemia, hypobetalipoproteinaemia and PANK2 mutations including the HARP syndrome. McLeod syndrome is associated with haemolysis and acanthocytes as well as dystonia, chorea, areflexia, tics, seizures and occasionally dementia and muscular dystrophy. The age of onset is older than in chorea-acanthocytosis and it is associated with mutations of the XK gene on chromosome Xp21.

*Rapid onset dystonia parkinsonism (RODP)*

RODP [54] is a very rare autosomal dominant disorder. There is abrupt onset of bulbar and upper limb dystonia with bradykinesia progressing over a few days followed by a relatively stable course. There is no response to l-dopa. Linkage has been found on chromosome 19 in two American families [55]. The clinical picture is usually dominated by dystonia, but the diagnosis should still be considered in cases of juvenile parkinsonism beginning acutely.

*Mitochondrial cytopathy and JP*

Idiopathic Parkinson's disease has been associated with reduced complex 1 activity in the mitochondrial oxidative phosphorylation chain and dystonia, myoclonus and chorea are the most frequently described movement disorders. Parkinsonian features have also been rarely reported in the mitochondrial cytopathies. Recently, a series of patients with mutations in complex III have been described, including one with juvenile onset aged 6 [56]. Between the ages of 6 and 16, the patient developed a lack of facial expression, decreased blink frequency, hypophonia, asymmetrically increased tone in the upper limbs and a resting tremor. The patient also had a flexed posture and a reduced arm swing. Pyramidal signs and stimulus sensitive myoclonus were evident. Cortical blindness secondary to stroke like episodes then ensued followed by status epilepticus.

*Neuronal Intranuclear Inclusion Body Disease (NIID)*

The first description of this very rare disorder occurred in 1968 [57]. The clinical manifestations of the disease are variable depending on the sites of neuronal loss. A multi-system degenerative process of the CNS is usually present, but the disorder may present as a visceral neuropathy. It is usually sporadic but hereditary forms have been described [58], where the pattern would fit with autosomal dominant inheritance. Several cases of NIID have been reported with juvenile l-dopa responsive parkinsonism [10, 59-61]. In most of these cases, there was rapid progression of the disease with the development of other neurological signs including neuropathies, dementia and pyramidal tract signs. The characteristic intranuclear inclusions can be identified on full thickness rectal biopsy.

Intranuclear inclusions have been identified in various CAG trinucleotide repeat disorders [62, 63] and also in chorea-acanthocytosis [64] where the inclusions were shown to contain polyglutamine repeats as described in NIID [65].

## Some other rare genetic neuro-metabolic disorders

Niemann-Pick type C (NPC) is an autosomal recessive neurovisceral lipoidosis. Mutations in the gene NPC1 on chromosome 18q have been identified [66]. The classical phenotype involves hepatosplenomegaly with progressive ataxia, dystonia and dementia and a vertical supranuclear gaze palsy. Whilst the onset is usually in late childhood with death in the second decade, a predominantly akinetic rigid syndrome in the second decade of life is a rare presentation [67]. The diagnosis is suggested by a reduced rate of cholesterol esterification in cultured skin fibroblasts. The presence of sea-blue histiocytes on bone marrow biopsy also supports the diagnosis.

Juvenile neuronal ceroid lipofuscinosis (JNCL) is an autosomal recessive lysosomal storage disorder. The gene is located on chromosome 16p [68]. The clinical picture includes visual failure, psychomotor retardation and epilepsy.

Extrapyramidal signs including parkinsonism may develop in adolescence [69]. In common with NIID, the parkinsonism in JNCL may respond well initially to dopaminergic therapy [70] and the diagnosis of this condition can be clinched by rectal or muscle biopsy.

Hallervorden Spatz syndrome is another rare disorder caused by mutations in the PANK2 gene coding for pantothenate kinase [71]. The clinical phenotype is varied but can include parkinsonism in juveniles [72]. Recently a 100% association between PANK2 mutations and "the eye of the tiger sign" on MRI has been reported [73] suggesting that the absence of this finding on MRI makes a PANK2 mutation highly unlikely. Lewy bodies in the cerebral cortex and basal ganglia are found in some cases at autopsy. Pantothenic acid is under trial as a potential therapy.

HARP [74] is a similar and related condition, consisting of hypoprebetalipoproteinaemia, acanthocytosis, retinal pigment abnormalities and MRI findings similar to those found in Hallervorden-Spatz syndrome, suggesting it may be the same genetic disorder.

Parkinsonism has also been reported in the autosomal dominant condition Dercum's disease [75], which consists of painful symmetrical lipomatosis. Necrotic cystic areas are described in the putamina.

Homocystinuria (the classical features of which are a marfanoid habitus, lens dislocation, a predisposition to arterial and vascular thrombosis) has also been reported as causing parkinsonism in a juvenile, as has an inborn error of folate metabolism, but in each case additional neurological signs were present [76, 77].

## ■ Infective causes

A number of neurotropic viruses have been associated with parkinsonism. These include Coxackie B-2 [78], Epstein Barr virus [79], Central European tick-borne encephalitis, Western Equine encephalitis, Polio [80], measles, Influenza, HIV [81], varicella zoster and Murray valley encephalitis [82]. L-dopa responsiveness in these cases is variable.

Japanese B encephalitis (JE) has received particular attention recently and it is one of the most frequent endemic encephalitic illnesses in South East Asia. It affects approximately 50,000 people annually with movement disorders being common sequelae. A recently published series of 50 cases of JE reported movement disorders in 35, with ages ranging from 2 to 64 years old [83]. Parkinsonism tended to appear 1-4 weeks after the onset of the illness as consciousness started to improve. On MRI, hypodense areas were seen in T2 weighted images, in the thalamus, basal ganglia, midbrain, pons, cerebral cortex and the cerebellum. Of these patients, those with a pure parkinsonian disorder tended to fare better than those with a mixed movement disorder.

SSPE is a slow virus infection of the CNS caused by measles. It is uncommon in the West due to vaccination programmes and less than 10 cases per year are reported in the USA [84]. There is usually a history of primary measles infection in early life, followed after a latency of 6-8 years, by a relentlessly progressive neurological disorder consisting of behavioural change, motor disturbances and periodic myoclonic jerks. SSPE can cause parkinsonism but usually with additional neurological features [85]. In one case, serial MRI revealed migratory basal ganglia lesions suggestive of axonal spread of the measles virus. This case demonstrated good initial, but an unsustained response to l-dopa. Diagnosis rests on CSF measles viral titres, local synthesis of immunoglobulin in the cerebrospinal fluid, reverse transcription PCR and EEG. There is no adequate therapy, but immunomodulatory treatments such as IVIg may prolong life beyond the usual mean survival of 18 months. Brain biopsy in early SSPE often reveals mild meningitis and encephalitis involving cortical and sub-cortical grey matter as well as white matter. Histological examination reveals gliosis, lymphocyte proliferation and demyelination. Neurofibrilliary tangles and inclusion bodies containing viral antigens may be seen at *post mortem*.

HIV infection can be associated with parkinsonism either in the context of opportunistic infection or as a direct effect of viral damage in HIV encephalopathy. A case of pure parkinsonism as the sole manifestation of HIV has been reported in an adult [81] with a clear improvement in the parkinsonian features on antiretroviral treatment. There was a mild improvement of symptoms with l-dopa suggesting that dopaminergic neurons were damaged as a consequence of the viral infection [86]. Although this case did not justify description as juvenile parkinsonism, the increase in HIV infection requires us to consider it as a cause of JP and an akinetic rigid syndrome has been reported in a 13 year-old with HIV associated progressive multifocal leukoencephalopathy [10]. In a recent series of 2460 HIV positive patients in South America [87], 28 had movement disorders and 14 of these had parkinsonism. In 12, direct HIV infection was presumed to be the cause. Antiretroviral drugs have also been rarely associated with an iatrogenic parkinsonian syndrome [88].

Post-vaccinal parkinsonism has been reported in a five year old, 18 days after a vaccination for measles [89]. The akinetic rigid syndrome developed after three days of fever and was associated with a CSF pleocytosis. MRI, three months after the onset, revealed clear-cut evidence of bilateral *substantia nigra* lesions, suggesting secondary gliosis. The parkinsonian features persisted for two years after onset and responded well to l-dopa albeit with early adverse reactions.

Atypical bacterial infections have also been associated with the development of parkinsonism and mycoplasma pneumoniae has been reported to cause hypophonia, hypomimia, bradykinesia and dystonia in a single case [90] or as a component of the neurological clinical picture in 4 further cases [91].

The exact pathological mechanism behind infection and subsequent parkinsonism is not clear. It may occur as a direct effect of the virus or bacteria on dopaminergic production or as a consequence of a parainfectious autoimmune process.

Some of these neurotropic infectious agents have at some point been implicated as aetiological agents in encephalitis lethargica (EL) or Von Economo's encephalitis [92]. Lethargic encephalitis has been known for centuries, having been described by

Hippocrates in the 5th century B.C and later in Europe in the 16th century (*mendossa* in Lisbon and *pestilence soporeuse* in Italy). Von Economo described the EL epidemic in Europe between 1916 and 1927. An association between influenza and EL has been postulated because of the temporal association with the 1918 influenza pandemic, (although Von Economo rejected this hypothesis at the time). This has now been effectively discounted on the basis of a failure to isolate influenza RNA in brains from the EL epidemic [93].

Cases of sporadic encephalitis lethargica still occur and can be a cause of parkinsonism in juveniles [94, 95] (Figure 1). The characteristic form of the disease starts with increasing drowsiness, pyrexia and confusion followed by sleep inversion, stupor and coma. The proposed diagnostic criteria comprise the presence of an acute or sub-acute encephalitic illness with three of the following: (1) signs of basal ganglia involvement, (2) oculogyric crises, (3) ophthalmoplegia, (4) obsessive-compulsive behaviour, (5) akinetic mutism, (6) central respiratory irregularities and (7) somnolence or sleep inversion [94].

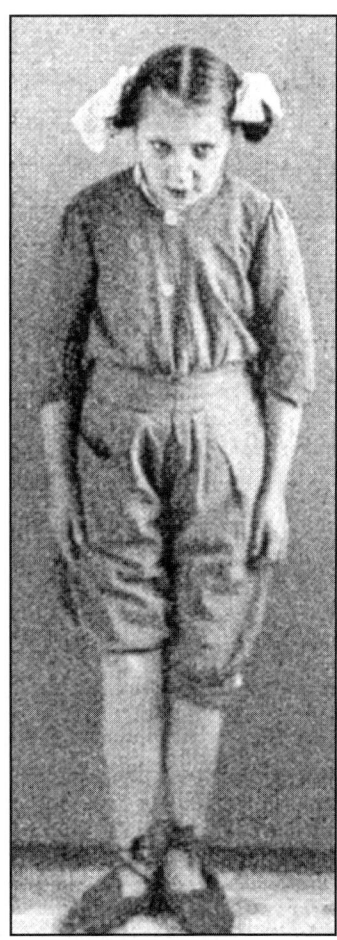

**Figure 1.** Postencephalitic parkinsonism in a child [92]
(reproduced with permission from Oxford University Press).

Encephalitis Lethargica is sometimes associated with the presence of CSF oligoclonal bands (OCB) and cases have recently been successfully treated with immunomodulatory therapy [96-98]. This has led to the proposition that EL is immune mediated. Immunological factors related to antibasal ganglia antibodies cross-reacting with beta-haemolytic streptococcus may be of importance [95, 99]. Interestingly, Von Economo noted that an EL like illness was induced in dogs after vaccination against streptococcus [92].

Dale et al. recently reported a series of 20 patients, 40% had MRI abnormalities in the deep grey matter (Figure 2), CSF examination revealed elevated protein and OCB in 75% and 69% respectively with no evidence of a viral infection. Anti Streptolysin O (ASO) titres were elevated in 65% of patients and Western immunoblotting showed that 95% of EL patients had autoantibodies reactive against human basal ganglia antigens.

Streptococcal infections, are well known to be related to the development of symptoms of basal ganglia dysfunction. The classic phenotype is Sydenhams chorea. More recently, motor tics in combination with a behavioural disorder have been termed paediatric autoimmune neuropsychiatric disorders associated with streptococcal infections (PANDAS) [100-102]. Parkinsonism in a 10 year-old female after a streptococcal throat infection has recently been reported [103] supporting the notion that a relatively pure parkinsonian syndrome can occur as a consequence of streptococcal infection. The cause of variability in the clinical presentations of these post streptococcal neurological syndromes is not clear, but it may be due to the genetics of the host or the streptococcal serotype involved. Quite why post-streptococcal CNS disease is predominantly localised to basal ganglia dysfunction is unclear.

In cases of suspected infectious causes of parkinsonism in juveniles, blood and CSF should be taken for bacteriological and virological studies including PCR. This should include PCR studies where possible. Serum for acute and convalescent antibody titres may be useful in diagnosing mycoplasma infection. Other investigations which may be helpful include ASO titre, antibasal ganglia antibodies, EEG and MR imaging of the brain.

## ■ Immune mediated or inflammatory causes

Systemic *lupus erythematosus* (SLE) commonly affects the central nervous system. The most frequent manifestations are psychiatric disturbance, seizures and cranial nerve disorders. Movement disorders are rare and the most common of these is chorea. A recent extensive review of the literature described 25 cases of parkinsonism associated with SLE [104]. Females were more commonly affected and the most frequent extrapyramidal signs were rigidity followed by akinesia then tremor. Of the 25 cases reported, 10 were in patients under the age of 21 (9 females and 1 male). In the 11 patients who had MRI scans, basal ganglia abnormalities were reported in 4 cases. All of the patients improved clinically with treatment for SLE and with anti-parkinsonian medication. In these cases, there were neurological features in addition to the akinetic rigid syndrome suggesting widespread CNS involvement in neurolupus. Vasculopathy, coagulopathy, emboli from cardiac disease and bleeding disturbances as well as circulating immune-complexes and autoantibody-induced pathology have all been suggested in neurolupus although the exact aetiology is unclear.

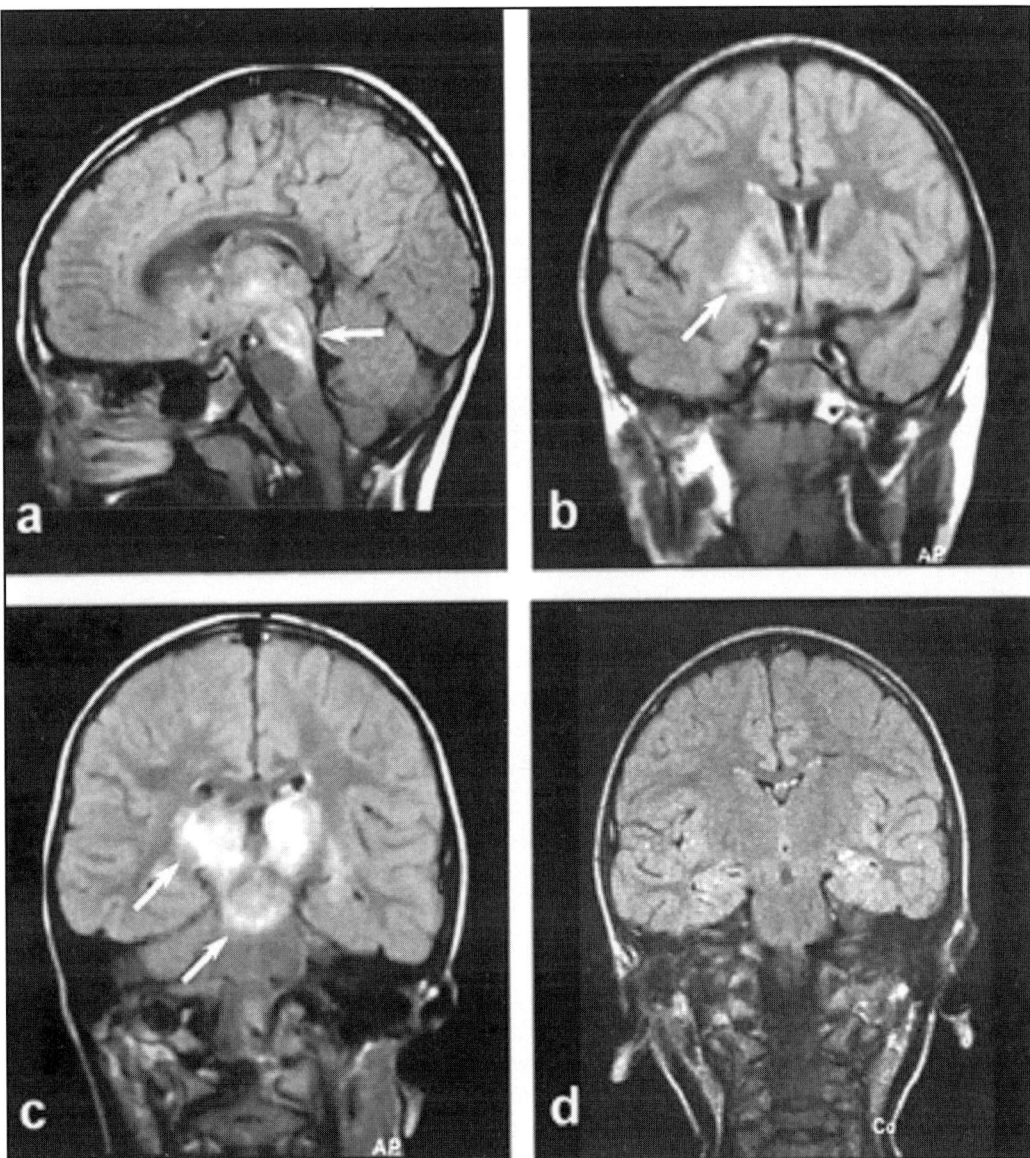

**Figure 2.** MRI of the brain in a somnolent patient with bradykinesia and rigidity, showing inflammatory lesions (arrows) in the (a) midbrain and periaqueductal grey matter, (b) right putamen and (c) bilateral thalami and midbrain. (d) Convalescent imaging showing resolution of the inflammatory changes in the thalami and midbrain. (Reproduced with permission from Oxford University Press) [95].

SLE should be excluded with inflammatory markers such as an ESR as well as serological testing including ANA, anti dsDNA, anti-cardiolipin antibodies and CSF examination, which may help exclude a CNS vasculitits.

## Drug-induced juvenile Parkinsonism

Neuroleptic drugs, calcium channel blockers [105-107] (cinnarizine, flunarizine, nifedipine and amplodipine) and antiemetic drugs, particularly metoclopramide and prochlorperazine, are common causes of iatrogenic parkinsonism in adults. When neuroleptic drugs provoke parkinsonism in juveniles, the picture is characteristically of a symmetrical, reversible, predominantly bradykinetic rigid syndrome which is responsive to anticholinergic drugs but not l-dopa. Acute dystonic reactions, akathisia and persistent dystonia may also be associated. These cases would not fulfil the Queen Square Brain Bank criteria for a diagnosis of PD and have normal nigrostriatal dopamine systems on functional imaging. Following withdrawal of the offending drug, neurological recovery may take up to 6 months. There are isolated case reports of drugs such as chloroquine (after prolonged use) [108], vincristine and adriamycin [109] and sodium valproate [110] causing parkinsonism in juveniles.

## Toxic insults

In a large series of 242 patients with CO poisoning [111], there were several patients with parkinsonian symptoms before the age of 21. The mean latency between the appearance of parkinsonism varied from two to 26 weeks, but was usually present within 1 month after the insult. All patients initially demonstrated encephalopathy and varying degrees of impaired consciousness and cognitive function. Abnormalities of the basal ganglia on MRI are usually present. L-dopa and anticholinergic drugs are ineffective but the prognosis in the 16 patients followed up was good, with 13 recovering spontaneously within 6 months.

Organophosphate (OP) insecticides consist of a group of chemical substances that noncompetitively inhibit acetylcholine esterase. Although very rare compared to the acute neurological symptoms of toxicity (meiosis, sweating, fasciculations, muscle weakness, confusion and eventually coma and seizures), parkinsonism has been described in a 17-year-old female presenting after attempted suicide with organophosphate (100 ml chlorpyrifos) ingestion [112]. Six days after recovering consciousness, she developed a rigid posture with a resting tremor and marked bradykinesia and cogwheel rigidity in the upper limbs. She was treated with amantadine and 9 months later she had fully recovered. The correct identification of OP poisoning is important as prompt treatment may facilitate a full recovery.

Cyanide induced parkinsonism with pathological follow up in a juvenile has also been reported [113]. Major destructive changes were found in the globus pallidus and putamen but the *substantia nigra* was intact with normal melaninisation.

Other toxic causes such as manganese, MPTP, toluene, carbon disulphide, methanol [114], *n*-hexane and MDMA (ecstasy) also need to be considered.

## A miscellany of other rare causes

Hypoxic or hypotensive insults in juveniles can result in a variety of neurological sequelae. Acute parkinsonism developed four days after open heart surgery for a VSD

Table II. Rare causes of juvenile parkinsonism; Useful investigations.

| | Important Investigations | Result |
|---|---|---|
| Dopa Responsive Dystonia | GTPCH-1 gene analysis. Phenylalanine loading test. Trial of L-dopa. | Not widely available. ↑ plasma phenylalanine, ↓ biopterin and tyrosine. |
| Wilson's Disease | Serum Copper/Caeruloplasmin. Slit lamp ophthalmoscopy. Liver biopsy. | ↓ caeruloplasmin, ↓ serum copper, ↑ serum "free copper" and urinary copper excretion. Kayser-Fleischer rings. ↑ dry weight copper concentration. |
| Neuro-acanthocytosis | At least three wet blood films for acanthocytes (some recommend six). | > 3% acanthocytes on blood film. |
| Hallervorden-Spatz (PANK-2 mutations) | T2 MRI. PANK-2 mutation analysis. | Specific pattern of hyperintensity within the hypointense medial globus pallidus. |
| HARP | MRI. Blood film. | May have similar appearances to cases with PANK-2 mutations. Acanthocytes present > 3%. |
| Mitochondrial cytopathies | Muscle biopsy (needle biopsy may not be sufficient), with mtDNA analysis and biochemical studies on extracted mitochondria. MRI. Serum and CSF lactate. | Ragged red fibres. Basal ganglia signal change. Raised CSF lactate. |
| NIID | Full thickness rectal biopsy. | Neuronal intranuclear eosinophilic inclusions. |
| Niemann-Pick C | Bone marrow biopsy. Skin biopsy with cultured fibroblasts. | Sea blue histiocytes. Defective cholesterol esterification. |
| Juvenile neuronal ceroid-lipofuscinosis | Skin/muscle biopsy. Blood smear/electron microscopy. | Fingerprint profile of lysosomal inclusions. Vacuolated lymphocytes. |

in an 8 year old, during which a significant hypotensive episode occurred [115]. A CT scan demonstrated symmetrical hypodensities in the basal ganglia and 99 m Tc HMPAO SPECT showed decreased regional cerebral blood flow. L-dopa administration resulted in a degree of improvement and the child completely recovered over 8 months.

A parkinsonian syndrome has been reported in three children undergoing allogenic bone marrow transplantation (BMT), treated with high doses of amphotericin B for pulmonary aspergillosis [116]. All were encephalopathic and had received cytosine, cyclophosphamide as well as total body irradiation prior to BMT. Another case of parkinsonism post BMT was described in a 21-year-old man who had received cyclosporin A [117]. Imaging revealed cerebellar, cerebral and basal ganglia atrophy as well as white matter involvement.

Table III. L-dopa responsiveness.

| L-Dopa responsive | L-Dopa Unresponsive |
|---|---|
| Parkin mutations | Neuro-acanthocytosis |
| Dopa responsive dystonia | Rapid onset dystonia parkinsonism |
| Tyrosine Hydroxylase deficiency/mutation | PANK2 mutations (neurodegeneration with brain iron accumulation) |
| Westphal variant of Huntington's disease | Hypobetalipoproteinaemia acanthocytosis retinitis pigmentosa pallidal degeneration (HARP) syndrome |
| SCA-2 | Niemann Pick type C |
| SCA-3 | Mitochondrial cytopathies |
| Neuronal intranuclear inclusion body disease | Wilson's disease |
| Juvenile neuronal ceroid lipofuscinosis | Carbon monoxide poisoning |
| Systemic lupus erythematosus | Cyanide poisoning |
| Sub-acute sclerosing pan-encephalitis | Bone marrow transplant |
| Post encephalitic parkinsonism/Encephalitis lethargica | Methanol poisoning |
| Post vaccine | Epstein Barr virus encephalitis |
| Extra pontine myelinolysis | Japanese encephalitis |
| Organophosphate poisoning | Mycoplasma |

Space occupying lesions can cause parkinsonism, either as a result of hydrocephalus [118] which probably involves variable sites of dysfunction in the nigrostriatal pathway and the cortico-striato-pallido-thalamo-cortical circuit, or as a direct result of the location of the tumour, causing distortion or destruction of the basal ganglia. Tumours directly invading the basal ganglia including arteriovenous malformations can also rarely cause parkinsonism [119]. Supratentorial fronto-parietal and posterior fossa tumours can also cause a parkinsonian syndrome [120] due to indirect pressure effects, as can damage secondary to radiotherapy [121].

Central pontine myelinolysis (CPM) is due to rapid correction of hyponatraemia. In approximately 10% of patients with CPM, lesions are found outside the pons (extra pontine myelinolysis: EPM) and the basal ganglia can be affected resulting in parkinsonism [122]. The few cases described in the literature in juveniles have responded well to l-dopa.

## ■ Other unusual possible causes

Hypo and hypercalcaemia as a consequence of hypoparathyroidism, pseudohypoparathyroidism and hyperparathyroidism have been reported as causes of parkinsonism in the literature [123-126]. In addition to these cases, familial idiopathic basal ganglia calcification has been associated with parkinsonism in patients in their 30's [127].

Whipple's disease should also be considered a possibility as parkinsonism reversed with antibiotics has been reported [128]. A case of paraneoplastic basal ganglia degeneration with parkinsonism [129] with no Lewy bodies and a poor response to l-dopa in a case of breast cancer has also been described. Other rare conditions such as adult onset Chediak-Higashi syndrome with or without oculo-cutaneous features [130, 131] and cerebrotendinous xanthomatosis [132], have been reported as causing young onset parkinsonism.

# Conclusion

The majority of the causes of JP discussed in this review would be excluded from the Queen Square Brain Bank (QSBB) clinical criteria of Parkinson's disease and we suggest therefore Juvenile Parkinson's Syndrome as a more appropriate term. There is very limited *post mortem* histopathological data available on the known genetic causes of parkinsonism and although Lewy bodies have been found in one case with a compound heterozygous parkin mutation with onset over 50 years [24], no other cases with Lewy bodies have been reported. The more commonly reported pathology in parkin mutations is of extensive neuronal loss and gliosis in the SNpc with the remaining neurons having a low melanin content. A normal population of neurons with no visible melanin and no evidence of a degenerative process such as Lewy body formation is also seen in DRD.

A case of juvenile parkinsonism with an age of onset at 6 years and death at 39 years has been reported with Lewy bodies present. It is unknown whether the patient had a parkin mutation. The pathology was independently reported [5, 6] with differing opinions as to the significance of the findings. Mizutani and colleagues suggested a different pathophysiological process to classical PD based on the decreased number of neurons, large proportion of immature neurons and the abnormally low melanin content. They suggested that Lewy bodies arose as a consequence of abnormal dopamine metabolism rather than a degenerative process. Gibb and colleagues however suggested that selective vulnerability of the SNpc, resulting in Lewy body formation, similar to that found in Parkinson's disease was responsible. The clinical features in this case were not typical of Parkinson's disease, but resembled those observed in some parkin cases. More clinico-pathological reports of JP are needed to determine whether cases clinically and pathologically indistinguishable from Parkinson's disease exist.

Very few causes of juvenile parkinsonism present a pure parkinsonian phenotype fulfilling QSBB operational criteria. In l-dopa responsive JP with few additional features, the chance of finding a genetic cause, particularly a parkin mutation, is extremely high. Wilson's disease and DRD need to be considered and positively excluded. In acute onset cases, infectious and autoimmune causes need to be eliminated. When confronted with additional atypical clinical signs outside the basal ganglia and with a negative response to l-dopa, further investigations are required to exclude some of the other uncommon conditions discussed in this chapter.

# References

1. de Rijk MC, Tzourio C, Breteler MM, et al. Prevalence of parkinsonism and Parkinson's disease in Europe: the EUROPARKINSON Collaborative Study. European Community Concerted Action on the Epidemiology of Parkinson's disease. J Neurol Neurosurg Psychiatry 1997; 62 (1): 10-5.
2. Quinn N, Critchley P, Marsden CD. Young onset Parkinson's disease. Mov Disord 1987; 2 (2): 73-91.
3. Ludecke B, Knappskog PM, Clayton PT, et al. Recessively inherited L-DOPA-responsive parkinsonism in infancy caused by a point mutation (L205P) in the tyrosine hydroxylase gene. Hum Mol Genet 1996; 5 (7): 1023-8.
4. Gibb WR, Lees AJ. A comparison of clinical and pathological features of young – and old – onset Parkinson's disease. Neurology 1988; 38 (9): 1402-6.
5. Mizutani Y, Yokochi M, Oyanagi S. Juvenile parkinsonism: a case with first clinical manifestation at the age of six years and with neuropathological findings suggesting a new pathogenesis. Clin Neuropathol 1991; 10 (2): 91-7.
6. Gibb WR, Narabayashi H, Yokochi M, Iizuka R, Lees AJ. New pathologic observations in juvenile onset parkinsonism with dystonia. Neurology 1991; 41 (6): 820-2.
7. Pranzatelli MR, Mott SH, Pavlakis SG, Conry JA, Tate ED. Clinical spectrum of secondary parkinsonism in childhood: a reversible disorder. Pediatr Neurol 1994; 10 (2): 131-40.
8. Ramsay Hunt J. Progressive Atrophy of the Globus Pallidus. Brain 1917; 40 (58): 923-75.
9. Schrag A, Ben Shlomo Y, Brown R, Marsden CD, Quinn N. Young-onset Parkinson's disease revisited-clinical features, natural history, and mortality. Mov Disord 1998; 13 (6): 885-94.
10. Gibb WR, Lees AJ. The relevance of the Lewy body to the pathogenesis of idiopathic Parkinson's disease. J Neurol Neurosurg Psychiatry 1988; 51 (6): 745-52.
11. Lucking CB, Durr A, Bonifati V, et al. Association between early-onset Parkinson's disease and mutations in the parkin gene. French Parkinson's Disease Genetics Study Group. N Engl J Med 2000; 342 (21): 1560-7.
12. Jeon BS, Kim JM, Lee DS, Hattori N, Mizuno Y. An apparently sporadic case with parkin gene mutation in a Korean woman. Arch Neurol 2001; 58 (6): 988-9.
13. Hattori N, Kitada T, Matsumine H, et al. Molecular genetic analysis of a novel Parkin gene in Japanese families with autosomal recessive juvenile parkinsonism: evidence for variable homozygous deletions in the Parkin gene in affected individuals. Ann Neurol 1998; 44 (6): 935-41.
14. Golbe LI, Di Iorio G, Sanges G, et al. Clinical genetic analysis of Parkinson's disease in the Contursi kindred. Ann Neurol 1996; 40 (5): 767-75.
15. Kitada T, Asakawa S, Hattori N, et al. Mutations in the parkin gene cause autosomal recessive juvenile parkinsonism. Nature 1998; 392 (6676): 605-8.
16. Periquet M, Latouche M, Lohmann E, et al. Parkin mutations are frequent in patients with isolated early-onset parkinsonism. Brain 2003; 126 (Pt 6): 1271-8.
17. Yamamura Y, Hattori N, Matsumine H, Kuzuhara S, Mizuno Y. Autosomal recessive early-onset parkinsonism with diurnal fluctuation: clinicopathologic characteristics and molecular genetic identification. Brain Dev 2000; 22 (suppl 1): S87-S91.
18. Portman AT, Giladi N, Leenders KL, et al. The nigrostriatal dopaminergic system in familial early onset parkinsonism with parkin mutations. Neurology 2001; 56 (12): 1759-62.
19. Leenders KL, Salmon EP, Tyrrell P, et al. The nigrostriatal dopaminergic system assessed in vivo by positron emission tomography in healthy volunteer subjects and patients with Parkinson's disease. Arch Neurol 1990; 47 (12): 1290-8.
20. Thobois S, Ribeiro MJ, Lohmann E, et al. Young-onset Parkinson disease with and without parkin gene mutations: a fluorodopa F 18 positron emission tomography study. Arch Neurol 2003; 60 (5): 713-8.

21. Khan NL, Brooks DJ, Pavese N, et al. Progression of nigrostriatal dysfunction in a parkin kindred: an [18F] dopa PET and clinical study. Brain 2002; 125 (Pt 10): 2248-56.
22. van de Warrenburg BP, Lammens M, Lucking CB, et al. Clinical and pathologic abnormalities in a family with parkinsonism and parkin gene mutations. Neurology 2001; 56 (4): 555-7.
23. Khan NL, Graham E, Critchley P, et al. Parkin disease: a phenotypic study of a large case series. Brain 2003; 126 (Pt 6): 1279-92.
24. Farrer M, Chan P, Chen R, et al. Lewy bodies and parkinsonism in families with parkin mutations. Ann Neurol 2001; 50 (3): 293-300.
25. Hayashi S, Wakabayashi K, Ishikawa A, et al. An autopsy case of autosomal-recessive juvenile parkinsonism with a homozygous exon 4 deletion in the parkin gene. Mov Disord 2000; 15 (5): 884-8.
26. Mori H, Kondo T, Yokochi M, et al. Pathologic and biochemical studies of juvenile parkinsonism linked to chromosome 6q. Neurology 1998; 51 (3): 890-2.
27. Nygaard TG, Marsden CD, Fahn S. Dopa-responsive dystonia: long-term treatment response and prognosis. Neurology 1991; 41 (2 Pt 1): 174-81.
28. Nygaard TG. Dopa-responsive dystonia. Delineation of the clinical syndrome and clues to pathogenesis. Adv Neurol 1993; 60: 577-85.
29. Swaans RJ, Rondot P, Renier WO, Van Den Heuvel LP, Steenbergen-Spanjers GC, Wevers RA. Four novel mutations in the tyrosine hydroxylase gene in patients with infantile parkinsonism. Ann Hum Genet 2000; 64 (Pt 1): 25-31.
30. Rijk-van Andel JF, Gabreels FJM, Geurtz, B, et al. L-dopa-responsive infantile hypokinetic rigid parkinsonism due to tyrosine hydroxylase deficiency. Neurology 2000; 55 (12): 1926-8.
31. Grattan-Smith PJ, Wevers RA, Steenbergen-Spanjers GC, Fung VS, Earl J, Wilcken B. Tyrosine hydroxylase deficiency: clinical manifestations of catecholamine insufficiency in infancy. Mov Disord 2002; 17 (2): 354-9.
32. Tassin J, Durr A, Bonnet AM, et al. Levodopa-responsive dystonia. GTP cyclohydrolase I or parkin mutations? Brain 2000; 123 (Pt 6): 1112-21.
33. O'Sullivan JD, Costa DC, Gacinovic S, Lees AJ. SPECT imaging of the dopamine transporter in juvenile-onset dystonia. Neurology 2001; 56 (2): 266-7.
34. Turjanski N, Bhatia K, Burn DJ, Sawle GV, Marsden CD, Brooks DJ. Comparison of striatal 18F-dopa uptake in adult-onset dystonia- parkinsonism, Parkinson's disease, and dopa-responsive dystonia. Neurology 1993; 43 (8): 1563-8.
35. Hyland K, Fryburg JS, Wilson WG, et al. Oral phenylalanine loading in dopa-responsive dystonia: a possible diagnostic test. Neurology 1997; 48 (5): 1290-7.
36. Bandmann O, Goertz M, Zschocke J, et al. The phenylalanine loading test in the differential diagnosis of dystonia. Neurology 2003; 60 (4): 700.
37. Walshe JM, Yealland M. Wilson's disease: the problem of delayed diagnosis. J Neurol Neurosurg Psychiatry 1992; 55 (8): 692-6.
38. Orth M, Schapira AH. Mitochondria and degenerative disorders. Am J Med Genet 2001; 106 (1): 27-36.
39. Walshe JM, Yealland M. Not Wilson's disease: a review of misdiagnosed cases. QJM 1995; 88 (1): 55-9.
40. Squitieri F, Berardelli A, Nargi E, et al. Atypical movement disorders in the early stages of Huntington's disease: clinical and genetic analysis. Clin Genet 2000; 58 (1): 50-6.
41. Young AB, Shoulson I, Penney JB, et al. Huntington's disease in Venezuela: neurologic features and functional decline. Neurology 1986; 36 (2): 244-9.
42. Jongen PJ, Renier WO, Gabreels FJ. Seven cases of Huntington's disease in childhood and levodopa induced improvement in the hypokinetic-rigid form. Clin Neurol Neurosurg 1980; 82 (4): 251-61.

43. Gwinn-Hardy K, Singleton A, O'Suilleabhain P, et al. Spinocerebellar ataxia type 3 phenotypically resembling parkinson disease in a black family. Arch Neurol 2001; 58 (2): 296-9.
44. Gwinn-Hardy K, Chen JY, Liu HC, et al. Spinocerebellar ataxia type 2 with parkinsonism in ethnic Chinese. Neurology 2000; 55 (6): 800-5.
45. Lee WY, Jin DK, Oh MR, et al. Frequency analysis and clinical characterization of spinocerebellar ataxia types 1, 2, 3, 6, and 7 in Korean patients. Arch Neurol 2003; 60 (6): 858.
46. Schols L, Peters S, Szymanski S, et al. Extrapyramidal motor signs in degenerative ataxias. Arch Neurol 2000; 57 (10): 1495-500.
47. Subramony SH, Hernandez D, Adam A, et al. Ethnic differences in the expression of neurodegenerative disease: Machado-Joseph disease in Africans and Caucasians. Mov Disord 2002; 17 (5): 1068-71.
48. Sasaki H, Wakisaka A, Sanpei K, et al. Phenotype variation correlates with CAG repeat length in SCA2 – A study of 28 Japanese patients. Journal of the Neurological Sciences 1998; 159 (2): 202-8.
49. Schols L, Gispert S, Vorgerd M, et al. Spinocerebellar ataxia type 2. Genotype and phenotype in German kindreds. Arch Neurol 1997; 54 (9): 1073-80.
50. Payami H, Nutt J, Gancher S, et al. SCA2 may present as levodopa-responsive parkinsonism. Mov Disord 2003; 18 (4): 425-9.
51. Hardie RJ, Pullon HW, Harding AE, et al. Neuroacanthocytosis. A clinical, haematological and pathological study of 19 cases. Brain 1991; 114 (Pt 1A): 13-49.
52. Peppard RF, Lu CS, Chu NS, Teal P, Martin WR, Calne DB. Parkinsonism with neuroacanthocytosis. Can J Neurol Sci 1990; 17 (3): 298-301.
53. Dobson-Stone C, Danek A, Rampoldi L, et al. Mutational spectrum of the CHAC gene in patients with chorea- acanthocytosis. Eur J Hum Genet 2002; 10 (11): 773-81.
54. Pittock SJ, Joyce C, O'Keane V, et al. Rapid-onset dystonia-parkinsonism: A clinical and genetic analysis of a new kindred. Neurology 2000; 55 (7): 991-5.
55. Kramer PL, Mineta M, Klein C, et al. Rapid-onset dystonia-parkinsonism: linkage to chromosome 19q13. Ann Neurol 1999; 46 (2): 176-82.
56. De Coo IF, Renier WO, Ruitenbeek W, et al. A 4-base pair deletion in the mitochondrial cytochrome b gene associated with parkinsonism/MELAS overlap syndrome. Ann Neurol 1999; 45 (1): 130-3.
57. Lindenberg R, Rubinstein LJ, Herman MM, Haydon GB. A light and electron microscopy study of an unusual widespread nuclear inclusion body disease. A possible residuum of an old herpesvirus infection. Acta Neuropathol (Berl) 1968; 10 (1): 54-73.
58. Kimber TE, Blumbergs PC, Rice JP, et al. Familial neuronal intranuclear inclusion disease with ubiquitin positive inclusions. J Neurol Sci 1998; 160 (1): 33-40.
59. O'Sullivan JD, Hanagasi HA, Daniel SE, Tidswell P, Davies SW, Lees AJ. Neuronal intranuclear inclusion disease and juvenile parkinsonism. Mov Disord 2000; 15 (5): 990-5.
60. Kish SJ, Gilbert JJ, Chang LJ, Mirchandani L, Shannak K, Hornykiewicz O. Brain neurotransmitter abnormalities in neuronal intranuclear inclusion body disorder. Ann Neurol 1985; 17 (4): 405-7.
61. Funata N, Maeda Y, Koike M, et al. Neuronal intranuclear hyaline inclusion disease: report of a case and review of the literature. Clin Neuropathol 1990; 9 (2): 89-96.
62. Greco CM, Hagerman RJ, Tassone F, et al. Neuronal intranuclear inclusions in a new cerebellar tremor/ataxia syndrome among fragile X carriers. Brain 2002; 125 (8): 1760-71.
63. Munoz E, Rey MJ, Mila M, et al. Intranuclear inclusions, neuronal loss and CAG mosaicism in two patients with Machado-Joseph disease. Journal of the Neurological Sciences 2002; 200 (1-2): 19-25.
64. Walker RH, Morgello S, Davidoff-Feldman B, et al. Autosomal dominant chorea-acanthocytosis with polyglutamine-containing neuronal inclusions. Neurology 2002; 58 (7): 1031-7.

65. Takahashi J, Fukuda T, Tanaka J, Minamitani M, Fujigasaki H, Uchihara T. Neuronal intranuclear hyaline inclusion disease with polyglutamine- immunoreactive inclusions. *Acta Neuropathol* (Berl) 2000; 99 (5): 589-94.
66. Carstea ED, Morris JA, Coleman KG, et al. Niemann-Pick C1 disease gene: homology to mediators of cholesterol homeostasis. *Science* 1997; 277 (5323): 228-31.
67. Coleman RJ, Robb SA, Lake BD, Brett EM, Harding AE. The diverse neurological features of Niemann-Pick disease type C: a report of two cases. *Mov Disord* 1988; 3 (4): 295-9.
68. Gardiner M, Sandford A, Deadman M, et al. Batten disease (Spielmeyer-Vogt disease, juvenile onset neuronal ceroid- lipofuscinosis) gene (CLN3) maps to human chromosome 16. *Genomics* 1990; 8 (2): 387-90.
69. Jarvela I, Autti T, Lamminranta S, Aberg L, Raininko R, Santavuori P. Clinical and magnetic resonance imaging findings in Batten disease: analysis of the major mutation (1.02-kb deletion). *Ann Neurol* 1997; 42 (5): 799-802.
70. Aberg LE, Rinne JO, Rajantie I, Santavuori P. A favourable response to antiparkinsonian treatment in juvenile neuronal ceroid lipofuscinosis. *Neurology* 2001; 56 (9): 1236-9.
71. Zhou B, Westaway SK, Levinson B, Johnson MA, Gitschier J, Hayflick SJ. A novel pantothenate kinase gene (PANK2) is defective in Hallervorden- Spatz syndrome. *Nat Genet* 2001; 28 (4): 345-9.
72. Galvin JE, Giasson B, Hurtig HI, Lee VMY, Trojanowski JQ. Neurodegeneration with brain iron accumulation, Type 1 is characterized by {alpha}-, {beta}-, and {gamma}-synuclein neuropathology. *Am J Pathol* 2000; 157 (2): 361-8.
73. Hayflick SJ, Westaway SK, Levinson B, et al. Genetic, clinical, and radiographic delineation of Hallervorden-Spatz syndrome. *N Engl J Med* 2003; 348 (1): 33-40.
74. Higgins JJ, Patterson MC, Papadopoulos NM, Brady RO, Pentchev PG, Barton NW. Hypoprebetalipoproteinemia, acanthocytosis, retinitis pigmentosa, and pallidal degeneration (HARP syndrome). *Neurology* 1992; 42 (1): 194-8.
75. Kyllerman M, Brandberg G, Wiklund LM, Mansson JE. Dysarthria, progressive parkinsonian features and symmetric necrosis of putamen in a family with painful lipomas (Dercum disease variant). *Neuropediatrics* 2002; 33 (2): 69-72.
76. Keskin S, Yurdakul F. Parkinsonian manifestations in a patient with homocystinuria. *J Child Neurol* 1996; 11 (3): 235-6.
77. Clayton PT, Smith I, Harding B, Hyland K, Leonard JV, Leeming RJ. Subacute combined degeneration of the cord, dementia and parkinsonism due to an inborn error of folate metabolism. *J Neurol Neurosurg Psychiatry* 1986; 49 (8): 920-7.
78. Poser CM, Huntley CJ, Poland JD. Para-encephalitic parkinsonism. Report of an acute case due to coxsackie virus type B 2 and re-examination of the etiologic concepts of postencephalitic parkinsonism. *Acta Neurol Scand* 1969; 45 (2): 199-215.
79. Hsieh JC, Lue KH, Lee YL. Parkinson-like syndrome as the major presenting symptom of Epstein-Barr virus encephalitis. *Arch Dis Child* 2002; 87 (4): 358.
80. Bickerstaff ER, Cloake PCP. Mesencephalitis and rhombencephalitis. *British Medical Journal* 1951; 2: 77-81.
81. Hersh BP, Rajendran PR, Battinelli D. Parkinsonism as the presenting manifestation of HIV infection: improvement on HAART. *Neurology* 2001; 56 (2): 278-9.
82. Bennett NM. Murray Valley encephalitis, 1974: clinical features. *Med J Aust* 1976; 2 (12): 446-50.
83. Misra UK, Kalita J. Prognosis of Japanese encephalitis patients with dystonia compared to those with parkinsonian features only. *Postgrad Med J* 2002; 78 (918): 238-41.
84. Garg RK. Subacute sclerosing panencephalitis. *Postgrad Med J* 2002; 78 (916): 63-70.
85. Sawaishi Y, Yano T, Watanabe Y, Takada G. Migratory basal ganglia lesions in subacute sclerosing panencephalitis (SSPE): Clinical implications of axonal spread. *Journal of the Neurological Sciences* 1999; 168 (2): 137-40.

86. Bennett BA, Rusyniak DE, Hollingsworth CK. HIV-1 gp120-induced neurotoxicity to midbrain dopamine cultures. *Brain Res* 1995; 705 (1-2): 168-76.
87. de Mattos JP, de Rosso ALZ, Correa RB, Novis SAP. Movement Disorders in 28 HIV- infected Patients. *Arq Neuro-Psiquiatr* 2002; 60 (3A).
88. Kelly DV, Beique LC, Bowmer MI. Extrapyramidal symptoms with ritonavir/indinavir plus risperidone. *Ann Pharmacother* 2002; 36 (5): 827-30.
89. Alves RS, Barbosa ER, Scaff M. Postvaccinal parkinsonism. *Mov Disord* 1992; 7 (2): 178-80.
90. Kim JS, Choi IS, Lee MC. Reversible parkinsonism and dystonia following probable mycoplasma pneumoniae infection. *Mov Disord* 1995; 10 (4): 510-2.
91. Smith R, Eviatar L. Neurologic manifestations of mycoplasma pneumoniae infections: diverse *spectrum of diseases. A report of six cases and review of the literature. Clin Pediatr* (Phila) 2000; 39 (4): 195-201.
92. Von Economo C. *Encephalitis lethargica. Its sequelae and treatment.* Translated by K.O. Newman. 1 ed. London: Oxford University Press, 1931.
93. McCall S, Henry JM, Reid AH, Taubenberger JK. Influenza RNA not detected in archival brain tissues from acute encephalitis lethargica cases or in postencephalitic Parkinson cases. *J Neuropathol Exp Neurol* 2001; 60 (7): 696-704.
94. Howard RS, Lees AJ. Encephalitis lethargica. A report of four recent cases. *Brain* 1987; 110 (Pt 1): 19-33.
95. Dale RC, Church AJ, Surtees RA, et al. Encephalitis lethargica syndrome: 20 new cases and evidence of basal ganglia autoimmunity. *Brain* 2004; 127 (Pt 1): 21-33.
96. Blunt SB, Lane RJ, Turjanski N, Perkin GD. Clinical features and management of two cases of encephalitis lethargica. *Mov Disord* 1997; 12 (3): 354-9.
97. Kiley M, Esiri MM. A contemporary case of encephalitis lethargica. *Clin Neuropathol* 2001; 20 (1): 2-7.
98. Williams A, Houff S, Lees A, Calne DB. Oligoclonal banding in the cerebrospinal fluid of patients with postencephalitic parkinsonism. *J Neurol Neurosurg Psychiatry* 1979; 42 (9): 790-2.
99. Dale RC, Church AJ, Surtees RA, Lees AJ, Neville BG, Giovannoni G. Re-emergence of encephalitis lethargica: new evidence of an autoimmune disease. *J Neurol Neurosurg Psychiatry* 2002; 73 (2): 213-36 (abstract).
100. Swedo SE, Leonard HL, Garvey M, et al. Pediatric autoimmune neuropsychiatric disorders associated with streptococcal infections: clinical description of the first 50 cases. *Am J Psychiatry* 1998; 155 (2): 264-71.
101. Bottas A, Richter MA. Pediatric autoimmune neuropsychiatric disorders associated with streptococcal infections (PANDAS). *Pediatr Infect Dis J* 2002; 21 (1): 67-71.
102. Dale RC, Church AJ, Surtees RA, Thompson EJ, Giovannoni G, Neville BG. Post-streptococcal autoimmune neuropsychiatric disease presenting as paroxysmal dystonic choreoathetosis. *Mov Disord* 2002; 17 (4): 817-20.
103. Ben Pazi H, Livne A, Shapira Y, Dale RC. Parkinsonian features after streptococcal pharyngitis. *J Pediatr* 2003; 143 (2): 267-9.
104. Garcia-Moreno JM, Chacon J. Juvenile parkinsonism as a manifestation of systemic lupus erythematosus: Case report and review of the literature. *Mov Disord* 2002; 17 (6): 1329-35.
105. Negrotti A, Calzetti S. A long-term follow-up study of cinnarizine- and flunarizine-induced parkinsonism. *Mov Disord* 1997; 12 (1): 107-10.
106. Teive HA, Germiniani FM, Werneck LC. Parkinsonian syndrome induced by amlodipine: case report. *Mov Disord* 2002; 17 (4): 833-5.
107. Padrell MD, Navarro M, Faura CC, Horga JF. Verapamil-induced parkinsonism. *Am J Med* 1995; 99 (4): 436.

108. Parmar RC, Valvi CV, Kamat JR, Vaswani RK. Chloroquine induced parkinsonism. *J Postgrad Med* 2000; 46 (1): 29-30.
109. Boranic M, Raci F. A Parkinson-like syndrome as side effect of chemotherapy with vincristine and adriamycin in a child with acute leukaemia. *Biomedicine* 1979; 31 (5): 124-5.
110. Alvarez-Gomez MJ, Vaamonde J, Narbona J, et al. Parkinsonian syndrome in childhood after sodium valproate administration. *Clin Neuropharmacol* 1993; 16 (5): 451-5.
111. Choi IS. Parkinsonism after carbon monoxide poisoning. *Eur Neurol* 2002; 48 (1): 30-3.
112. Shahar E, Andraws J. Extra-pyramidal parkinsonism complicating organophosphate insecticide poisoning. *Eur J Paediatr Neurol* 2001; 5 (6): 261-4.
113. Uitti RJ, Rajput AH, Ashenhurst EM, Rozdilsky B. Cyanide-induced parkinsonism: a clinicopathologic report. *Neurology* 1985; 35 (6): 921-5.
114. Davis LE, Adair JC. Parkinsonism from methanol poisoning: benefit from treatment with anti-Parkinson drugs. *Mov Disord* 1999; 14 (3): 520-2.
115. Straussberg R, Shahar E, Gat R, Brand N. Delayed parkinsonism associated with hypotension in a child undergoing open-heart surgery. *Dev Med Child Neurol* 1993; 35 (11): 1011-4.
116. Mott SH, Packer RJ, Vezina LG, et al. Encephalopathy with parkinsonian features in children following bone marrow transplantations and high-dose amphotericin B. *Ann Neurol* 1995; 37 (6): 810-4.
117. Pirker W, Baumgartner C, Brugger S, et al. Severe akinetic syndrome resulting from a bilateral basal ganglia lesion following bone marrow transplantation. *Mov Disord* 1999; 14 (3): 525-8.
118. Curran T, Lang AE. Parkinsonian syndromes associated with hydrocephalus: case reports, a review of the literature, and pathophysiological hypotheses. *Mov Disord* 1994; 9 (5): 508-20.
119. Krauss JK, Nobbe F, Wakhloo AK, Mohadjer M, Vach W, Mundinger F. Movement disorders in astrocytomas of the basal ganglia and the thalamus. *J Neurol Neurosurg Psychiatry* 1992; 55 (12): 1162-7.
120. Pohle T, Krauss JK. Parkinsonism in children resulting from mesencephalic tumors. *Mov Disord* 1999; 14 (5): 842-6.
121. Skiming JA, McDowell HP, Wright N, May P. Secondary parkinsonism: an unusual late complication of craniospinal radiotherapy given to a 16-month child. *Med Pediatr Oncol* 2003; 40 (2): 132-4.
122. Nagamitsu S, Matsuishi T, Yamashita Y, Yamada S, Kato H. Extrapontine myelinolysis with parkinsonism after rapid correction of hyponatremia: high cerebrospinal fluid level of homovanillic acid and successful dopaminergic treatment. *J Neural Transm* 1999; 106 (9-10): 949-53.
123. Derex L, Trouillas P. Reversible parkinsonism, hypophosphoremia, and hypocalcemia under vitamin D therapy. *Mov Disord* 1997; 12 (4): 612-3.
124. Hirooka Y, Yuasa K, Hibi K, et al. Hyperparathyroidism associated with parkinsonism. *Intern Med* 1992; 31 (7): 904-7.
125. Kovacs CS, Howse DC, Yendt ER. Reversible parkinsonism induced by hypercalcemia and primary hyperparathyroidism. *Arch Intern Med* 1993; 153 (9): 1134-6.
126. Pearson DW, Durward WF, Fogelman I, Boyle IT, Beastall G. Pseudohypoparathyroidism presenting as severe parkinsonism. *Postgrad Med J* 1981; 57 (669): 445-7.
127. Manyam BV, Walters AS, Keller IA, Ghobrial M. Parkinsonism associated with autosomal dominant bilateral striopallidodentate calcinosis. *Parkinsonism & Related Disorders* 2001; 7 (4): 289-95.
128. Uldry PA, Bogousslavsky J. Partially reversible parkinsonism in Whipple's disease with antibiotherapy. *Eur Neurol* 1992; 32 (3): 151-3.
129. Golbe LI, Miller DC, Duvoisin RC. Paraneoplastic degeneration of the substantia nigra with dystonia and parkinsonism. *Mov Disord* 1989; 4 (2): 147-52.
130. Pettit RE, Berdal KG. Chediak-Higashi syndrome. Neurologic appearance. *Arch Neurol* 1984; 41 (9): 1001-2.

131. Hauser RA, Friedlander J, Baker MJ, Thomas J, Zuckerman KS. Adult Chediak-Higashi parkinsonian syndrome with dystonia. *Mov Disord* 2000; 15 (4): 705-8.
132. Grandas F, Martin-Moro M, Garcia-Munozguren S, Anaya F. Early-onset parkinsonism in cerebrotendinous xanthomatosis. *Mov Disord* 2002; 17 (6): 1396-7.
133. Leroy E, Anastasopoulos D, Konitsiotis S, Lavedan C, Polymeropoulos MH. Deletions in the Parkin gene and genetic heterogeneity in a Greek family with early onset Parkinson's disease. *Hum Genet* 1998; 103 (4): 424-7.
134. Tassin J, Durr A, de Broucker T, *et al*. Chromosome 6-linked autosomal recessive early-onset parkinsonism: linkage in European and Algerian families, extension of the clinical spectrum, and evidence of a small homozygous deletion in one family. The French Parkinson's Disease Genetics Study Group, and the European Consortium on Genetic Susceptibility in Parkinson's Disease. *Am J Hum Genet* 1998; 63 (1): 88-94.
135. Maruyama M, Ikeuchi T, Saito M, *et al*. Novel mutations, pseudo-dominant inheritance, and possible familial affects in patients with autosomal recessive juvenile parkinsonism. *Ann Neurol* 2000; 48(2): 245-50.
136. Klein C, Pramstaller PP, Kis B, *et al*. Parkin deletions in a family with adult-onset, tremor-dominant parkinsonism: expanding the phenotype. *Ann Neurol* 2000; 48(1): 65-71.
137. Nisipeanu P, Inzelberg R, Abo Mouch S, *et al*. Parkin gene causing benign autosomal recessive juvenile parkinsonism. *Neurology* 2001; 56 (11): 1573-5.
138. Hedrich K, Marder K, Harris J, *et al*. Evaluation of 50 probands with early-onset Parkinson's disease for parkin mutations. *Neurology* 2002; 58(8): 1239-46.
139. Munoz E, Tolosa E, Pastor P, *et al*. Relative high frequency of the c.255delA parkin gene mutation in Spanish patients with autosomal recessive parkinsonism. *J Neurol Neurosurg Psychiatry* 2002; 73 (5): 582-4.
140. West A, Periquet M, Lincoln S, *et al*. Complex relationship between parkin mutations and Parkinson disease. *Am J Med Genet* 2002; 114 (5): 584-91.
141. Hoenicka J, Vidal L, Morales B, *et al*. Molecular findings in familial Parkinson's disease in Spain. *Arch Neurol* 2002; 59 (6): 966-70.
142. Illarioshkin SN, Periquet M, Rawal N, *et al*. Mutation analysis of the parkin gene in Russian families with autosomal recessive juvenile parkinsonism. *Mov Disord* 2003; 18(8): 914-9.
143. Lohmann E, Periquet M, Bonifati V, *et al*. How much phenotypic variation can be attributed to parkin genotype? *Ann Neurol* 2003; 54 (2): 176-85.
144. Rawal N, Periquet M, Lohmann E, *et al*. New parkin mutations and atypical phenotypes in families with autosomal recessive parkinsonism. *Neurology* 2003; 60(8): 1378-81.

# Benign hereditary chorea

### Ángeles Schteinschnaider

*Pediatric Neurology Department, Raúl Carrea Institute for Neurological Research (FLENI), Buenos Aires, Argentina*

---

Benign Hereditary Chorea (BHC) is an autosomal dominant disorder presenting with childhood-onset chorea, no dementia, and little or no progression. Since the first reports of this disease in the mid-1960s [1-3], a large number of families have been described [4-6].

## Clinical Features

Chorea is the only clinical manifestation of the disease and it may present with a significant degree of clinical variability from one patient to another, which may even be observed among members of the same family [4, 5]. In fact, the variation in clinical features is such that its very existence has been doubted [6, 7]. In some subjects, the movement disorder may be so subtle that it may only be perceived by an experienced examiner. In others, its severity may preclude proper drinking from a cup.

Such movements are worsened by anxiety but not by voluntary movements, exercise, startle, caffeine, or alcohol [8]. There is absence of chorea during sleep.

The syndrome manifests as early childhood onset of sudden choreiform movements of small amplitude, generally involving the distal parts of the upper limbs, but also involving the feet, shoulders, head, and face. The onset of the disease is insidious, usually during the first year of life or later infancy, although in many cases a precise age at onset cannot be determined.

The movement disorder becomes obvious by the stage in which the child is supposed to acquire independent walking. In the following years, the chorea is characterized by initial progression of the movement disorder, followed by a plateau stage in which individual adaptation suggests an apparent clinical improvement [9]. Regression of the movement disorder is exceptional.

Clinical evaluations reveal sudden, brief, continuous, non-paroxysmal (though fluctuating) irregular jerky movements of small amplitude involving the distal parts of the upper limbs. Any body region may be affected (face, tongue, neck, trunk or limbs), while similar movements have on occasion been noted in the shoulder, feet, head, and face. Some cases are described as having grimacing or dysarthria due to laryngeal muscle involvement. Usual findings on physical examination in these patients include diffuse and mild low tone, motor clumsiness, inability to perform tandem walk properly, and wide-based gait. Cranial nerve testing results are normal. The remainder of the coordination, gait, muscle strength, muscle tone, and sensation is normal.

Patients usually seek medical evaluation due to motor delay, lack of independent walking being the main concern.

These patients are "clumsy walkers" with a history of frequent falls. Scarring may be present at the level of elbows and knees.

A positive family history is suggestive towards early diagnosis.

Although the condition is not associated with dementia or a decrease in life span, it can be socially disabling. Several children have had difficulties at school, but it is unclear whether this is a direct consequence of the CNS disease or related to problems with social interaction. Several were unable to finish school and experienced serious social isolation. There are isolated reports of concomitant low IQ [8].

Some BHC families show atypical additional features, such as dysarthria and gait disturbances [10], mental impairment [11], or axial dystonia and progression in adulthood [12]. The latter report could describe a variant of the disorder, but might as well be an entirely separate entity, considering the progressiveness of the chorea in that family [13]. Other variants have been described as well, such as BHC associated with sensorineural deafness [14] and BHC with intention tremor [3].

## ■ Pathophysiology

Pathophysiology remains obscure. Because the clinical features in BHC patients appear before the first year, a disturbance in maturation of glia cells might be part of the pathogenic process, although so far no major cerebral abnormalities, as detectable by MRI studies, have been found in BHC [4, 5]. At a later patient age, delayed maturation may be partly overcome by other factors consistent with the reduction of symptoms.

PET studies remain inconclusive with findings ranging from caudate hypometabolism to normal metabolism in the striatum and the cortex [15-18].

### Neuropathological findings

One patient died at age 59 years of leukemia. Apart from mild frontal-parietal-temporal atrophy, gross examination showed no abnormalities including a normal appearing striatum and pigmented *substantia nigra*. On routine sections and particularly with glial fibrillary acidic protein immunohistochemistry, the globus pallidus, thalamus, hippocampus, and periaqueductal gray matter demonstrated nonspecific astrocytosis and hyperplasia without noticeable neuronal loss. Staining of selected blocks with Bielschowsky stain and antibodies to β-amyloid, synuclein, tau, ubiquitin, and TITF failed to disclose any abnormalities [15].

# Diagnosis

The diagnosis of the disease is based on clinical grounds and is made by exclusion. All ancillary testing are negative (MR or CT imaging of the brain, DNA screening for HD, urinary organic acid screening to exclude glutaricaciduria, determination of serum copper and ceruloplasmin levels and uric acid levels, search for acanthocytes, routine hematologic and blood chemistry testing, thyroid function tests, serum lipid profile, and ophthalmologic examination, EEG, CSF examination).

This entity should be borne in mind whenever a child presents with nonprogressive chorea with lack of other neurological manifestations. A negative family history does not exclude the diagnosis.

## Differential diagnosis

The phenotype of BHC is most commonly confused with two other causes of chorea, namely Huntington's disease (HD) and Sydenham's chorea. BHC differs from HD in that the onset of choreiform movements is in early childhood, it is nonprogressive [19] and life expectancy is normal, does not involve deteriorating cognitive or behavioral changes, does not have caudate atrophy on neuroimaging, and has a normal-sized CAG repeat in the HD gene [20].

Although many subjects have been thought to have Sydenham's chorea, BHC is present for years or even decades, is not associated with rheumatic fever, and has a family history.

A particularly difficult distinction is between "BHC" and hereditary essential myoclonus (which may be the same as hereditary myoclonic dystonia) [21]. Age of onset of both conditions is reported to be early childhood, they are both dominantly inherited with variable penetrance, progression may be mild, other neurological abnormalities are absent, and additional dystonia may occur in both. Chorea is thought to be distinguished from hereditary essential myoclonus by "flitting" unpredictable jerks, frequent involvement of gait, which is rare in hereditary essential myoclonus, and by the lack of response to alcohol. It is when the jerks predominate in the fingers and hands that the distinction is most difficult, and electrophysiological investigations are unhelpful because a mixture of short and long bursts with and without co-contraction may occur in both conditions.

Others differential diagnoses includes Cerebral Palsy, Familial Cerebellar Ataxia, Ataxia telangiectasia and hereditary forms of dystonia.

## Diagnostic criteria of Benign Hereditary Chorea

Characteristic movement disorder.
Nonprogressive nature of the disease.
Lack of cognitive involvement.
No history of drug exposure.
Positive family history.
Negative ancillary testing.

## Genetics

The mode of inheritance is autosomal dominant (vertical, with numerous male-to-male transmissions) with incomplete penetrance and variable expression [3, 10]. X-Linked inheritance appears to be excluded by the apparent transmission through an unaffected male [3].

Through studies of locus D4S10, BHC has been excluded as an allelic variant of Huntington's chorea [20].

In a large Dutch kindred with BHC, de Vries et al. [19] found strong evidence for linkage between the disorder and markers on 14q (maximum lod score of 6.32 at recombination fraction 0.0). The BHC locus in this family was located between markers D14S49 and D14S1064, a region spanning approximately 20.6 cM and containing several candidate genes involved in the development and/or maintenance of the central nervous system, including glia maturation factor-beta (GMFB; 601713), GTP cyclohydrolase I (GCH1; 600225), and SMN-interacting protein-1 (SIP1; 602595).

Fernandez et al. [8] reported a 4-generation family with BCH showing linkage to 14q. Haplotype analysis defined a 6.93-cM critical region between D14S1068 and D14S1064, excluding SIP1 as a candidate gene. Direct sequencing of the GCH1 gene in this family revealed no mutations.

Breedveld et al. [22] reported clinical and genetic heterogeneity in 6 families with BHC and the large Dutch family reported by de Vries et al. [19]. Three of the 7 families showed linkage to chromosome 14 between markers D14S49 and D14S278, and haplotype analysis narrowed the critical interval for the BHC locus to 8.4 cM. In the remaining 4 families, linkage to 14q was excluded. The 3 families with linkage to 14q had a similar clinical phenotype including onset in infancy and childhood, chorea, and absence of mental deterioration. Other variable features in these families included gait difficulties, pyramidal signs, slow saccades, and abnormal reflexes. The 4 unlinked families had a slightly later age at onset and other signs besides chorea, including myoclonic jerks, dystonia, tremor, and tics.

## Treatment

Although treatment with haloperidol, chlorpromazine, and prednisone led to improvement for some patients [5], and phenobarbital and diazepam in others [8], a general curative treatment is not available and to date, there are no proven benefits from any pharmacological agent.

## Conclusion

Benign Familiar chorea is an inherited disorder characterized by nonprogressive but persistent choreic movements with early onset and no cognitive involvement.

Despite the lack of proven pharmacological therapies to date, early recognition of this condition prevents unnecessary testing as well as prolonged hospitalizations and the possibility of prompt genetic counselling.

Benign hereditary chorea is a clinically and genetically heterogeneous disorder, with one well-defined clinical syndrome mapping to chromosome 14q.

## References

1. Haerer AF, Currier RD, Jackson JF. Hereditary nonprogressive chorea of early onset. *Neurology* 1966; 16: 307.
2. Haerer AF, Currier RD, Jackson JF. Hereditary nonprogressive chorea of early onset. *N Engl J Med* 1967; 276: 1220-4.
3. Pincus JH, Chutoria A. Familial benign chorea with intention tremor: a clinical entity. *J Pediatr* 1967; 70: 724-9.
4. Bruyn GW, Myrianthopoulos NC. Chronic juvenile hereditary chorea (benign hereditary chorea of early onset). In: Bruyn GW, Vinken PJ, Klawans HL, eds. *Handbook of clinical neurology. Vol 5. Extrapyramidal disorders.* Amsterdam: Elsevier Science, 1986: 335-48.
5. Wheeler PG, Weaver DD, Dobyns WB. Benign hereditary chorea. *Pediatr Neurol* 1993; 9: 337-40.
6. Schrag A, Quinn NP, Bhatia KP, et al. Benign hereditary chorea: entity or syndrome? *Mov Disord* 2000; 15: 280-8.
7. Quinn N, Schrag A. Huntington's disease and other choreas. *J Neurol* 1998; 245: 709-16.
8. Fernandez M, Raskind W, Matsushita M, Wolff J, Lipe H, Bird T. Hereditary benign chorea: clinical and genetic features of a distinct disease. *Neurology* 2001; 57: 106-10.
9. Harper PS. Benign hereditary chorea: clinical and genetic aspects. *Clin Genet* 1978; 13: 85-95.
10. Chun RWM, Daly RF, Mansheim BJ, et al. Benign familial chorea with onset in childhood. *JAMA* 1973; 225: 1603-7.
11. Leli DA, Furlow TW, Falgout JC. Benign familial chorea: an association with intellectual impairment. *J Neurol Neurosurg Psychiatric* 1984; 47: 471-4.
12. Schady W, Meara RJ. Hereditary Progressive chorea without dementia. *Journal of Neurology, Neurosurgery and Psychiatry* 1998; 51: 295-7.
13. Wheeler PG, Weaver DD, Dobyns WB. Benign hereditary chorea. *Pediatric Neurology* 1993; 9: 337-40.
14. Damasio H, Antunes L, Damasio AR. Familial nonprogressive involuntary movements of childhood. *Ann Neurol* 1977; 1: 602-3.
15. Kleiner-Fisman G, Rogaeva E, Halliday W, et al. Benign hereditary chorea: clinical, genetic, and pathological findings. *Ann Neurol* 2003; 54: 244-7.
16. Martin WRW, Hayden MR, Suchowersky O, Beckman J, Adam M. Striatal Metabolism in Huntington's disease and in benign hereditary chorea. *Annals of Neurology* 1984; 1 (16): 126.
17. Suchowersky O, Hayden MR, Martin WRW, Stoessl Aj, Hildebrand AM, Pate BD. Cerebral metabolism of glucose in benign hereditary chorea. *Mov Disord* 1986; 1: 33-4.
18. Hosokawa S, Ichiya Y, Kuwabara Y, et al. Positron emission tomography in cases of chorea with different underlying disease. *Journal of Neurology, Neurosurgery and Psychiatry* 1987; 50: 1284-7.
19. deVries BB, Arts WF, Breedveld GJ, et al. Benign hereditary chorea of early onset maps to chromosome 14q. *Am J Hum Genet* 2000; 66: 136-42.
20. Yapijakis C, Kapaki E, Zournas C, et al. Exclusion mapping of the benign hereditary chorea gene from Huntington's disease locus: report of a family. *Clin Genet* 1995; 47: 133-8.
21. Quinn NP. Essential myoclonus and myoclonic dystonia. *Mov Disord* 1996; 11: 119-24.
22. Breedveld GJ, Percy AK, MacDonald ME, et al. Clinical and genetic heterogeneity in benign hereditary chorea. *Neurology* 2002; 59: 579-84.

# Opsoclonus-myoclonus-ataxia syndrome

**Michael R. Pranzatelli**

*National Pediatric Myoclonus Center and the Departments of Neurology and Pediatrics, Southern Illinois University School of Medicine, Springfield, Illinois, USA*

## ■ Definition

Opsoclonus-myoclonus syndrome (OMS), also called Kinsbourne syndrome, dancing eyes syndrome (DES), and myoclonic encephalopathy, is a rare, pervasive, neurobehavioral disorder [1]. *Opsoclonus* denotes chaotic darting eye movements and *myoclonus* indicates brief involuntary muscle jerks. The tremorous appearance of the myoclonus has been called polyminimyoclonus. Although opsoclonus and myoclonus are the only obligate features, most children also exhibit ataxia, behavioral problems, and developmental delay [2].

## ■ Epidemiology

OMS typically afflicts toddlers, but can appear throughout childhood [3]. Neuroblastoma or ganglioneuroblastoma, the only commonly associated tumor [4], is found in 7-46% of the cases [5-7]. This neural-crest-derived tumor is usually benign in children with OMS: INSS Stage I or II, aneuploid DNA content, no MYCN amplification [8]. OMS may accompany 1-3% of neuroblastoma cases [8, 9]. Its presence triggers the search for an occult tumor, but on occasion OMS follows tumor detection and treatment. Paradoxically, presence of the paraneoplastic syndrome with its attendant neurodevelopmental morbidity augers excellent tumor survival [10].

Absence of a tumor poses a diagnostic challenge. Several different neurotropic viruses have been described in OMS [11-13], but there are no large epidemiologic studies of viral OMS in children. Modern techniques to document the presence of a specific virus in the CNS are not routinely employed or reported, so a "viral" diagnosis is often made on purely clinical grounds due to the presence of a viral-like prodrome. However, even paraneoplastic cases can have a "viral" prodrome [14], making it a less than reliable differentiating factor.

The true incidence of OMS is unknown, because many cases are often misdiagnosed as acute cerebellar ataxia [15] and neuroblastoma may involute and resolve spontaneously [16, 17]. In the world literature, children from all races, major socioeconomic groups, and geographic regions are affected [2]. OMS occurs in males and females with roughly equal frequency. No occurrence in multiple family members has been reported.

## ■ Clinical Course

### Prodromal phase

In the prodromal phase, symptoms of an apparent upper respiratory or gastrointestinal illness may appear [14]. Extreme irritability is a hallmark feature – the children may be inconsolable and sleepless. Occasionally, OMS follows immunization.

### Acute neurological phase

In the acute neurological phase, incoordination and falling often precede opsoclonus or myoclonus [15]. Over a few days to several weeks, there is progressive neurological deterioration, with inability to sit or stand, and speech becomes slurred or ceases. The myoclonus is primarily action-evoked, but also may occur spontaneously. It has subcortical features, interferes with fine motor coordination, is worse on waking, and may persist during sleep [2]. Opsoclonus is not time-locked with myoclonus and also may continue during sleep. Gait ataxia is characteristic. Rage attacks and hypotonia are common, and some children have head tilt, Horner's syndrome, deep tendon reflex abnormalities, or seizures [2].

### Chronic neurological phase

In mild cases, OMS may be monophasic (Figure 1). With more severe presentation, however, it is typically multiphasic [7]. In this group, neurological relapse can be triggered by infections, immunizations, and premature tapering of immunotherapy. Occurrence of a few relapses is still compatible with remission, but multiple relapses, especially if severe, augers for chronic relapsing-remitting disease. In a small percentage of cases, progressive deterioration occurs. The classification of this subgroup, which might represent another paraneoplastic syndrome, is unclear.

Whether OMS progresses to a chronic phase depends on disease severity and timeliness and effectiveness of treatment. If it does, cognitive function is usually impaired, and IQ may drop into the 80-60 range [6, 18]. Attention deficit disorder (ADD) – with or without hyperactivity – obsessive-compulsive disorder (OCD), mood disorders, and oppositional-defiant disorder (ODD) are common [19]. Most children have speech articulation and fluency problems, and ataxia is usually more apparent than myoclonus [20]. Over time, opsoclonus transforms to ocular flutter. Strabismus is common.

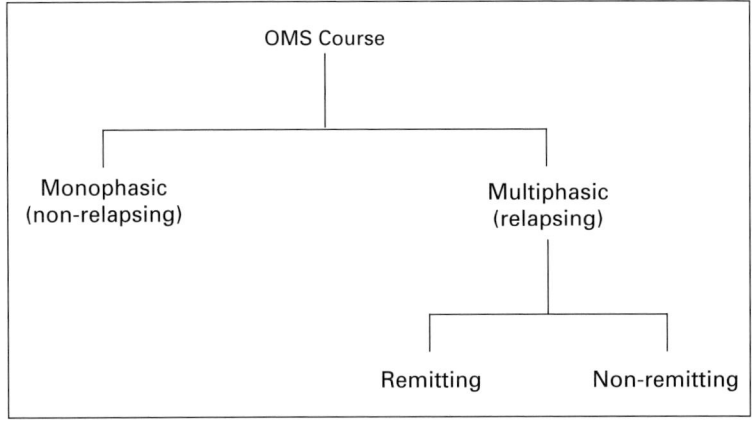

**Figure 1.** Clinical course of OMS. The primary differentiation is between monophasic and multiphasic. The more relapses that occur, the greater the likelihood of a chronic disorder. This wide clinical spectrum raises the possibility that OMS is more than one disorder.

# ■ Pathophysiology

## Immunology

OMS is a putative autoimmune disorder *(Figure 2)*, a "friendly fire" attack of the immune system on the brain [21]. Induction of the autoimmune disease takes place in the periphery and crosses into the central nervous system (CNS). No one antibody marker for childhood OMS has been identified, but the search for onconeural antigens continues.

*Autoantibodies*

Several circulating antibodies *(Table I)* have been reported in childhood OMS [22-24]. Low serum titers of anti-Hu antibodies found in research labs occur as often in neuroblastoma without OMS [22, 23, 25] and do not correlate with neurological outcome [9]. Autoantibodies to post-synaptic densities or other unidentified brain antigens can be seen on Western blots, but they are heterogeneous [24]. Both serum IgG [26] and IgM [27] antineurofilament antibodies have been reported in OMS, but they are not specific, having been found in widely divergent disorders [28-30].

A role for paraneoplastic antibodies in the developmental of brain dysfunction has not been established in the majority of cases [31]. Autoantibodies are not found in all children and there is autoantigen diversity in OMS [24]. Attempts to cause OMS in experimental animals by passive transfer of Ig have not been successful [32, 33]. As a result, attention has turned to clarifying the role of cellular immunity in the pathogenesis of OMS. Tumors from children with OMS are more highly infiltrated with lymphocytes than those from non-OMS counterparts [34], and both B-cells and T-cells congregate in immune nodules [35]. Tumor-infiltrating lymphocytes may trigger the immune surveillance that promotes lymphocyte permeation into the brain, which occurs in normals only at a low level by "trafficking" [36].

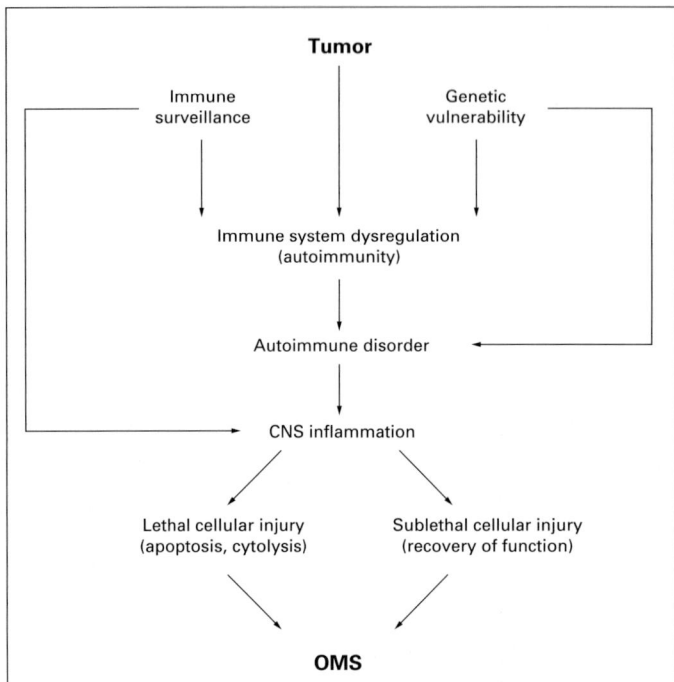

**Figure 2.** Schema of proposed pathogenesis in OMS. Genetic and environmental factors probably conspire to misdirect the immune system from tumor surveillance to autoimmune disease. The transition from autoimmunity to autoimmune disease leads to injury of the nervous system, which may or may not be reversible.

Table I. Autoantibodies in pediatric OMS.

| Antibody Nomenclature | Ig Class | Protein Antigen | MW (kd) | Neural Target | Subcellular Organelle | Ref. |
|---|---|---|---|---|---|---|
| Anti-Hu (ANNA-1; type 11a) | IgG | HuD, HuC, Hel-N1 Hel-N2 (Elav proteins) | 35-40 | Purkinje cell, granule cell, nerve | Nuclei (not nucleoli) | [22,23] |
| Unnamed | IgG | Unknown | – | Purkinje cell | Nuclei | [23] |
| Anti-NF | IgG | Neurofilament | 210 | Purkinje cell, granule cell, nerve | Cytoplasm | [26] |
| Unnamed | IgM | Unknown | 34, 55, 68, 80, 84 | Purkinje cell | – | [27] |
| Unnamed | IgG* | Protein phosphate-1 Proteins associated with nucleic acids** Unknown proteins | – | Post-synaptic densities | – | [24] |

In adult women with breast cancer and other gynecological cancers, anti-Ri (ANNA-2; type 11b) antibodies have been reported to both 55 KDa (NOVA 1) and 70 KDa (NOVA 2) Purkinje cell proteins [68, 69]. They have not been found in children.
\* Besides enzyme-linked immunoadsorption assays (ELISA) and Western blots, the technique of using sera to probe a cDNA library has been employed recently to isolate target neuronal antigens.
\*\* Zinc-finger proteins, RNA binding protein

*CNS lymphocyte recruitment*

Recent immunophenotyping studies of cerebrospinal fluid (CSF) lymphocytes in pediatric OMS by flow cytometry [37] support the hypothesis that both B-cells and T-cells are recruited to the CNS *(Figure 3)* [38], as occurs in multiple sclerosis [39].

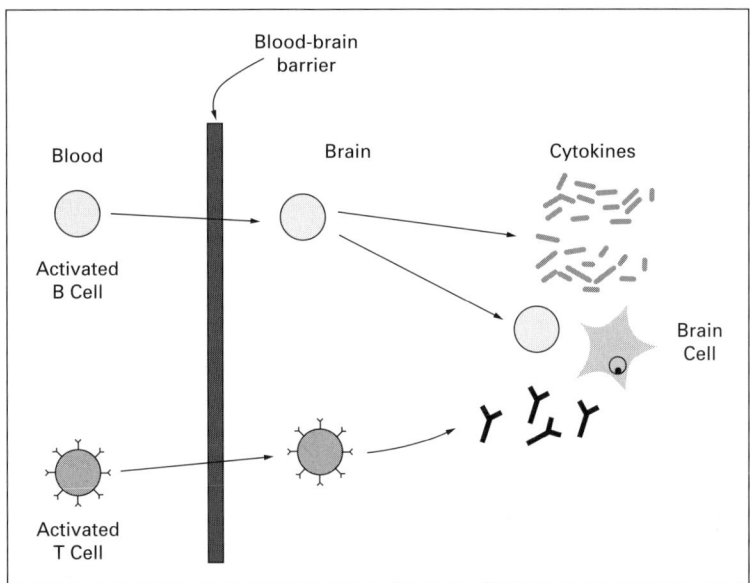

**Figure 3.** CNS lymphocyte recruitment and potential mechanisms of immune-mediated neural injury. Antibodies could cause destruction of receptors or cells, blocking of receptors, or stimulation of receptors. Cytokines, several of which have actions on both immune cells and neural cells, could result in cross-talk, with effects on neuronal signalling, neural modulation, and promotion of inflammation. Reactive or cytotoxic immune cells could cause direct neural cytotoxicity by membrane permeation, cross-linking, and other means. Both conventional ($\alpha\beta$) and unconventional ($\gamma\sigma$) T-cells are involved. Some lymphocytes may be regulatory and anti-inflammatory.

The characteristic pattern is an increased percentage of $CD19^+$ B-cells, $HLA-DR^+$ (activated) T-cells, and $\gamma\sigma$ T-cells, with reduced $CD4^+$ helper/inducer T-cells. Both the $CD5^+$ and $CD5^-$ B-cell subsets are involved [40]. The CSF concentration of neopterin, an inflammatory cellular immune activation marker, is also increased [41]. This intrathecal lymphocyte "expansion" and increased T-cell activation persists in children with lingering symptoms and signs of OMS despite conventional immunotherapy. There is a positive correlation between B-cell and T-cell expansion and neurological severity and a negative correlation with OMS duration. Recruitment of lymphocytes into the CNS introduces several potential mechanisms of neural injury in OMS *(Figure 3)*. Because most children with OMS do not die from their disorder, there is little neuropathologic information. The few autopsy studies have found no consistent abnormality, although inflammatory cells and cerebellar cell loss are sometimes identified [42-44].

*CNS target*

The focus of the attack is elusive and may involve more than one neural site. Cerebellar vermian atrophy was found in an ataxic adult whose severe OMS presented in infancy [45]. A small group of children with neuroblastoma and residual neurological deficits had cerebellar atrophy several years after onset of OMS [46]. Whether cerebellar dysfunction alone is sufficient to account for cognitive and neurobehavioral consequences of OMS is uncertain [2]. Non-motor functions of the cerebellum are now well accepted [47] and the cerebellum plays an important role in language acquisition [48]. However, the anatomic substrate of opsoclonus appears to be the brainstem [49], with mesencephalic and pontine ocular gaze centers containing the burst and omnipause cells that control saccadic eye movements [50]. Also, the seat of myoclonus can be wide-ranging within the CNS, with the nucleus *gigantocellularis reticularis* in caudal medulla being closest to a "myoclonus center" [2].

There may be particular cerebellar vulnerability in childhood OMS. The human cerebellum continues to develop postnatally [51]. Even in toddlers, there is inward migration of granule cells from the external to internal granular layers, refinements to the formation of cerebellar circuitry, and further cerebellar differentiation. Perhaps a diffuse neural network originating in the cerebellum with brainstem and frontal connections becomes dysfunctional in OMS [2]. Purkinje neurons, the main cerebellar outflow to deep cerebellar nuclei, may play a crucial role.

## Pharmacology

The puzzle of how immunologic abnormalities in OMS translate to abnormal neurotransmission is unsolved. Several different neurotransmitters, such as serotonin, γ-aminobutyric acid (GABA), and glycine, have been implicated in myoclonus [52], however, myoclonus and other neurological features of OMS are unlikely to be a single neurotransmitter proposition. Despite the rare enthusiastic case study [53-55], an array of more than 30 antiepileptic drugs and neuroceptor-active drugs are not effective in treating myoclonus or opsoclonus [2, 56].

*CSF neurotransmitter studies*

In a subgroup of children with OMS, CSF concentrations of the serotonin metabolite 5-hydroxyindoleacetic acid (5-HIAA) and the dopamine metabolite homovanillic acid (HVA) are low [57] and remain so despite treatment [58]. CSF levels of the monoamine precursor tetrahydrobiopterin [41] and free choline [59] are normal. It has been speculated that serotonin receptors, which are found in neuroblastoma [60], may be one target of immunological injury [2]. Mood problems and OCD in OMS could relate to serotonin, too. However, neuroblastoma is replete with other neurotransmitter receptors as well.

# Diagnostic Testing

## Screening for neuroblastoma

Differentiation of tumor and non-tumor etiologies of OMS is a fundamental diagnostic goal *(Figure 4)*. Perhaps the most definitive diagnostic tool for neuroblastoma is computerized tomography (CT) of neck, chest, abdomen, and pelvis [61]. Urinary catecholamines, a tumor by-product, are helpful when elevated, but normal levels do not rule out a tumor [62]. Serum neuron-specific enolase also may be elevated [63]. Total body scintigraphy with $^{131}$I-MIBG (metaiodobenzylguanidine) or $^{111}$In-penetreotide (somatostatin receptor ligand) is sensitive but also gives rise to false positives [62, 64-66].

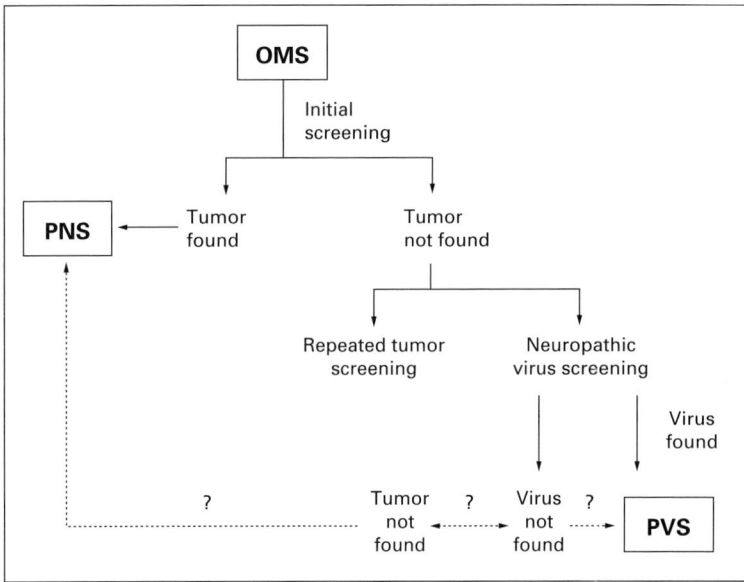

**Figure 4.** Decision-making schema in OMS. PNS, paraneoplastic syndrome; PVS, paraviral syndrome. Controversy surrounds the evaluation of OMS when no tumor is found. There is no consensus on how often a child should be screened for neuroblastoma, but it is a common practice to retest at least once or twice over the period of a year or two. The screening for viruses needs to be done during the acute illness and is too often neglected.

## Screening for viruses

In the absence of tumor, and when the history does not indicate the presence of a major childhood viral exanthem, screening for enteroviruses and Epstein-Barr virus (EBV) should be done [11-13]. Other infections are rare and easily identified by their clinical presentations [2]. Routine CSF studies, such as leukocyte count, protein, and glucose, are typically normal.

## Antibody screening

There is no confirmatory laboratory test for OMS [67-69]. Children with OMS are usually seronegative by commercial testing [7] for "paraneoplastic" autoantibodies found in adults, such as anti-Ri, anti-Yo, and anti-Hu. Increased CSF immunoglobulins, IgG synthesis rate, and oligoclonal bands are not typical [2].

## Neurodiagnostic studies

Brain imaging studies, such as magnetic resonance imaging (MRI) and computerized tomography (CT) are usually normal early in the course of OMS. Later, only a small subgroup of children develops cerebellar atrophy [45, 46]. The electroencephalogram (EEG) may show slowing, but is typically normal. Epileptiform features are rare [2].

# ■ Treatment

## Overview

No cure for OMS exists, and treatment strategies are still being optimized. Although it has been stated that early treatment does not alter outcome [9, 20], few children with OMS receive treatment within days or even a few weeks of onset [15]. Treatment should be directed at achieving fast and complete neurologic remission as well as addressing immunologic abnormalities. Children with OMS may require long-term therapy. The rarity of OMS has precluded controlled trials, so therapies derive from small open-label studies or are largely anecdotal.

The National Pediatric Myoclonus Center introduced multi-modal immunotherapy for pediatric OMS in 1992, and chemotherapy as one component shortly thereafter. Its premise is that treatment must be early and sufficient, guided by CSF lymphocyte immunophenotyping to make it evidence-based [37]. The development of a specific rating scale for OMS [70] should aid clinical trials. Beyond the following discussion, more treatment information is available at: www.omsusa.org.

## Tumor therapy

Although there is overlap between treatment for the paraneoplastic syndrome and the neoplasm, it is best to consider the tumor and the paraneoplastic syndrome as separate entities with different therapeutic end-points. Surgical treatment alone is associated with improvement of OMS in only about one-third of cases, and the response is usually incomplete [2]. Paradoxically, some patients worsen after surgery. Children with moderate and severe symptoms at the onset of OMS will not improve on their own and require immunotherapy. The "wait and watch" approach in this group following tumor resection is ill-advised [71].

When the tumor is large and wraps around vital structures, chemotherapy is often used to shrink the tumor for later gross total resection. For high tumor stages, multi-agent chemotherapy, including cyclophosphamide, adriamycin, cisplatin, doxorubicin, and etoposide, is administered, and retinoic acid promotes tumor maturation [63]. Another approach is radioactive MIBG, which is selective for neuroblastoma [72]. Overly aggressive tumor resection can result in unnecessary disability.

## Neuromodulation

If the exact basis of altered neurotransmission in OMS were known, more direct neuromodulation might be possible. For now, there are two main approaches.

*ACTH (corticotropin)*

ACTH has the highest likelihood of inducing a neurological remission [38]. It binds to CNS melanocortin receptors [73], and has a multiplicity of effects on neurotransmission and brain development [74]. The efficacy of $ACTH_{1-39}$, available as Acthar gel® in the US, was reported first by Kinsbourne [1] and many others since [2]. A high-dose protocol, starting with 150 IU/m² by intramuscular or subcutaneous injection, is quite efficacious [58]. Other than the first two weeks of daily injections, this regimen calls for alternate day dosing, with tapering over several months. Relapse on withdrawal from ACTH is common unless other immunotherapies have been instituted. In Europe, $ACTH_{1-24}$ is sometimes used instead [75, 76]. In infants and young children, prophylaxis with trimethoprim/sulfamethoxazole and ranitidine as well as salt restriction is recommended. Some children become transiently hypertensive on ACTH therapy and require short-term antihypertensive treatment.

*Symptomatic therapy*

While treatment with neuropsychotrophic drugs to modulate neurotransmission is not successful for the motor features of OMS, it is very useful for ADD (stimulants), rage attacks (risperidone), and sleep disturbance (trazodone). Symptomatic treatment to some degree is required for severe OMS and can be used safely in combination with immunotherapy.

## Immunomodulation

Broad categories of immunotherapy for OMS encompass cytotoxic agents and those that modulate immune cell numbers and distribution without causing cell death. Each includes drugs and biologicals *(Table II)*. Besides its neuromodulatory effects, ACTH is also immunomodulatory [38], but has already been discussed.

Table II. Immunotherapies for OMS*.

| Biologicals | Drugs | Pheresis |
|---|---|---|
| ACTH (corticotropin) | Corticosteroids | Plasmapheresis |
| IVIG | Azathioprine | Immunoadsorption |
| Rituximab | Mycophenolate<br>Cyclophosphamide<br>6-Mercaptopurine<br>Methotrexate | Leukocytopheresis |

* Treatments from different classes or within the same class may be combined.

## Corticosteroids

Oral corticosteroids, such as prednisone, and pulse doses of intravenous steroids, such as methyprednisolone or dexamethasone, are commonly used in OMS [77] for convenience of administration but are much less efficacious than ACTH [78]. Cushingoid side-effects are common. Children on chronic steroid therapy should undergo annual screening for cardiovascular, opthalmologic, and bone metabolism side effects.

## IVIG

Intravenous immunoglobulin (IVIG) was first tried in OMS a decade ago [79]. Treatment successes have since been reported [80]. The presumed mechanism of IVIG action is immunomodulation by interfering with or down-regulating components of the immune attack [38]. IVIG also may reduce infections, which otherwise can provoke a relapse. No one brand has been shown to be more effective than another. In IgA deficient children, IgA-depleted IVIG should be used to prevent a hypersensitivity reaction.

## Azathioprine

Azathioprine, a slow-acting purine antimetabolite [81], can be used chronically for immunosuppression [21]. Its slow onset of action, which may take months, is a disadvantage. Drug levels are commercially available and the absolute lymphocyte count should be kept in the target zone of about 1000. There is no need to make the patient neutropenic. Immunosuppressant effects can persist for a few months after discontinuation of therapy.

## Mycophenolate

Mycophenolate has a similar profile of immunosuppression [82], acting on both B-cells and T-cells by inhibiting proliferation [83]. It may be more rapidly acting. Drug levels are commercially available and absolute lymphocyte counts should be followed.

## Chemotherapy

Of all cytotoxic agents, cyclophosphamide is most often used in paraneoplastic OMS, adopted from neuroblastoma therapy [72]. However, it is not routine, and tumor therapy is the usual indication. The standard immunological dosing is six cycles: 1 g/kg IV monthly for six consecutive months. Cyclophosphamide can be given concurrently with ACTH and IVIG. The use instead of 6-mercaptopurine (6-MP) and methotrexate is under evaluation at the National Pediatric Myoclonus Center.

## Rituximab

Of the new cell-specific agents, rituximab, a chimeric monoclonal antibody against $CD20^+$ B-cells [84], is the most promising. Rituximab reduces or eliminates CSF B-cells [85], so children with CSF B-cell expansion are the best candidates. The dose-dependent effect of this intravenously administered agent lasts for several months [86].

*Plasma exchange*

Experience with pheresis in pediatric OMS is limited. Plasmapheresis not only removes humoral factors but modulates cellular immunity [87]. A case report suggests efficacy [88], but steroids and azathioprine were co-administered. Immunoadsorption, in which plasma is passed over a staphylococcus A protein column, was of some benefit in a few adults with paraneoplastic disorders [89], but has not been evaluated in children. Antibody rebound is a potential risk [38].

## Adjunctive therapy

Speech therapy, early intervention programs, and contact with normal healthy children of the same age are tenets of adjunctive therapy for OMS. Besides improving speech articulation, speech therapy should include speech fluency training. Physical therapy may be of benefit in the early stages of OMS.

Neuropsychological testing is useful in determining optimal educational venues for children with OMS [18]. A small classroom setting with more one-on-one teaching is advantageous for those with ADD or ADHD. IQ also should be monitored for insidious decline [20], a possible indication of reactivated autoimmune disease.

## Other issues

*Immunization*

Immunization is hazardous in OMS because it activates T-cells, which are already activated [37]. No live-virus immunizations should be given, and groupings of multiple vaccines are best avoided even after immunotherapy is completed. Children exposed to varicella while on immunotherapy should be treated with antiviral drugs, and it may be necessary to interrupt immunotherapy during that time.

*Problems with sedation*

Children with OMS undergo many procedures requiring sedation, but sedatives, such as midazolam, fentanyl, ketamine, chloral hydrate, or diphenhydramine, are often ineffective, cause paradoxical excitation, or sometimes worsen symptoms [90]. Intravenous propofol is a short-acting efficacious alternative, but larger than normal doses are needed.

*Intercurrent illnesses*

Parents should be vigilant about infections and seek treatment early. For relapse caused by an overwhelming infection, an extra dose of IVIG is prudent. Large day-care facilities or those with poor reporting of sick children should be avoided, especially during immunotherapy.

*Tapering of medications*

Relapse can be triggered by premature tapering of immunotherapy, creating a "yo-yo effect" of dose decreases and increases. When multiple agents are used together, they should not be tapered simultaneously. Also, tapering during winter months, when the infection rate is high, is not recommended.

*Prevention of further cerebellar insults*

Because of the vulnerability of Purkinje cells to hyperthermia, fevers in children with OMS should be aggressively managed with antipyretics, and heat stroke (sun stroke) should be avoided. Use of agents with potential CNS toxicity, such as cyclosporine and tacrilimus, is not advised. Children with OMS and seizures should not be placed on phenytoin or related drugs.

*Family issues*

OMS is a family disorder. It has far-reaching effects on normal siblings, who are often the target of the affected child's aggressive behavior, and the marital stress it engenders contributes to a high divorce rate. Early recognition of this fact and individual and family counselling can be helpful.

## ■ Summary

Opsoclonus-myoclonus syndrome (OMS) is a prototypic autoimmune movement disorder. It is often multiphasic, triggered by neuroblastoma or viral infections. Principal motor features, such as opsoclonus, myoclonus, and ataxia, are subcortical in origin, emanating from brainstem and cerebellum. Cognitive impairment and behavioral problems, the most serious long-term consequences, may have a broader neural basis.

Detection of circulating autoantibodies to diverse autoantigens supports a humoral component to OMS. However, antibodies are not found in all cases, do not correlate with neurological severity, and have not induced OMS in experimental animals when passively transferred from humans. As a result, T-cells are probably also critical. Immunophenotyping studies of CSF lymphocytes in OMS directly confirm both B-cell and T-cell recruitment to the CNS, which increases with neurologic severity and decreases with disease duration. These new disease biomarkers will allow evidence-based selective therapies.

Lack of concern about the tumor due to low tumor stage and excellent tumor survival should not carryover to management of the paraneoplastic syndrome. Late recognition and treatment of OMS are responsible for poor outcome – misdiagnosis as acute cerebellar ataxia is the norm – and inadequate immunotherapy is a setup for relapse. Tumor resection usually is not a sufficient treatment for OMS and should not delay immunotherapy. Combination immunotherapy has decided advantages over monotherapy. Corticotropin, which is more effective than steroids, and IVIG are the standard agents for mild cases, but steroid sparers or single-agent chemotherapy should be added for others. An innovative approach is the use of cell-specific agents, such as rituximab. Pheresis is usually reserved for severe refractory cases due to its infeasibility in toddlers. Symptomatic therapies are adjunctive, alleviating co-morbid behavioral and sleep problems. Recognition that children with OMS often require comprehensive therapy for years helps families, schools, and medical providers work toward the best possible long-term outcome.

**Acknowledgements:** *Supported in part by the American Medical Association Research and Education Foundation, the Children's Miracle Network, and the Southern Illinois University School of Medicine.*

# References

1. Kinsbourne M. Myoclonic encephalopathy of infants. *J Neurol Neurosurg Psychiatry* 1962; 25: 221-76.
2. Pranzatelli MR. The neurobiology of opsoclonus-myoclonus. *Clin Neuropharmacol* 1992; 15 (3): 186-228.
3. Pranzatelli MR. Paraneoplastic syndromes: An unsolved murder. *Sem Ped Neurol* 2000; 7 (2): 118-30.
4. Solomon GE, Chutorian AM. Opsoclonus and occult neuroblastoma. *N Engl J Med* 1968; 279: 475-7.
5. Talon P, Stoll C. Opso-myoclonus syndrome of infancy. New observations. Review of literature (110 cases). *Pédiatrie* 1985; 40: 441-9.
6. Pohl KRE, Pritchard J, Wilson J. Neurological sequelae of the dancing eye syndrome. *Eur J Pediatr* 1996; 155: 237-44.
7. Pranzatelli MR, Tate ED, Wheeler A, et al. Screening for autoantibodies in children with opsoclonus-myoclonus-ataxia. *Ped Neurol* 2002; 27 (5): 384-7.
8. Gambini C, Conte M, Bernini G, et al. Neuroblastic tumors associated with opsoclonus-myoclonus syndrome: histological, immunohistochemical and molecular features of 15 Italian cases. *Virchows Arch* 2003; 442 (6): 555-62.
9. Rudnick E, Khakoo Y, Antunes NL, et al. Opsoclonus-myoclonus-ataxia syndrome in neuroblastoma: clinical outcome and antineuronal antibodies – a report from the Children's Cancer Group Study. *Med Pediatr Oncol* 2001; 36: 612-22.
10. Altmann AJ, Baehner RL. Favorable prognosis for survival in children with coincident opso-myoclonus and neuroblastoma. *Cancer* 1976; 37: 846-52.
11. Kuban KC, Ephros MA, Freeman RL, Laffell LB, Bresnan MJ. Syndrome of opsoclonus-myoclonus caused by Coxsackie B3 infection. *Ann Neurol* 1983; 13: 69-71.
12. Sheth RD, Horwitz SJ, Aronoff S, Gingold M, Bodensteiner JB. Opsoclonus myoclonus syndrome secondary to Epstein-Barr virus infection. *J Child Neurol* 1995; 10 (4): 297-9.
13. McMinn P, Stratov I, Nagarajan L, Davis S. Neurological manifestations of enterovirus 71 infection in children during an outbreak of hand, foot, and mouth disease in Western Australia. *Clin Infect Dis* 2001; 32: 236-42.
14. Bolthauser E, Deonna T, Hirt HR. Myoclonic encephalopathy of infants or "dancing eyes syndrome". *Helv Paediatr Acta* 1979; 34: 119-33.
15. Tate ED, Pranzatelli MR, Allison T, Verhulst SJ. Neuroepidemiologic trends in 88 cases of pediatric opsoclonus-myoclonus. *Neurology* 2003; 60 (5) (suppl 1) A447.
16. Everson TC, Cole WH. *Spontaneous regression of neuroblastoma*. In: Everson TC, Cole WH, eds. *Spontaneous Regression of Cancer*. Philadelphia: WB Saunders, 1966.
17. Nishihara H, Toyoda Y, Tanaka Y, et al. Natural course of neuroblastoma detected by mass screening: a 5-year prospective study at a single institution. *J Clin Oncol* 2000; 18: 3012-7.
18. Papero PH, Pranzatelli MR, Margolis CJ, Tate E, Wilson LA, Glass P. Neurobehavioral and psychosocial functioning of children with opsoclonus-myoclonus syndrome. *Dev Med Child Neurol* 1995; 37: 915-32.
19. Koh PS, Raffensperger JG, Berry S, et al. Long-term outcome in children with opsoclonus-myoclonus and ataxia and coincident neuroblastoma. *J Pediatr* 1994; 125: 712-6.
20. Mitchell WG, Davalos-Gonzalez Y, Brumm VL, et al. Opsoclonus-ataxia caused by childhood neuroblastoma: developmental and neurologic sequelae. *Pediatrics* 2002; 109: 86-98.
21. Pranzatelli MR. Friendly Fire. *Discover* 2000; April: 35-6.
22. Dalmau J, Graus F, Cheung H-k, et al. Major histocompatibility (MHC) proteins, anti-Hu antibodies and paraneoplastic encephalomyelitis in neuroblastoma and small cell lung cancer. *Cancer* 1995; 75: 99-109.

23. Antunes NL, Khakoo Y, Matthay KK, et al. Antineuronal antibodies in patients with neuroblastoma and paraneoplastic opsoclonus-myoclonus. *J Pediatr Hematol Oncol* 2000; 22: 315-20.
24. Bataller L, Rosenfeld MR, Graus F, Vilchez JJ, Cheung NK, Dalmar J. Autoantigen diversity in the opsoclonus-myoclonus syndrome. *Ann Neurol* 2003; 53: 347-53.
25. Fisher PG, Wechsler DS, Singer HS. Anti-Hu antibody in a neuroblastoma-associated paraneoplastic syndrome. *Pediatr Neurol* 1994; 10: 309-12.
26. Noetzel M, Cawley LP, James VL, Minard BJ, Agrawal HC. Anti-neurofilament protein antibodies in opsoclonus-myoclonus. *J Neuroimmunol* 1987; 15: 137-45.
27. Connolly AM, Pestronk A, Mehta S, Pranzatelli MR, Noetzel MJ. Serum autoantibodies in childhood opsoclonus-myoclonus syndrome: an analysis of antigenic targets in neural tissues. *J Pediatr* 1997; 130: 878-84.
28. Plioplys AV, Greaves A, Yoshida W. Anti-CNS antibodies in childhood neurologic diseases. *Neuropediatrics* 1989; 20: 93-102.
29. Sadiq SA, van den Berg LH, Thomas FP, Kilidireas K, Hays AP, Latov N. Human monoclonal antineurofilament antibody cross-reacts with a neuronal surface protein. *J Neurosci Res* 1991; 29: 319-25.
30. Stubbs EB Jr, Lawlor MW, Richards MP, et al. Anti-neurofilament antibodies in neuropathy with monoclonal gammopathy of undetermined significance produce experimental motor nerve conduction block. *Acta Neuropathol (Berl)* 2003; 105: 109-16.
31. Sutton I. Paraneoplastic neurological syndromes. *Curr Opin Neurol* 2002; 15: 685-90.
32. Graus F, Illa I, Agusti M, Ribalta T, Cruz-Sanchez F, Juarez C. Effect of intraventricular injection of an anti-Purkinje cell antibody (anti-Yo) in a guinea pig model. *J Neurol Sci* 1991; 106: 82-7.
33. Smitt S, Manley GT, Posner JB. High titer antibodies but no disease in mice immunized with the paraneoplastic antigen HuD [abstract]. *Neurology* 1994; 44: A378.
34. Martin EF, Beckwith JB. Lymphoid infiltrates in neuroblastoma: Their occurrence and prognostic significance. *J Pediatr Surg* 1968; 3: 161-4.
35. Cooper R, Khakoo Y, Matthay KK, et al. Opsoclonus-myoclonus-ataxia syndrome in neuroblastoma: histopathologic features – a report from the children's cancer group. *Med Pediatr Oncol* 2001; 36: 623-9.
36. Hickey WF. Leukocyte traffic in the central nervous system: the participants and their roles. *Semin Immunol* 1999; 11: 125-37.
37. Pranzatelli MR, Travelstead A, Tate ED, et al. B- and T-cell markers in opsoclonus-myoclonus syndrome: immunophenotyping of CSF lymphocytes. *Neurology* 2004; 62: 1526-32.
38. Pranzatelli MR. The immunopharmacology of the opsoclonus-myoclonus syndrome. *Clin Neuropharmacol* 1996; 19: 1-47.
39. Sun JB. Autoreactive T and B cells in nervous system diseases. *Acta Neurol Scand Suppl* 1993; 142: 1-56.
40. Pranzatelli MR, Travelstead AL, Tate ED, Allison TJ, Verhulst SJ. CSF B-cell expansion in opsoclonus-myoclonus syndrome: a biomarker of disease activity. *Mov Disord* 2004; 19: 770-7.
41. Pranzatelli MR, Hyland K, Tate ED, et al. Evidence of cellular immune activation in children with opsoclonus-myoclonus: cerebrospinal fluid neopterin. *J Child Neurol* 2004; 19: 919-24.
42. Ziter FA, Bray PF, Cancilla PA. Neuropathological findings in a patient with neuroblastoma and myoclonic encephalopathy. *Arch Neurol* 1979; 36: 51.
43. Tuchman RF, Alvarez LA, Kantrowitz AB, Moser FG, Llena J, Moshe SL. Opsoclonus-myoclonus syndrome: correlation of radiographic and pathologic observations. *Neuroradiology* 1989; 31: 250-2.
44. Clerico A, Tenore A, Bartolozzi S, et al. Adrenocorticotropic hormone-secreting ganglioneuroblastoma associated with opso-myoclonic encephalopathy: A case report with immunohistochemical study. *Med Pediatr Oncol* 1993; 21: 690-4.
45. Pranzatelli MR, Tate ED, Kinsbourne M, Caviness VS Jr, Mishra B. Forty-one year follow-up of childhood-onset opsoclonus-myoclonus: cerebellar atrophy, multiphasic relapses, response to IVIG. *Mov Disord* 2002; 17 (6): 1387-90.

46. Hayward K, Jeremy RJ, Jenkins S, et al. Long-term neurobehavioral outcomes in children with neuroblastoma and opsoclonus-myoclonus-ataxia syndrome: relationship to MRI findings and antineuronal antibodies. *J Pediatr* 2001; 139: 552-9.
47. Schmahmann JD, Sherman JC. The cerebellar cognitive affective syndrome. *Brain* 1998; 121: 561-79.
48. Lieberman P. On the nature and evolution of the neural bases of human language. *Am J Phys Anthropol* 2002; 35 (suppl): 36-62.
49. Fuchs AF, Kaneko CRS, Seudder CA. Brainstem control of saccadic eye movements. *Annu Rev Neurosci* 1985; 8: 307-37.
50. Enderle JD. Neural control of saccades. *Prog Brain Res* 2002; 140: 21-49.
51. ten Donkelaar HJ, Lammens M, Wesseling P, Thijssen HO, Renier WO. Development and developmental disorders of the human cerebellum. *J Neurol* 2003; 250 (9): 1025-36.
52. Pranzatelli MR. The pharmacology of antimyoclonic drugs. *Clin Neurosci* 1996; 3: 246-52.
53. Fowler GW. Propranolol treatment of infantile polymyoclonia. *Neuropadiatric* 1976; 7: 443-9.
54. Papini M, Pasquinelli A, Filippini A. Steroid-dependent form of Kinsbourne syndrome: successful treatment with trazodone. *Ital J Neurol Sci* 1992; 13: 369-72.
55. Morretti R, Torre P, Antonello RM, Nasuelli D, Cazzato G. Opsoclonus-myoclonus syndrome: gabapentin as a new therapeutic proposal. *Eur J Neurol* 2000; 7: 455-6.
56. Pranzatelli MR, Tate E, Baldwin M. Clinical responses to 5-hydroxy-L-tryptophan in chronic pediatric opsoclonus-myoclonus suggest biochemical heterogeneity: a double-blinded placebo crossover pilot study. *Clin Neuropharmacol* 1994; 17: 103-16.
57. Pranzatelli MR, Huang Yy, Tate E, et al. Cerebrospinal fluid 5-hydroxyindoleacetic acid and homovanillic acid in the pediatric opsoclonus-myoclonus syndrome. *Ann Neurol* 1995; 37: 189-97.
58. Pranzatelli MR, Huang Y, Tate E, et al. Effect of high dose corticotropin on cerebrospinal fluid monoaminergic neurotransmitters or metabolites in corticotropin-responsive pediatric opsoclonus-myoclonus. *Mov Disord* 1998; 13: 522-8.
59. Pranzatelli MR, Hanin I, Tate E, et al. Cerebrospinal fluid free choline in movement disorders of pediatric onset. *Eur J Ped Neurol* 1998; 1: 33-9.
60. Pranzatelli MR, Balletti J. Serotonin receptors in human neuroblastoma: A possible biologic tumor marker. *Exp Neurol* 1992; 115: 423-7.
61. Shapiro B, Shulkin BL, Hutchinson RJ, Bass JC, Gross MD, Sisson JC. Locating neuroblastoma in the opsoclonus-myoclonus syndrome. *J Nucl Biol Med* 1994; 38 (4): 545-55.
62. Swart JF, de Kraker J, van der Lely N. Metaiodobenzylguanidine total-body scintigraphy required for revealing occult neuroblastoma in opsoclonus-myoclonus syndrome. *Eur J Pediatr* 2002; 161 (5): 255-8.
63. Weinstein JL, Katzenstein HM, Cohn SL. Advances in the diagnosis and treatment of neuroblastoma. *Oncologist* 2003; 8: 278-92.
64. Parisi MT, Hattner RS, Matthay KK, Berg BO, Sandler ED. Optimized diagnostic strategy for neuroblastoma in opsoclonus-myoclonus. *J Nucl Med* 1993; 34 (11): 1922-6.
65. Posada JC, Tardo C. Neuroblastoma detected by somatostatin receptor scintigraphy in a case of opsoclonus-myoclonus-ataxia syndrome. *J Child Neurol* 1998; 13 (7): 345-6.
66. Schilling FH, Bihl H, Jacobsson H, et al. Combined (111) In-pentetreotide scintigraphy and (123) I-mIBG scintigraphy in neuroblastoma provides prognostic information. *Med Pediatr Oncol* 2000; 35 (6): 688-91.
67. Szabo A, Dalmau J, Manley G, et al. HuD, a paraneoplastic encephalomyelitis antigen, contains RNA-binding domains and is homologous to elav and sex-lethal. *Cell* 1991; 67: 325-33.
68. Buckanovich RJ, Posner JB, Darnell RB. Nova, the paraneoplastic Ri antigen, is homologous to an RNA-binding protein and is specifically expressed in the developing motor system. *Neuron* 1993; 11: 657-72.
69. Dropcho EJ, Kline LB, Riser J. Antineuronal (Anti-Ri) antibodies in a patient with steroid-responsive opsoclonus-myoclonus. *Neurology* 1993; 43: 207-11.

70. Pranzatelli MR, Tate ED, Galvan I, Wheeler A. Controlled pilot study of piracetam for pediatric opsoclonus-myoclonus. *Clin Neuropharmacol* 2001; 24: 352-7.
71. Blaes F. Immunotherapeutic approaches to paraneoplastic neurological disorders. *Expert Opin Biol Ther* 2002; 2 (4): 419-30.
72. Mastrangelo R, Troncone L, Lasorella A, Riccardi R, Montemaggi P, Rufini V. $^{131}$I-metaiodobenzylguanidine in the treatment of neuroblastoma at diagnosis. *Am J Pediatr Hematol Oncol* 1989; 11 (1): 28-31.
73. Wilberg JE, Muceniece R, Mandrika I, et al. New aspects on the melanocortins and their receptors. *Pharmacol Res* 2000; 42: 393-420.
74. Pranzatelli MR. On the molecular mechanism of adrenocorticotrophic hormone: neurotransmitters and receptors. *Exp Neurol* 1994; 125: 142-61.
75. Robin A, Vallat M, Tapie P, Vallat J-N. Opsoclonus et troubles neurologiques associés. Opsoclonus and associated neurological disorders. *Arch Ophthalmol* 1976; 36: 645-56.
76. Corrias A, Nurchi AM, Rossi G, Sorcinelli R, Pusceddu G, Corda R. Opsoclonic encephalopathy in childhood (Kinsbourne syndrome). *Pediatr Med Chir* 1985; 7: 437-41.
77. Emir S, Akyuz C, Buyukpamukcu M. Correspondence: treatment of the neuroblastoma-associated opsoclonus-myoclonus-ataxia (OMA) syndrome with high-dose methylprednisolone. *Med Pediatr Oncol* 2003; 40 (2): 139.
78. Hammer MS, Larsen MB, Stack CV. Outcome of children with opsoclonus-myoclonus regardless of etiology. *Pediatr Neurol* 1995; 13 (1): 21-4.
79. Sugie H, Sugie Y, Akimoto H, Endo K, Shirai M, Ito M. High-dose IV human immunoglobulin in a case with infantile opsoclonus polymyoclonia syndrome. *Acta Paediatr* 1992; 18: 371-2.
80. Petruzzi JM, DeAlarcon PA. Neuroblastoma-associated opsoclonus-myoclonus treated with intravenously administered immune globulin G. *J Pediatr* 1995; 127: 328-9.
81. Hoffman M, Rychlewski J, Chrzanowska M, Hermann T. Mechanism of activation of an immunosuppressive drug: azathioprine. Quantum chemical study on the reaction of azathioprine with cysteine. *J Am Chem Soc* 2001; 123 (26): 6404-9.
82. Colic M, Stojic-Vukanic Z, Pavlovic B, Jandric D, Stefanoska I. Mycophenolate mofetil inhibits differentiation, maturation and allostimulatory function of human monocyte-derived dendritic cells. *Clin Exp Immunol* 2003; 134 (1): 63-9.
83. Jonsson CA, Carlsten H. Mycophenolic acid inhibits inosine 5'-monophosphate dehydrogenase and suppresses immunoglobulin and cytokine production of B cells. *Int Immunopharmacol* 2003; 3 (1): 31-7.
84. Cerny T, Borisch B, Introna M, Johnson P, Rose AL. Mechanism of action of rituximab. *Anticancer Drugs* 2002; 13 (suppl 2): S3-10.
85. Pranzatelli MR, Tate ED, Travelstead AL, Verhulst SJ. CSF B-cell expansion in opsoclonus-myoclonus: Effect of rituximab, an anti-B-cell monoclonal antibody. *Neurol* 2003; 60 (5) (suppl 1): A395.
86. Smith MR. Rituximab (monoclonal anti-CD20 antibody): mechanisms of action and resistance. *Oncogene* 2003; 22 (47): 7359-68.
87. Hehmke B, Salzsieder E, Matic GB, Winkler RE, Tiess M, Ramlow W. Immunoadsorption of immunoglobulins alters intracytoplasmic type 1 and type 2 T cell cytokine production in patients with refractory autoimmune diseases. *Ther Apher* 2000; 4 (4): 296-302.
88. Yiu VW, Kovithavongs T, McGonigle LF, Ferreira P. Plasmapheresis as an effective treatment for opsoclonus-myoclonus syndrome. *Pediatr Neurol* 2001; 24 (1): 72-4.
89. Batchelor TT, Platten M, Hochberg FH. Immunoadsorption therapy for paraneoplastic syndromes. *J Neurooncol* 1998; 40 (2): 131-6.
90. Tate ED, Pranzatelli MR, Huang Yy, Kaplan R. An innovative approach to the problem of sedating children with opsoclonus-myoclonus syndrome: effects of myoclonus and CSF monoamine metabolites. *Ann Neurol* 1994; 36: 543-4.

# Movement disorders in paediatric inherited ataxias

**Agathe Roubertie, Bernard Echenne**
Service de Neuropédiatrie, Hôpital Gui de Chauliac, Montpellier, France

Inherited ataxias represent a clinically, genetically and pathologically heterogeneous group of diseases. According to their mode of inheritance, they can be classified in autosomal recessive disorders or autosomal dominant disorders; X-linked forms are very rare [1]. Cerebellar ataxia is the core feature of these disorders, and other neurological or extraneurological symptoms are frequently associated. Despite the recent genetic characterisation of several types of hereditary ataxias (HA), the delineation of their clinical phenotype is still discussed. Growing interest in this matter provided clues for the occurrence of abnormal movements in various forms of HA; in a Spanish study, movement disorders were observed in 23 out of 38 patients with childhood-onset HA [2]. Actually, movement disorders are common in some types of autosomal dominant HA with adult onset (SCA3, SCA6); in some forms of childhood-onset HA, they are not unusual (ataxia telangiectasia); in other forms of HA, they were recognised only recently, and their description is usually scarce. In this paper we focused our attention on the phenomenology of abnormal movements in childhood-onset hereditary ataxias (summarized in Table I).

## ■ Autosomal Recessive Ataxias

### Friedreich's ataxia

Friedreich's ataxia (FA) is the most frequent recessive HA (30% of the autosomal recessive ataxia) with an estimated prevalence of 3-4 per 100 000 [3]. Onset of the disease usually occurs between 5 and 15 years of age. Neurological features include gait and limb ataxia, dysarthria, lower limb areflexia, loss of proprioception, pyramidal tract signs. Other manifestations of the disease include hypertrophic cardiomyopathy, diabetes mellitus, scoliosis, mild mental impairment, sensorineural hearing loss.

Tremor can be the presenting symptom of Friedreich's ataxia or can appear later when the disease progresses [4, 5]. Postural tremor with a slow amplitude can be observed in some patients when the upper limbs are held in an outstretched position. Upper limb involvement might also be represented by low-amplitude kinetic tremor with terminal amplification. Axial tremor manifests as a low-frequency postural truncal sway; also termed "titubation", this sway is omnidirectional, has a large amplitude, and is presumably caused by hypotonia of the axial muscles [6].

Dystonia might concern the upper limbs (with sometimes a writer's cramp), the lower limbs, the cervical region with dystonic head tremor. Generalized dystonia has also been described. It has been suggested that axial muscles dystonia might be partly implicated in the scoliosis frequently associated in patients with FA [6].

Chorea is a rare manifestation of FA, but it has been the presenting symptom in five patients reported in the literature [7].

The frequency of abnormal movements in FA is difficult to assess; in Garcia Ruiz's study, abnormal movements were observed in 14 out of 21 FA patients with onset before 18 years of age [2]; nevertheless, other published series provide poor data concerning movement disorders. Various types of abnormal movements are often mixed in the same patient; according to Garcia Ruiz, dystonia is the most frequent abnormal movement in FA patients with onset before 18 years (observed in 12/21 subjects), although tremor is more often cited in the literature [2].

## Ataxia with vitamin E deficiency

Ataxia with vitamin E deficiency (AVED) is a rare neurodegenerative disorder clinically characterized by Friedreich-like phenotype, whose symptoms can be improved after vitamin E supplementation.

Tremor and head titubation, as described in FA, are not uncommon in patients with AVED [8].

The occurrence of dystonia when the disease progresses and before vitamin E supplementation has been reported in some patients with AVED. Recently, Angelini described a patient whose first symptoms at 8 years of age were myoclonic dystonia of the head; dystonia and myoclonic jerks progressively worsened, before development of ataxia and other symptoms of the disease a couple of years later [9]. We reported the case of a Moroccan boy with AVED who presented torticollis 3 years after onset of vitamin E supplementation that had drastically improved the other cardinal features of the disease. Increase of the doses of vitamin E was ineffective on abnormal movements, as dystonia progressively became generalized within 3 years; other symptoms remained stabilized. Dystonia was finally improved by trihexiphenidyl and torticollis was alleviated by botulinum toxin injections [10].

| | |
|---|---|
| AVED: | Ataxia with vitamin E deficiency |
| AOA: | Ataxia with oculomotor apraxia |
| IOSCA: | Infantile onset spinocerebellar ataxia |
| DRPLA: | Dentatorubral-pallidoluysian atrophy |
| SCA: | Spinocerebellar ataxia |

Table I. Abnormal movements in hereditary ataxias.

| | Disorder | Locus | Gene, type of mutation | Type of abnormal movement |
|---|---|---|---|---|
| Early onset | Friedreich's Ataxia | 9q13 | Frataxin<br>Trinucleotide repeat (GAA)/Point mutation | Postural tremor ⎫ in more than 60%<br>Kinetic tremor ⎭ of the patients<br>Dystonia<br>Chorea |
| | AVED | 8q13.1-13.3 | α-Tocopherol transfer protein<br>Point mutation | Tremor and head titubation<br>Dystonia<br>Myoclonic jerks |
| | AOA1 | 9p13 | Aprataxin<br>Point mutation, insertion, deletion | Chorea<br>Dystonia |
| | AOA2 | 9q34 | ? | Chorea |
| | Ataxia telangiectasia | 11q22 | ATM<br>Point mutations | Chorea<br>Dystonia<br>Rest tremor<br>Myoclonus |
| | IOSCA | 10q | ? | Athetoid movements |
| | DRPLA | 12p13 | Atrophin-1<br>CAG repeat (62-79 for juvenile onset) | Chorea, Tremor |
| | SCA3 | 14q24.3-q31 | Ataxin-3<br>CAG repeat (54-89) | Dystonia<br>Chorea (facial involvement)<br>Rigidity<br>L-dopa responsive dystonia or parkinsonism in adult-onset cases |
| | SCA7 | 3p21.1-p12 | Ataxin-7<br>CAG repeat (37-306) | Cervical or limb dystonia |
| | SCA12 | 5q31-q33 | PPP2R2B<br>CAG repeat (55-78) | Head and arms tremor |
| | SCA14 | 19q13.4 | PRKCG<br>Point mutation | Involuntary tremulous movement and axial myoclonus |
| Adult onset | SCA2 | 12q24 | Ataxin-2<br>CAG repeat (32-77) | Dystonia<br>Chorea<br>L-dopa responsive parkinsonism<br>Action tremor |
| | SCA1 | 6p23 | Ataxin-1<br>CAG repeat (39-83) | Chorea |
| | SCA6 | 19p13 | CACNA1A gene<br>Alpha12 subunit calcium channel<br>CAG repeat (20-33) | Dystonia<br>Chorea<br>Parkinsonism<br>Postural tremor |
| | SCA17 | 6q27 | TATA box binding Protein<br>CAG repeat (44-63) | Parkinsonism |

## Early-onset ataxia with oculomotor apraxia

AOA type 1 was initially described in Japanese patients; in the Caucasian population, AOA1 represents 9% of progressive cerebellar ataxia with autosomal recessive inheritance and with onset before 25 years of age [11]. AOA1 is clinically characterized by early-onset cerebellar ataxia, oculomotor apraxia, peripheral neuropathy and mental deficiency. Hypercholesterolemia and hypoalbuminemia are often associated; brain imaging visualizes cerebellar atrophy in all the patients [12].

Chorea and dystonia are common in patients with AOA1; they represent the predominant symptom at onset of the disease in half of the patients [11]. Chorea is observed at onset of the disease in 79% of the patient in Le Ber study (14 Caucasian patients); its localization includes the limbs, but also the face with grimacing; its course is noteworthy, as it tends to spontaneously decrease (choreiform movements are only observed in 43% of the patients at follow-up in Le Ber study). Dystonia was noticed in two thirds of the patients in the Caucasian study; generalized dystonia as a presenting symptom has recently been reported in a Japanese girl [13].

AOA type 2 phenotype is very similar to AOA1's. Chorea is also very frequent. Genetic localisation is distinct [14].

## Ataxia-telangiectasia

The frequency of ataxia-telangiectasia (AT) is estimated around 1 per 40000 newborns. Patients present in early childhood with progressive cerebellar ataxia and later develop conjunctival telangiectases, other progressive neurologic degeneration, immune defects with sinopulmonary infection, and predisposition to malignancies. Brain imaging shows cerebellar atrophy. Biological features include increased serum alpha-fetoprotein and carcinoembryonic antigen levels; chromosomal breakage is common.

Dystonia and chorea are observed in more than half of the patients with AT [15]. Dystonic and choreiform or choreoathetoid movements might be isolated or more often mixed together. Dystonia might involve the extremities, or might be more widespread with dysarthria and generalized abnormal movements. Dystonic movements usually develop as a late manifestation of the disease, but they can also be the presenting and predominant symptom [16, 17] Hypokinetic-rigid syndrome is often associated, with an impassive face, and a stereotyped smile.

Tremor is not common, but resting tremor as a predominating symptom has been described in two patients with AT [18].

## Infantile onset spinocerebellar ataxia with sensory neuropathy (IOSCA)

Infantile onset spinocerebellar ataxia with sensory neuropathy has been described in the Finnish population. It is a progressive neurological disorder that severely affects the sensory system. The first symptoms of IOSCA appear between one and two years of age in previously healthy infants; they include cerebellar ataxia, hypotonia, hearing deficit and ophthalmoplegia. Slowly progressive optic atrophy, sensory neuropathy, female hypogonadism and epilepsy are later manifestations of the disease. Neuroradiological investigations disclose cerebellar atrophy. Athetoid jerky movements in arms and face are commonly observed early in the course of the disease [19].

## Other Autosomal recessive inherited ataxia

To our knowledge, abnormal movements have not been reported in autosomal recessive spastic ataxia of Charlevoix-Saguenay, neither in autosomal recessive ataxia with hearing impairment and optic atrophy linked to chromosome 6p.

Autosomal recessive ataxia with onset in childhood include disorders not clearly classified, or not genetically characterized. In Garcia Ruiz study of 28 cases with early onset recessive cerebellar ataxia, 6 cases were unclassified; the phenotype of 4 of these 6 patients included mixed abnormal movements (tremor, dystonia, chorea, tics) [2].

# ■ Autosomal Dominant Ataxias

Although classically adult-onset disorders, autosomal dominant ataxias can also present before 18 years of age; in Garcia Ruiz study, onset occurred before 18 years in 10 out of 38 patients [2].

Although brain imaging shows a more or less widespread cerebellar atrophy, clinical phenotype is heterogeneous. Harding classified autosomal dominant cerebellar ataxias (ADCA) in three groups. In ADCA I, cerebellar ataxia of gait and limbs is invariably associated with supranuclear ophthalmoplegia, pyramidal or extrapyramidal signs, mild dementia, and peripheral neuropathy. In ADCA II, macular and retinal degeneration are added to the features. ADCA III is a pure form of late-onset cerebellar ataxia [20]. In the last few years, some of the causative genes implicated in various forms of autosomal dominant ataxia have been identified, leading to new classifications; importantly, many of the AD ataxia are genetically characterized by unstable repeat expansions with anticipation phenomenon [3].

## Dentatorubral-pallidoluysian atrophy

The prevalence of DRPLA is high in Japan, but this neurodegenerative disorder is rare in the Caucasian population [21]. DRPLA symptoms depend on the age of onset and the number of CAG trinucleotide repeats.

Adult-onset phenotype is characterized by variable combination of clinical manifestations including ataxia, myoclonus, seizures, dementia, and choreic movements; dystonia has also been reported (cervical dystonia). Patients with juvenile-onset develop symptoms of progressive myoclonic epilepsy, with myoclonus, seizures of various types, ataxia, mental deterioration. Tremor or facial choreiform movements can also be noticed in patients with juvenile onset [22].

## SCA 3 (Machado-Joseph disease)

Machado-Joseph disease (MJD) or SCA3 (ADCAI) is the most frequent form of dominantly inherited ataxia in the Caucasian population. Variations in repeat lengths substantially influence age of onset as well as phenotype. MJD is clinically characterized by cerebellar ataxia, external ophthalmoplegia, pyramidal signs, extrapyramidal signs and sometimes distal muscular atrophy. In patients with young onset (type 1 MJD), extrapyramidal symptoms can overshadow the other manifestations of the disease. These symptoms include dystonic movements, facial chorea, rigidity [23]. Munchau described a German woman who presented with severe generalized dystonia beginning at the age of 18 years when she noticed involuntary twisting and cramping of her right hand and twisting of both feet shortly thereafter. Symptoms worsened when she was stressed. At the age of 19 years, she began to grimace when talking and laughing, and her speech became difficult to understand. Over a period of 2 years her symptoms deteriorated, and she became unable to walk without support [24].

In patients with adult onset of the disease, dystonia, chorea or myoclonus are also very common; phenotypes mimicking L-dopa responsive dystonia or parkinsonism have been reported [25, 26].

## SCA7 (ADCAII)

Clinical features are anticipation, onset age varying from 1 to 50 years, early blue-yellow colour blindness, macular degeneration due to cone dystrophy progressing to photoreceptor dystrophy over the entire retina, cerebellar signs followed by ophtalmoplegia. Cervical dystonia or limb dystonia have been described in childhood-onset cases [27]. Orofacial dyskinesia, choreoathetosis, dystonia can occur in the course of adult-onset disease [28].

## SCA12

SCA12 is a very slowly progressive disorder leading over several decades to gait ataxia, dysmetria, dysdiadokinesis, hyperreflexia, paucity of movement, abnormal eye movements, and, in the oldest subjects, dementia. Most individuals present in the fourth decade with upper extremity tremor; nevertheless, early age of onset has been reported (up to 8 years); upper extremities tremor can be a presenting symptom; action tremor of the head and arms is the most distinguishing feature in comparison to other dominant SCAs [29].

## SCA14

SCA 14 was initially reported in a Japanese family; patients with a late onset (greater than or equal to 39 years) exhibited pure cerebellar ataxia, whereas those with an early onset (in their teens) first showed tremulous involuntary movements and intermittent axial myoclonus followed by ataxy [30].

## Other autosomal dominant spinocerebellar ataxias

Together, SCA1 and SCA2 constitute around 20% of the mutations leading to autosomal cerebellar ataxia in the Caucasian population (adult or childhood onset together). Symptoms of SCA1 and SCA2 usually begin in the third or fourth decade of life. Infantile or juvenile onset have rarely been reported in the literature, with scarce clinical data [31, 32].

Dystonia, chorea, and L-dopa responsive parkinsonism have been described in adult-onset patients with SCA2 [33, 34]. Slow saccades, myoclonus, and action tremor also suggest SCA2. Chorea or athetoid movements have been described occasionally in adult-onset patients with SCA1 [35].

Other genetically identified AD ataxia are characterized by the possible association of extrapyramidal manifestations, but onset of the disease occur in adulthood.

SCA 6 is a late onset progressive ataxia (onset in the fifties). Patients with a prolonged clinical course show other accompanying clinical features including dystonic postures, parkinsonism, postural tremor, chorea [36].

SCA17 is a severe but rare form of AD ataxia; most individuals present in the third decade with gait ataxia and dementia; extrapyramidal symptoms (mainly parkinsonian features) are not uncommon [37].

The genetic basis of AD ataxias are not fully elucidated; in theses "unidentified" cases with young-onset abnormal movement can be noticed; in Garci Ruiz study 7 out of 10 cases with onset before 18 years of age were unclassified; 4 patients displayed postural tremor [2].

## ■ Comments and Conclusion

Hereditary ataxias are an heterogeneous group of disorders whose phenotypes overlap extensively. The description of various types of abnormal movements in patients with HA enlarges the clinical spectrum of such genetically distinct disorders, and help refining their clinical pattern. Postural tremor and dystonia are the most common abnormal movements described in childhood onset HA; parkinsonism is not uncommon in adult-onset HA (especially in patients with SCA2, SCA1, or SCA6); to our knowledge, parkinsonism has not been described in young-onset HA. Movement disorders in HA are characterized by a great heterogeneity, as different types of abnormal movements have been described among patients with the same genetically identified disorder (for example, postural tremor, dystonia, chorea have been reported in patients with Friedreich's ataxia). Furthermore, abnormal movements in HA are characterized by a great intrafamilial heterogeneity without phenotype-genotype correlation (especially no correlation with the size of the expansion in expansion related disorders).

Awareness of movement disorders existence in HA is relevant for accurate diagnosis. Actually, abnormal movements, especially when they are the first or predominant symptoms might mislead the diagnosis; in such cases, careful neurological examination and meticulous family history analysis are very important. Erroneous diagnosis of juvenile Huntington disease, Sydenham chorea or hereditary benign chorea have been reported at the initial phase of the disease in patients with AOA1 [11]; on the other hand, early-onset chorea with oculomotor apraxia strongly suggests the diagnosis of ataxia telangiectasia or AOA1, even before cerebellar symptoms. Chorea and myoclonus have also been reported as the unusual first symptoms of Friedreich's ataxia [7].

The clinical significance of the abnormal movements varies greatly among the various types of HA, and among patients with the same genetically defined disorder. Abnormal movements might be unnoticed by the patient or their relatives and recorded only by an advised examiner; on the other hand, abnormal movements might be the predominant and more disabling feature of the disease (generalized dystonia in ataxia telangiectasia) [17]. Abnormal movements might be improved by medical treatment (for example the dystonic manifestations of our patient with AVED were drastically improved by trihexiphenidyl and botulinum toxin), although poor benefit is usually obtained on cerebellar symptoms. Nevertheless, the prognosis impact of abnormal movements in young onset ataxia remains to be clarified.

Although abnormal movements in HA are probably underregognized, their description has broadened the clinical spectrum of HA, but also raises many pathophysiological questions. Actually, the pathophysiological significance of abnormal movements in HA is probably multiple. In certain types of HA, direct clues for basal ganglia dysfunction were provided by neuropathological examination: basal ganglia abnormalities have been identified by post-mortem studies of patients with SCA2 or SCA3 [38]. Lesions in the basal ganglia have been visualized by brain imaging in some ataxia telangiectasia patients with abnormal movements [39]. In one chorea-dystonic patient with AOA1, brain functional imaging showed hypoperfusion of the caudate nucleus; Le ber *et al.* suggested that since aprataxin is expressed in the caudate nuclei, aprataxin mutations might be hypothesized to compromise the function of this brain structure [11].

Recently, Deonna's group reported 8 unrelated children who presented in the first year of life with an unusual pattern of abnormal movements of the head, consistent with head stereotypies; the patients also displayed hypotonia, axial ataxia and language delay; follow-up only showed persistent head abnormal movements. In two of these patients, brain imaging disclosed cerebellar abnormalities. Deonna proposed that such abnormal movement were related to pathology of the development of the cerebellum [40]. Quite similarly, abnormal movements in hereditary ataxias might be hypothesized as the consequence of cerebellar or cerebello-striatal pathway dysfunction, which might open new fields of understanding concerning the role of the cerebellum.

# References

1. Gasser T, Bressman S, Durr A, Higgins J, Klockgether T, Myers RH. State of the art review: molecular diagnosis of inherited movement disorders. Movement Disorders Society task force on molecular diagnosis. *Mov Disord* 2003; 18: 3-18.
2. Garcia Ruiz PJ, Mayo D, Hernandez J, Cantarero S, Ayuso C. Movement disorders in hereditary ataxias. *J Neurol Sci* 2002; 202: 59-64.
3. Albin RL. Dominant ataxias and Friedreich ataxia: an update. *Curr Opin Neurol* 2003; 16: 507-14.
4. De Michele G, Di Maio L, Filla A, *et al*. Childhood onset of Friedreich ataxia: a clinical and genetic study of 36 cases. *Neuropediatrics* 1996; 27: 3-7.
5. Pilch J, Jamroz E, Marszal E. Friedreich's ataxia. *J Child Neurol* 2002; 17: 315-9.

6. Hou JG, Jankovic J. Movement disorders in Friedreich's ataxia. *J Neurol Sci* 2003; 206: 59-64.
7. Zhu D, Burke C, Leslie A, Nicholson GA. Friedreich's ataxia with chorea and myoclonus caused by a compound heterozygosity for a novel deletion and the trinucleotide GAA expansion. *Mov Disord* 2002; 17: 585-9.
8. Cavalier L, Ouahchi K, Kayden HJ, et al. Ataxia with isolated vitamin E deficiency: heterogeneity of mutations and phenotypic variability in a large number of families. *Am J Hum Genet* 1998; 62: 301-10.
9. Angelini L, Erba A, Mariotti C, Gellera C, Ciano C, Nardocci N. Myoclonic dystonia as unique presentation of isolated vitamin E deficiency in a young patient. *Mov Disord* 2002; 17: 612-4.
10. Roubertie A, Biolsi B, Rivier F, Humbertclaude V, Cheminal R, Echenne B. Ataxia with vitamin E deficiency and severe dystonia: report of a case. *Brain Dev* 2003; 25: 442-5.
11. Le Ber I, Moreira MC, Rivaud-Pechoux S, et al. Cerebellar ataxia with oculomotor apraxia type 1: clinical and genetic studies. *Brain* 2003; 126: 2761-72.
12. Aicardi J, Barbosa C, Andermann E, et al. Ataxia-ocular motor apraxia: a syndrome mimicking ataxia-telangiectasia. *Ann Neurol* 1988; 24: 497-502.
13. Sekijima Y, Hashimoto T, Onodera O, et al. Severe generalized dystonia as a presentation of a patient with aprataxin gene mutation. *Mov Disord* 2003; 18: 1198-200.
14. Nemeth AH, Bochukova E, Dunne E, et al. Autosomal recessive cerebellar ataxia with oculomotor apraxia (ataxia-telangiectasia-like syndrome) is linked to chromosome 9q34. *Am J Hum Genet* 2000; 67: 1320-6.
15. Woods CG, Taylor AM. Ataxia telangiectasia in the British Isles: the clinical and laboratory features of 70 affected individuals. *Q J Med* 1992; 82: 169-79.
16. Bodensteiner JB, Goldblum RM, Goldman AS. Progressive dystonia masking ataxia in ataxia telangiectasia. *Arch Neurol* 1980; 37: 464-5.
17. Goyal V, Behari M. Dystonia as presenting manifestation of ataxia telangiectasia: a case report. *Neurol India* 2002; 50: 187-9.
18. Hiel JA, Weemaes CM, Smeets DF, Van de Vlasakker CJ, Horstink MW. Late-onset ataxia telangiectasia in two brothers presenting with juvenile resting tremor. *Mov Disord* 1994; 9: 460-2.
19. Koskinen T, Santavuori P, Sainio K, Lappi M, Kallio AK, Pihko H. Infantile onset spinocerebellar ataxia with sensory neuropathy: a new inherited disease. *J Neurol Sci* 1994 121: 50-6.
20. Harding AE. The clinical features and classification of the late onset autosomal dominant cerebellar ataxias. A study of 11 families, including descendants of 'the Drew family of Walworth'. *Brain* 1982; 105: 1-28.
21. Le Ber I, Camuzat A, Castelnovo G, et al. Prevalence of dentatorubral-pallidoluysian atrophy in a large series of white patients with cerebellar ataxia. *Arch Neurol* 2003; 60: 1097-9.
22. Licht DJ, Lynch DR. Juvenile dentatorubral-pallidoluysian atrophy: new clinical features. *Pediatr Neurol* 2002; 26: 51-4.
23. Schols L, Peters S, Szymanski S, Kruger R, Lange S, Hardt C, Riess O, Przuntek H. Extrapyramidal motor signs in degenerative ataxias. *Arch Neurol* 2000; 57: 1495-500.
24. Munchau A, Dressler D, Bhatia KP, Vogel P, Zuhlke C. Machado-Joseph disease presenting as severe generalised dystonia in a German patient. (Letter) *J Neurol* 1999; 246: 840-2.
25. Wilder-Smith E, Tan EK, Law HY, Zhao Y, Ng I, Wong MC. Spinocerebellar ataxia type 3 presenting as an L-DOPA responsive dystonia phenotype in a Chinese family. *J Neurol Sci* 2003; 213: 25-8.
26. Gwinn-Hardy K, Singleton A, O'Suilleabhain P, et al. Spinocerebellar ataxia type 3 phenotypically resembling Parkinson disease in a black family. *Arch Neurol* 2001; 58: 296-9.
27. Modi G, Modi M, Martinus I, Rodda J, Saffer D. The clinical and genetic characteristics of spinocerebellar ataxia type 7 (SCA 7) in three black South African families. *Acta Neurol Scand* 2000; 101: 177-82.

28. Benton CS, de Silva R, Rutledge SL, Bohlega S, Ashizawa T, Zoghbi HY. Molecular and clinical studies in SCA-7 define a broad clinical spectrum and the infantile phenotype. *Neurology* 1998; 51: 1081-6.
29. O'Hearn E, Holmes SE, Calvert PC, Ross CA, Margolis RL. SCA-12: Tremor with cerebellar and cortical atrophy is associated with a CAG repeat expansion. *Neurology* 2001; 56: 299-303.
30. Yamashita I, Sasaki H, Yabe I, et al. A novel locus for dominant cerebellar ataxia (SCA14) maps to a 10.2-cM interval flanked by D19S206 and D19S605 on chromosome 19q13.4-qter. *Ann Neurol* 2000; 48: 156-63.
31. Moretti P, Blazo M, Garcia L, Armstrong D, Lewis RA, Roa B, Scaglia F. Spinocerebellar ataxia type 2 (SCA2) presenting with ophthalmoplegia and developmental delay in infancy. *Am J Med Genet* 2004; 124A: 392-6.
32. Ranum LP, Chung MY, Banfi S, et al. Molecular and clinical correlations in spinocerebellar ataxia type I: evidence for familial effects on the age at onset. *Am J Hum Genet* 1994; 55: 244-52.
33. Pareyson D, Gellera C, Castellotti B, et al. Clinical and molecular studies of 73 Italian families with autosomal dominant cerebellar ataxia type I: SCA1 and SCA2 are the most common genotypes. *J Neurol* 1999; 246: 389-93.
34. Lu CS, Wu Chou YH, Yen TC, Tsai CH, Chen RS, Chang HC. Dopa-responsive parkinsonism phenotype of spinocerebellar ataxia type 2. *Mov Disord* 2002; 17: 1046-51.
35. Namekawa M, Takiyama Y, Ando Y, et al. Choreiform movements in spinocerebellar ataxia type 1. *J Neurol Sci* 2001; 187: 103-6.
36. Sethi KD, Jankovic J. Dystonia in spinocerebellar ataxia type 6. *Mov Disord* 2002; 17: 150-3.
37. De Michele G, Maltecca F, Carella M, et al. Dementia, ataxia, extrapyramidal features, and epilepsy: phenotype spectrum in two Italian families with spinocerebellar ataxia type 17. *Neurol Sci* 2003; 24: 166-7.
38. Rub U, Del Turco D, Del Tredici K, et al. Thalamic involvement in a spinocerebellar ataxia type 2 (SCA2) and a spinocerebellar ataxia type 3 (SCA3) patient, and its clinical relevance. *Brain* 2003; 126: 2257-72.
39. Koepp M, Schelosky L, Cordes I, Cordes M, Poewe W. Dystonia in ataxia telangiectasia: report of a case with putaminal lesions and decreased striatal '123I' iodobenzamide binding. *Mov Disord* 1994; 9: 455-9.
40. Hottinger-Blanc PM, Ziegler AL, Deonna T. A special type of head stereotypies in children with developmental (?cerebellar) disorder: description of 8 cases and literature review. *Eur J Paediatr Neurol* 2002; 6: 143-52.

# Abnormal movements in alternating hemiplegia of childhood

**Jean Aicardi**

*Child Neurology and Metabolic Diseases Department,
Hôpital Robert Debré, Paris, France*

---

Alternating hemiplegia of childhood (AHC) is a rare disorder of unknown cause first reported in 1971 by Verret and Steele [1]. It is characterized by the recurrence of transient episodes of hemiplegia affecting either side of the body. The hemiplegic attacks are associated with a remarkable constellation of symptoms and signs of which movement abnormalities are a major component and have a considerable diagnostic significance [2-7]. Hemiplegic attacks become associated after a few years with the emergence of chronic neurological and cognitive difficulties.

The major clinical features of AHC include: 1) an early onset, almost always before 18 months of age; 2) repeated episodes of hemiplegia lasting from minutes to days or weeks, remarkable by an unusual symptomatology with absence of pyramidal tract signs in most cases, rapid variations in the severity of the paralysis that may transiently disappear; the hemiplegia is frequently associated with dystonic features that may alternate with epochs of profound paralysis; 3) episodes of bilateral paralysis, either when a hemiplegia shifts from one side of the body to the opposite one, with a transient phase of diplegia, or bilateral involvement from the start; 4) eye movement abnormalities and/or autonomic phenomena; 5) a progressive course with an initial phase of paroxysmal attacks, variably associating these various disturbances, separated by intervals of complete or relative normality and eventually followed by the development of a fixed neurological impairment almost invariably featuring mental retardation and, in most cases, a chronic movement disorder. Epilepsy seems often associated although its relationship to the rest of the picture is unclear.

## ∎ The movement disorder of alternating hemiplegia

Abnormalities of movement are an almost constant feature of AHC. Importantly, abnormal movements are an early manifestation, often the first symptom and may occur in some infants even in the neonatal period. In a personal series of 29 patients [2, 5], hemiplegia was the initial manifestation in only 12 of them and was often delayed until over one year of age, whereas attacks of unilateral or bilateral tonic contraction and/or eye movement disturbances were the first symptom observed in 10 infants under 6 months of age.

Involvement of the skeletal muscles is the major component of the movement disorder. However, it seems justifiable to include in this description of the movement disturbances, abnormalities of eye movements, even though their mechanism is poorly known [3, 5] as their diagnostic value is considerable and that at least some of them are similar to what is seen in recognized movement disorders. Likewise, some autonomic manifestations of AHC, such as episodes of dyspnea and especially apneas, probably result in part from paroxysmal contractions of the pharyngolaryngeal muscles even though this mechanism is clearly not the only possible one [6, 8]. We will therefore describe successively these three different groups of manifestations, recognizing that they likely have partially different mechanisms.

## Abnormal movements of skeletal muscles

They present with different characteristics, depending on the evolutive period of the disease.

During the initial period (Figure 1), they are mostly *paroxysmal* and occur at the same time as a hemiplegia, either in association with episodes of abnormal eye movements or in isolation. As already mentioned, the flaccid paralysis of the limbs may even be interrupted partially for brief periods by dystonic attitudes or movements that predominate in the upper limbs and may recur many times in a single paralytic attack.

*Tonic or dystonic attacks* are present in over 90% of cases [7]. They may occur as early as a few days of age. They seldom first appear after 3.5 years of age although they may continue for several years or even to adult age. Unilateral attacks are most frequent, marked by a stiffening of one side of the body that may be extreme, sometimes resulting in a vibratory tremor. There may be incurvation of the trunk towards the affected side. Often the head is turned forcibly to one side, usually but not necessarily that of the tonic contracture. Bilateral tonic attacks feature arching of the back and upward or downward deviation of gaze. Stiffness may change side during a same attack. The onset of attacks is sudden, associated with fussiness and crying as if in pain. In some cases, a premonitory feeling has been noted [7]. Dystonic attacks are brief, usually lasting only a few minutes but may recur in rapid succession for up to a few hours [8, 9]. EEG recorded in a few cases of dystonic attacks have not shown paroxysmal activity.

More severe episodes of bilateral dystonia in the form of opisthotonos may be the initial symptom of attacks of diplegia not preceded by hemiplegia. These are often severe with marked distress and intense autonomic changes. Fusco and Vigevano [4] pointed out the presence of amimia and severe hypotonia at onset of such attacks.

At a later period of the disease (Figure 2), *permanent* abnormalities of movement tend to appear, while hemiplegic/dystonic attacks continue. Choreoathetosis is the commonest chronic movement disorder in AHC, occurring in 50% [7] to 100% [2] of cases. Such discrepancies in frequency of symptoms are probably due to the fact that the movement disorder is usually complex as ataxia, severe hypotonia, dystonia, tremor and spasticity are frequently associated and make precise classification of the

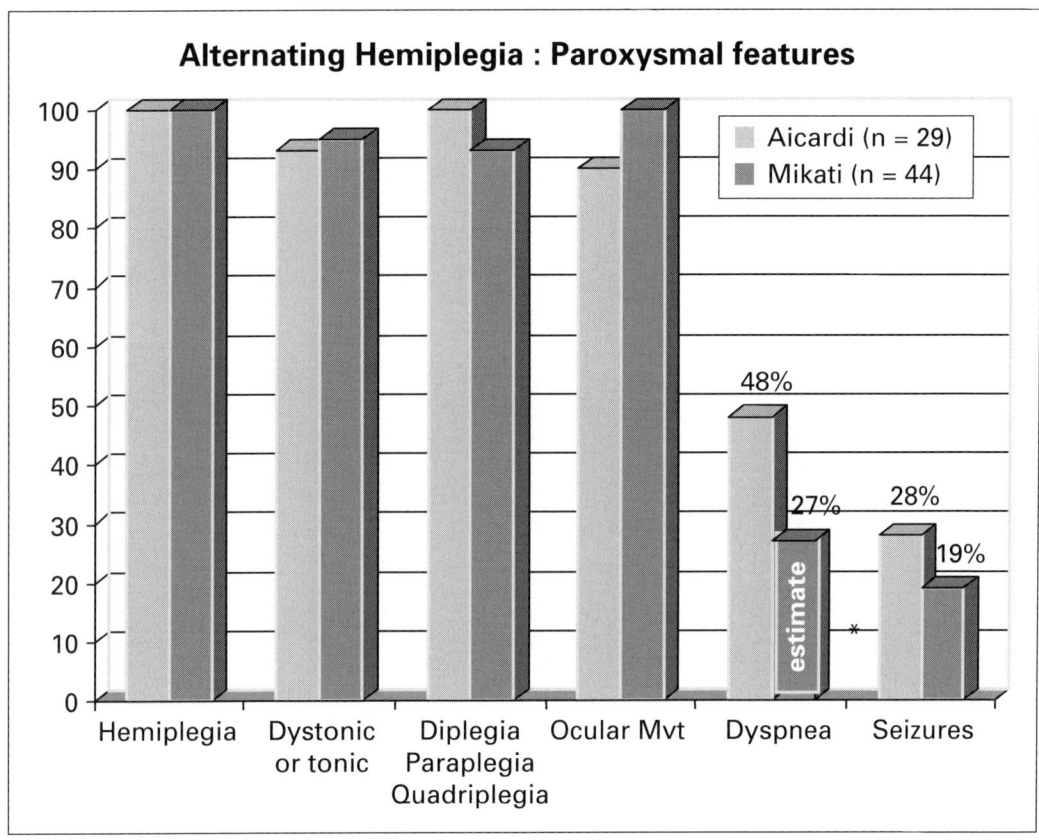

Figure 1. Alternating Hemiplegia: Paroxysmal features.

movement disorder difficult. The choreic component seems prominent and is associated with marked hypotonia that may significantly contribute to difficulties with standing and ambulation. The choreo-athetosis is of variable severity from hardly detectable clumsiness to extreme with ballistic movements. In many cases, the movement disorder at this stage represents the most disturbing abnormality especially in those few children who have no mental retardation or only mild learning disability. There seems to be some proportionality between the severity of the movement disorder and that of mental retardation [7] After an initial period of insidious progression, the movement disorder tends to stabilize although no systematic follow-up study is available.

Dystonia is often associated with choreoathetosis and may be prominent although it is usually only of less severity than the choreoathetosis. It is rarely isolated or predominant.

Ataxia was present in 68%-93% of patients in two large series [2, 8, 9] at the chronic stage. It is probably mainly of cerebellar origin and contributes significantly to the overall disability. It also seems to be stable. In one case, cerebellar atrophy was demonstrated by imaging in one adult [10].

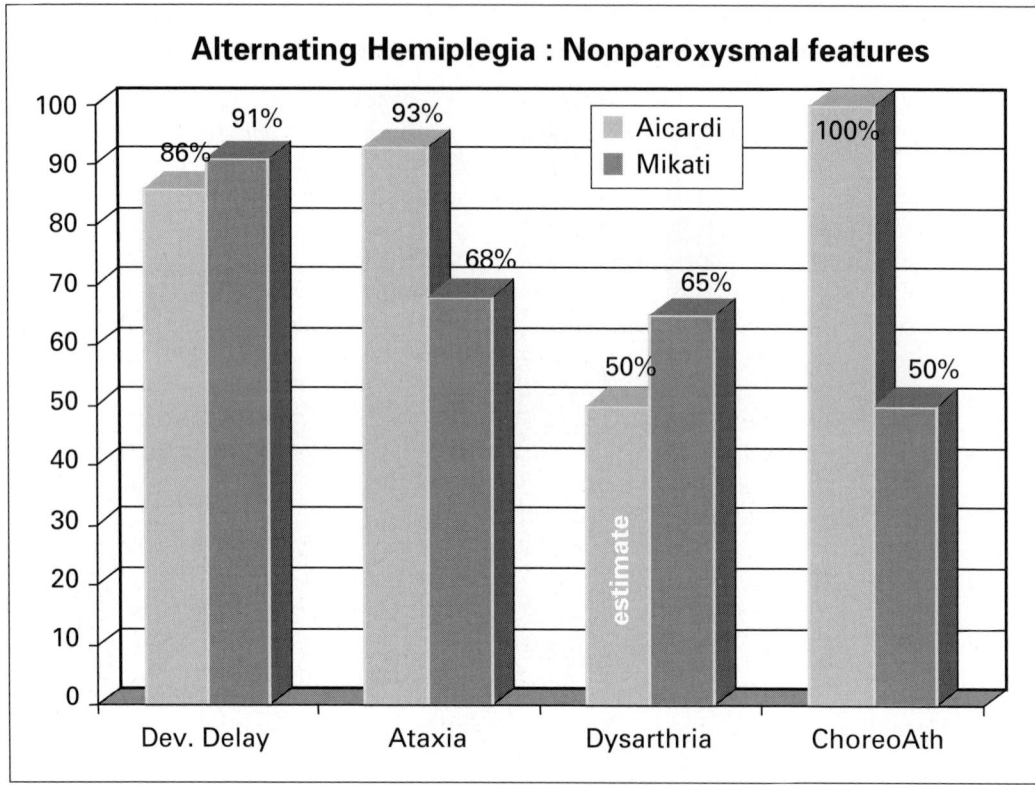

**Figure 2.** Alternating Hemiplegia: Nonparoxysmal features.

Dysarthria, present in 50% to 65% of cases, is a consequence of both choreoathetosis, dystonia and cerebellar disturbances and is often of such a degree that language is unintelligible and severely restricted or absent.

Other disturbances of movement in AHC are less common. Tremor is relatively uncommon but I saw it as an isolated movement disorder in one child. Myoclonus is rare [7].

Different types of movement abnormalities are often seen in the same patient and contribute to the overall disability. They also make precise qualification of the movement disorder difficult and may explain the differences in frequency of the different types in different series [11-14].

AHC has many similarities with other paroxysmal movement disorders such as the episodic character, the frequency of triggering factors, the effect of sleep, the alternance of paralytic episodes and the relatively frequent association with epilepsy thus suggesting the possibility of similar mechanisms.

## Abnormalities of eye movements

They usually occur early often in association with dystonic episodes but may be the only symptoms of an attack. They constitute a common and striking manifestation of AHC. Some of them are similar to what is observed in other movement disorders. One example is the occurrence of paroxysmal episodes of upward or downward deviation of the eyes reminiscent of oculogyric crises. However, the most common ocular abnormalities are probably the result of several mechanisms including paralysis of individual muscles or of gaze in addition to disturbances in the control of movement. Paroxysmal nystagmus is by far the most common [2, 6, 7, 15-17]. It is usually monocular as in 14 of 18 children for whom ocular movements could be documented in one series [2]. The nystagmus is of large amplitude and appears pendular in most cases but no oculographic recording is available. The eye involved is that on the side of the hemiplegic or dystonic attack; it can change with that of the attack. According to Fusco and Vigevano [4], in at least some cases the nystagmus is part of a complex abnormality that also includes impairment of movement of the contralateral eyeball that remains fixed in the lateral direction with neither abduction nor adduction but can move vertically. The eye that shows nystagmus is partially or completely abducted with lateral jerking. This type of eye dysfunction is usually brief, lasting only one or a few minutes. This phenomenon is reminiscent of the one-and-a half gaze disturbance observed with lesions of the central longitudinal bundle in the brainstem [17]. Other oculomotor symptoms may include ocular deviation to one side not necessarily towards the involved side, large amplitude jerks of the eyes in both horizontal and vertical directions, which in rare cases can persist for several days, up to 2 weeks, up-rolling or fixed downward deviation of both eyes, and various forms of paroxysmal strabismus [2, 8, 15].

## Respiratory difficulties. Apneas

Respiratory difficulties frequently accompany severe, especially bilateral, attacks. They are variably described as shallow respiratory movements or a labored breathing. *Apneic episodes* are frequent, occurring together either with other paroxysmal manifestations or in isolation. Some of these episodes are extremely spectacular with a complete arrest of respiration and the development of extreme cyanosis. Stridor and intercostal retraction, as well as sudden onset and absence of evidence of organic airway obstruction suggest the probable role of spasmodic contraction of the laryngeal muscles. In one patient, tonsillectomy suppressed frightening apneic episodes for several months, but eventually the episodes returned. It seems likely that some extreme episodes can result in death (see below). Although apnea is somehow related to the movement disorder, it is also clearly a part of the autonomic disturbances often present in AHC patients such as vasomotor and cardiac rhythm changes, fever, and skin color changes that can be unilateral.

## Outcome of AHC

The overall course of AHC can be divided into three successive phases [2, 5] significantly overlapping. *The first phase* is mostly marked by paroxysmal episodes often initially consisting of ocular motor abnormalities and/or dystonic attacks but featuring also, often slightly later, hemiplegic episodes. During *the second period*, the full gamut of paroxysmal manifestations is present. During this period, cognitive difficulties and often behavioral manifestations become progressively more apparent. *The third period*, which merges insensibly with the second, is that of fixed cognitive and neurological impairment in which movement abnormalities play an increasing role in disability whilst hemiplegic episodes continue.

The overall course tends to be severe although with considerable variations. Some patients are unable to walk, to talk and may even die after a few years as a result of pulmonary complications [5, 7]. Most children can walk and talk but with limitations due to the mental retardation and to abnormal movements. A few children are not or only mildly limited intellectually and can follow an adapted schooling.

However, in these children, the choreo-athetosis remains a severe disability mostly preventing a fully independent life. Epileptic seizures seem to become more frequent with the passing of time. In one series [2] epilepsy that was present initially in 19% of patients was present in 40% of those followed for 5 years or more.

Whether the AHC is a progressive condition has not been properly determined. Most authors think that there is some degree of intellectual deterioration during the initial phase of the disorder with later stability. However, the complete normality of patients at onset is hard to certify because of the early age of onset. Clearcut deterioration of skills can occur following severe bilateral attacks in some children. Some recovery is usually observed at a distance of the episodes but whether sequelae of such sever attacks remain has not been clarified and neuropsychological follow-up studies are clearly necessary.

## Atypical forms and variants of AHC

Despite a generally homogeneous clinical picture, a few cases of AHC present with unusual features that differ, to a variable extent, from the typical aspect described above.

*Late onset of the syndrome* is observed in some cases. Onset may be up to the age of 8 years [8] but otherwise the symptoms and signs are the same as in the classical form, although there may be a trend for the manifestations to be less severe. Dystonic episodes may have preceded the hemiplegia. This also applies to the rare *familial forms*. The onset of dominantly inherited cases is often after one year of age and may be as late as 4-6 years. Although the clinical picture is unmistakable, in some cases with less severity, major diagnostic characteristics are present such as bilateral attacks and the effect of sleep [18, 19]. In one familial case [19], in one of the affected children, there was a very late onset at 7 years and a number of unusual features. However this case was later shown to be associated to a mutation in the sodium/potassium ATPase APT12A gene (mapping to chromosome 1), raising the question of an atypical form of hemiplegic migraine. Other familial cases have been observed in siblings born to unaffected parents, but few details on the symptomatology are available. To my knowledge, at least 3 families in which a probably recessive inheritance was present (2 siblings in 3 families) are known. In addition, two pairs of affected identical twins are known and in two families two half siblings from the same mother are also on record [20].

Thus, although the majority of reported cases have been sporadic, a genetic factor may be operative in at least some cases and more research on this aspect is of obvious importance.

*Other rare syndromes* clearly show significant differences in their symptomatology that can put into question their relationship to AHC. These include cases in which infantile hypotonia with paroxysmal bilateral dystonic episodes are the major manifestation as reported in two unrelated patients by Andermann et al. [21]. One of these children developed choreoathetosis, lateralized dystonic attacks and eventually, at age 14 years, paroxysmal episodes of hemiplegia. Otherwise typical forms of AHC but in which paroxysmal episodes were predominantly dystonic were also observed by Mikati et al. [8].

A syndrome of *benign familial nocturnal alternating hemiplegia* in which episodes of hemiplegia arise from sleep and are unassociated with mental retardation or fixed neurologic deficits was initial described by Andermann et al. [22] and has since been reported in 6 patients [23]. This may well be a different condition to AHC.

An infant who developed suggestive symptoms (paroxysmal eye movement abnormalities, dystonic attacks, other movement anomalies and episodes of apnea) has been described by Saltik et al. [9]. This child died before age one year during an apneic attack and this case suggests that "non hemiplegic AHC" may possibly exist in infants.

## ■ Diagnostic Criteria

The diagnosis of AHC is purely clinical as no laboratory test or biological marker is currently available.

The EEG is of importance by showing the absence of paroxysmal activity during typical episodes. Ictal tracings show only slowing of the activity on the side corresponding to the hemiplegia without any spike [24]. Interestingly, typical seizure discharges were demonstrated in a few patients during clinically characteristic epileptic seizures, thus indicating the differences in mechanism between epilepsy and AHC episodes.

Biochemical investigations have been consistently unhelpful [2, 8]. Morphologic studies gave essentially normal results and a limited number of functional imaging studies have been somewhat difficult to interpret. Overall, SPECT suggested a decrease in blood flow during attacks with a compensatory increased perfusion at the end of the paralytic episodes [25, 26].

Positron emission tomography (PET) has given inconsistent results, probably because the of the long time necessary for image acquisition [27]. Recently, Pfund et al. [28] found an increased uptake of $\alpha$-methyl tryptophan by PET in both parietal regions, a finding not yet fully explained.

The clinical physionomy of the disease on the contrary is highly suggestive, once the condition is known [2, 8]. Although there are multiple causes of alternating hemiplegia, some features are highly distinctive. Hemiplegic episodes in AHC never remain isolated but are variably combined with dystonia, eye movement abnormalities, and respiratory or autonomic phenomena. The occurrence of shifting hemiplegia and of bilateral attacks is almost pathognomonic [2]. The effect of sleep is also very characteristic. As soon as the child falls asleep, hemiplegia and associated phenomena disappear and the movements of the involved side reappear in minutes, which can be easily appreciated even in sleep. Even more characteristic is the fact that, in prolonged attacks, there is resumption of the paralysis within 10 to 40 minutes of awakening, a phenomenon not known to occur, to my knowledge, in any other condition. Parents often volunteer the information that they take advantage of this period to feed the child.

## ■ Differential Diagnosis

Although the clinical symptomatology of AHC in its typical forms is quite distinctive, difficulties may arise in cases with incomplete or atypical features. This is especially the case at onset of the disorder, when no hemiplegias have yet occurred.

When hemiplegic episodes have occurred, a number of differential diagnoses should be discussed and a long list of conditions have to be discussed. The most common difficulty is separating AHC from epileptic seizures as the occurrence of unilateral tonic motor events, sometimes in association with a vibratory tremor, followed by transient hemiplegia is easily misdiagnosed for post-ictal Todd's paralysis.

Inhibitory seizures are a rare occurrence [29]. The frequent association of true epileptic seizures and mental and neurological deterioration with AHC may superficially resemble some cases of epileptic encephalopathy.

Hemiplegic migraine may be difficult to separate from AHC [30]. Indeed, the initial publication of Verret and Steele [1] included both genuine cases of AHC and others of hemiplegic migraine. However, the symptoms accompanying hemiplegic episodes are different from those in AHC and the two disorders are distinct.

Paroxysmal dyskinesias of the kinesigenic or non kinesigenic types are not followed by hemiplegia and not accompanied by the other paroxysmal phenomena described above.

Other conditions that may raise diagnostic difficulties are listed in the table but are relatively easy to distinguish from AHC, even though rare cases of vascular accidents (e.g. in Sneddon syndrome) may raise difficulties.

In the late, chronic stage, choreoathetosis or dystonia, although their symptomatology may be typical of a movement disorder, differ by the antecedent history of acute hemiplegic episodes.

**Differential diagnosis of alternating hemiplegia of childhood.**

- Epilepsy
  - Postictal (Todd's) paralysis
  - Inhibitory seizures
  - Epileptic encephalopathies
- Migraine and related conditions
  - Hemiplegic migraine
  - Basilar migraine
  - Migraine – coma and atypical forms
- Paroxysmal dyskinesias
  - Atypical kinesigenic dyskinesias
  - Paroxysmal choreoathetosis (Mount and Reback)
  - Paroxysmal torticollis of infancy
  - Paroxysmal episodic ataxias (type 2)
- Metabolic diseases
  - Mitochondrial disorders, especially mitochondrial
  - Encephalomyopathy with lactic acidosis and stroke-like episodes (MELAS)
  - Leigh's subacute encephalomyelopathy
  - Pyruvate dehydrogenase deficiency
  - Ornithine transcarbamylase and other ammonia cycle enzyme deficiencies
  - Intermittent forms of organic acids and aminoacids disorders
- Vascular diseases and blood coagulation abnormalities
  - Vascular (arteriovenous) malformations
  - Multiple emboli, *e.g.* atrial myxomas
  - Hereditary hemorrhagic telangiectasia (Osler-Weber-Rendu disease)
  - Cutis marmorata, livedo reticularis, Sneddon's disease
  - Homocystinuria
  - Thrombocythemia
- Demyelinating diseases
  - Acute disseminated encephalomyelitis (chronic forms)
  - Multiple sclerosis
  - Schilder's disease

# ■ Treatment

No satisfactory therapy for AHC is currently available. Antiepileptic agents are ineffective, except against true epileptic seizures when present. Flunarizine, a calcium channel blocker, has proved to be of some value [31, 32] in 50 to 85% of patients at doses of 5 to 15 mg/day. The main effect seems to be a reduction in severity and duration of the attacks rather than a decrease in their frequency [32]. In some cases, a highly significant reduction of the time with paralysis is obtained. However, total disappearance of the attacks is very rare. Whether successful treatment with flunarizine continued for years protects the patients against neurodevelopmental sequelae is yet unknown. It has not prevented the late appearance of cerebellar ataxia and atrophy in the case of Saito *et al.* [11]. Undesirable side-effects, especially extrapyramidal symptoms and signs that have been reported in adults, have not been observed to our knowledge in the treatment of AHC in children.

Other agents such as haloperidol [33], memantine [34], amantadine [35] have been reported in case reports to reduce the frequency of attacks but no controlled study is available.

Intermittent therapy by acute administration of chloral hydrate [36] or of naprizine [37] to induce sleep at onset of an attack may be temporarily effective.

## ■ Etiology and Physiopathology

The etiology of AHC is not known. Only a limited number of cases have been familial with different possible modes of inheritance but [5, 19, 20] the overwhelming majority of cases appear to be sporadic.

The *pathophysiology* of AHC also remains obscure. An epileptic mechanism can be excluded because of the absence of seizures and EEG abnormalities in a majority of cases. A relationship to hemiplegic migraine has often been suggested [30, 38] but the associated paroxysmal as well as nonparoxysmal disturbances are distinct and mental retardation especially strongly argues against such a mechanism. No linkage to chromosome 19 has been found in several patients [38]. The possibility of a mitochondrial disorder has been seriously considered [7] but no confirmation of this hypothesis has been found [39].

Many characteristics of AHC, such as the presence of paroxysmal episodes followed later by fixed neurological abnormalities, similarities of AHC with other conventional entities, the association in many cases with epilepsy and, to some extent, the therapeutic effects of the calcium-blocking agent flunarizine, suggest the possibility of a ionic channel disorder. However, this is, so far, only an hypothesis which is not supported by any hard data.

## ■ Conclusions

AHC remains a mysterious disorder but one with quite distinctive clinical characteristics, allowing a firm diagnosis, even in the absence of confirmatory laboratory test, once the condition is known. Even though the treatment of the disorder remains far from satisfactory, the calcium blocking agent flunarizine has a significant ameliorating effect in about half the cases, so the diagnosis is of practical significance.

It is not yet clear whether AHC is a single disease or if subgroups (*e.g.* familial cases and some atypical forms) with different causes or mechanisms exist. Genetic studies have so far failed to find any gene abnormalities or linkage to a locus. The current hypotheses are thus far unsupported by facts and it is clear that further studies and hypotheses are necessary. Likewise, a search for pharmaceuticals more active than flunarizine should be pursued. Further follow-up studies of affected children are also warranted, especially to determine the degree of progressivity of the condition and to what extent it is influenced by currently available treatment, especially with regard to mental deterioration and movement disorder.

# References

1. Verret S, Steele C. Alternating hemiplegia in childhood: A report of eight patients with complicated migraine beginning in infancy. *Pediatrics* 1971; 47: 675-80.
2. Bourgeois M, Aicardi J, Goutières F. Alternating hemiplegia of childhood. *J Pediatr* 1993; 122: 673-9.
3. Dittrich J, Havlova M, Nevsimalova S. Paroxysmal hemiparesis of childhood. *Dev Med Child Neurol* 1979; 21: 800-7.
4. Fusco L, Vigevano F. Alternating hemiplegia of childhood: clinical findings during attacks. In: Andermann F, Aicardi J, Vigevano F, eds. *Alternating hemiplegia of childhood*. New York: Raven Press, 1995: 29-41.
5. Aicardi J. Alternating hemiplegia of childhood. In: Guerrini R, Aicardi J, Andermann F, Hallett M, eds. *Epilepsy and Movement Disorders*. Oxford: Cambridge University Press, 2002: 379-92.
6. Krägeloh I, Aicardi J. Alternating hemiplegia in infants. Report of 5 cases. *Dev Med Child Neurol* 1980; 22: 794-801.
7. Hosking GP, Cavanagh MPC, Wilson J. Alternating hemiplegia: complicated migraine beginning in infancy. *Arch Dis Childh* 1978; 53: 655-9.
8. Mikati MA, Kramer U, Zupanc M, Shanahan R. Alternating hemiplegia of childhood: Clinical manifestations and long term outcome. *Pediatr Neurol* 2000; 23: 134-41.
9. Saltik S, Cokar O, Uslu T, Uluduz D, Dervent A. Alternating hemiplegia of childhood: presentation of two cases regarding the extent of variability. *Epileptic Disord* 2004, in press.
10. Philipps SG. Alternating hemiplegia of childhood – earlier features misdiagnosed as epilepsy. *Dev Med Child Neurol* 2004; 46 (suppl 98): 30 (abstract).
11. Saito Y, Sakuragawa M, Sasaki M, Sugai K, Hashimoto T. A case of alternating hemiplegia of childhood with cerebellar atrophy. *Pediatr Neurol* 1998; 19: 65-8.
12. Campistol Plana J, Capovilla G, Trevisan E, *et al.* Alternating hemiplegia of infants. In: Andermann F, Lugaresi E, eds. *Migraine and Epilepsy*. London: Butterworth, 1987: 189-201.
13. Dalla Bernardina B, Sans Fito A, Pineda M, Fernandez-Alvarez E. Hemiplegia alternante en la infancia: forma de presentacion, evolucion y tratamiento. *Ann Espan Pediatria* 1990; 332: 336-8.
14. Sakuragawa N. Alternating hemiplegia in childhood: 23 cases in Japan. *Brain Dev* 1992; 14: 283-8: 22; 99-101.
15. Egan RA. Ocular motor features of alternating hemiplegia of childhood. *J Fr Ophtalmol* 2002.
16. Bursztin J, Mikaeloff Y, Kaminska A, *et al.* Hémiplégie alternante de l'enfant et anomalies oculomotrices. *J Fr Ophtalmol* 2000: 23: 161-4.
17. Pierrot-Desailigny C, Chain F, Serdarn M, Gray F, Lhermitte F. The "one-and a half syndrome": electro-oculographic analysis of five cases with deductions about the physiological mechanisms of lateral gaze. *Brain* 1981: 104: 665-99.
18. Mikati M, Maguire H, Barlow CF. A syndrome of autosomal dominant alternating hemiplegia; clinical presentation mimicking intractable epilepsy; chromosomal studies and physiologic investigations. *Neurology* 1998; 42: 2251-7.
19. Kanavakis E, Xaidora A., Papathanasiou-Kloutza, Papadimitriou A, Valentsa S. Youroukos S. Alternating hemiplegia of childhood: a syndrome inherited with an autosomal dominant trait. *Dev Med Child Neurol* 2003; 45: 833-6.
19A. Suroboda KJ, Kanavakis E, Xaidora A, *et al.* Alternating hemiplegia of childhood or familial hemiplegic migraine? A novel ATP1 A2 mutation. *Ann Neurol* 2004; 55: 884-7.
20. Kramer U, Nevo Y, Margalit D, Shorer Z, Harel S. Alternating hemiplegia of childhood in half-sisters. *J Child Neurol* 2000; 15: 128-30.

21. Andermann F, Ohtahara S, Andermann E, Camfield P, Kobayashi K. Infantile hypotonia and paroxysmal dystonia: a variant of alternating hemiplegia in childhood. In: Andermann F, Aicardi J, Vigevano F, eds. *Alternating hemiplegia of childhood*. New York: Raven Press, 1995: 151-7.
22. Andermann E, Andermann F, Silver K, Levin S, Arnold DS. Benign familial nocturnal hemiplegia of childhood. In: Andermann F, Aicardi J, Vigevano F, eds. *Alternating hemiplegia of childhood*. New York: Raven Press, 1995: 145-9.
23. Chavez-Vicher V, Picard F, Andermann E, Della Bernardina B, Andermann F. Benign nocturnal alternating hemiplegia of childhood: six patients and long-term follow-up. *Neurology* 2001; 57: 1491-3.
24. Dalla Bernardina B, Fontana E, Colamaria V, et al. Alternating hemiplegia of childhood: epilepsy and electroencephalographic investigations. In: Andermann F, Aicardi J, Vigevano F, eds. *Alternating hemiplegia of childhood*. New York: Raven Press, 1995: 75-87.
25. Zupanc ML, Dobkin JA, Prelman SR. $^{123}$Iodoamphetamine SPECT brain imaging in alternating hemipegia. *Pediatr Neurol* 1991; 7: 35-8.
26. Zupanc ML, Perlman SB, Rust RS. Single photon emission computed tomography studies in alternating hemiplegia of childhood. In: Andermann F, Aicardi J, Vigevano F, eds. *Alternating hemiplegia of childhood*. New York: Raven Press, 1995: 99-107.
27. Mikati MA, Fishman AJ. Positron emission tomography in children with alternating hemiplegia of childhood. In: Andermann F, Aicardi J, Vigevano F, eds. *Alternating hemiplegia of childhood*. New York: Raven Press, 1995: 109-14.
28. Pfund Z, Chugani DC, Muzik O, et al. Alpha [11 C] methyl-L-triptophan positron emission tomography in patients with alternating hemiplegia of childhood. *J Child Neurol* 2002; 17: 253-60.
29. Shirazakia Y, Ito M, Okuno T, Mikawa H, Yamori Y. Epileptic seizures difficult to differentiate from alternating hemiplegia in infants: a case report. *Brain Dev* 1990; 12: 521-4.
30. Lance JW. Is alternating hemiplegia of childhood a variant of migraine? *Cephalalgia* 2000: 20: 685.
31. Casaer P. Flunarizine in alternating hemiplegia in childhood. An international study of 12 children. *Neuropediatrics* 1987; 18: 191-5.
32. Silver K, Andermann F. Alternating hemiplegia of childhood. Treatment with flunarizine. In Andermann F, Aicardi J, Vigevano F, eds. In: *Alternating hemiplegia of childhood*. New York: Raven Press, 1995: 195-8.
33. Wilson J. Treatment of alternating hemiplegia of childhood: the effect of haloperidol. In: Andermann F, Aicardi J, Vigevano F, eds. *Alternating hemiplegia of childhood*. New York: Raven Press, 1995: 201.
34. Korinthenberg R. Is alternating hemiplegia mediated by glutamate toxicity and can it be treated with memantine? *Neuropediatrics* 1996; 27: 277-8.
35. Sone K, Oguni H, Katsumori H, Funatsuka M, Tanaka T, Osawa M. Successful trial of amantadine hydrochloride for two patients with alternating hemiplegia of childhood. *Neuropediatrics* 2000; 31: 307-8.
36. Siemes H. Rectal chloral hydrate for alternating hemiplegia of childhood. *Dev Med Child Neurol* 1990; 32: 927-31.
37. Veneselli E, Biancheri R. Alternating hemiplegia of childhood; treatment of attacks with chloral hydrate and Niaprizine. *Europ J Pediatr* 1997; 156: 157-8.
38. Haan J, Kors EE, Terwindt GM, et al. Alternating hemiplegia of childhood: no mutations in the familial hemiplegia migraine CADNA 1 A gene. *Cephalalgia* 2000; 20: 696-700.
39. De Stefano N, Silver K, Andermann F, Arnold DL. Mitochondrial dysfunction in patients with alternating hemiplegia of childhood: Fluctuations over time in relation to clinical states. In: Andermann F, Aicardi J, Vigevano F, eds. *Alternating hemiplegia of childhood*. New York: Raven Press, 1995: 115-22.

# Movement disorders in children and calcification of the basal ganglia

**Victoria San Antonio, Alexis Arzimanoglou**

*Child Neurology and Metabolic Diseases Dpt.,
University Hospital Robert Debré, Paris, France*

---

First described in 1850 by Delacour [1], calcification of the basal ganglia has attracted the interest of pathologists and neuroscientists since the middle of the 19th century. Subsequently, many other reports followed, including the study by Fahr in 1930 [2], based on a collection of different disorders that had little in common. The rather confusing terms [3] "Fahr's syndrome" or "Fahr's disease" are still commonly used to describe calcification of the basal ganglia of unknown etiology, but it is now well recognized that the use of these terms is not specific.

With the introduction of modern neuroimaging techniques, especially computed tomography (CT) scanning, asymptomatic intracranial calcification has become a common finding. CT scanning is highly sensitive in detecting calcification and is considered as a current gold standard over magnetic resonance imaging (MRI). On MRI, signal intensity of the calcified foci varies depending on the calcium contents in the lesion. Densely calcified lesions show hypointensity on both T1- and T2-weighted sequences. But finely calcified foci are hyperintense on T1-weighted and isointense, to slightly hypointense, on T2-weighted images. On gradient echo sequences, calcified foci produce a hypointensity signal, because of increased magnetic susceptibility.

Large population studies have shown that about 0.7% of all patients submitted to routine CT scan have basal ganglia calcifications [4, 5]. The majority of these individuals were elderly people and had no clinical evidence of basal ganglia dysfunction. These findings, and the fact that 72% of routine autopsies show perivascular ferrocalcium deposits on microscopic study of the basal ganglia, suggest that calcification of the basal ganglia on CT scan in most individuals over the age of 50 may be the result of normal, age-related, vascular changes. Contrariwise, physiological calcification of the basal ganglia is rare in children – it occurred in only 0.03% of 18000 pediatric CT scans reported by Kendall and Cavanagh [6] – so that it can be considered abnormal in virtually all cases. With the larger use of the MRI signal abnormalities of the basal ganglia, other than calcifications, have been related to a great many pathological conditions in childhood.

In this chapter, we provide an extensive review of existing data on neuroimaging abnormalities of the basal ganglia in different pathological entities, with emphasis given to calcification of the basal ganglia and to those clinical entities manifesting with movement disorders. The main causes of calcification of the basal ganglia in infants and children [7-9] are given in Table I. A general list of pathological conditions resulting in various neuroimaging abnormalities of the basal ganglia is provided in Table II. Detailed discussion on other types of basal ganglia abnormal signals (lucencies, etc.), are out of the scope of this chapter and are only mentioned briefly, whenever necessary.

The role of the basal ganglia dysfunction in the origin of movement disorders is relatively well known and the presence of basal ganglia calcifications in children must always suggest searching for a pathological cause. However, the present review clearly demonstrates that the presence of calcifications is not necessarily related to a movement disorder. The opposite is also true; many of these pathological conditions can exhibit movement disorders independently of the presence or the absence of basal ganglia calcifications [9, 10].

## ■ Inflammatory causes

In infancy and childhood, inflammatory processes constitute a prominent cause of neuroimaging abnormalities of the basal ganglia. They may occasionally present with movement disorders, although in most of the cases these are not the main symptom. Several mechanisms may be involved, the most frequent being *vasculitic ischemia*. Other proposed mechanisms include direct neuronal injury by the infecting organism or through cytotoxins, and autoimmune cross reactivity with basal ganglia. Movement disorders, when present, usually develop during the acute phase of the illness and may be transient. Infections, that do not represent a major cause of secondary movement disorders in industrial countries, still are in underdeveloped countries where prophylactic and therapeutic measures are not yet generalized [11].

Congenital infections, such as *toxoplasmosis, rubella, cytomegalovirus* and *HIV* infection, are the first cause of basal ganglia calcifications in the newborn and their early presence is a strong argument but not decisive in favour of a clastic process, rather than a genetic condition. A disorder of movement is rarely in the forefront, the usual clinical picture combining meningo-encephalitis to other neurological and extra-neurological symptoms [7]. Neurological symptomatology with a predominant movement disorder has been reported in cases of cerebral toxoplasmosis and cytomegalovirus infection in children, and adults, with **acquired immunodeficiency syndrome** (AIDS). A special mention should be made regarding brain calcification in children with AIDS, a common disease than can mimic any progressive central nervous system disorder. Calcification of the basal ganglia and, to a lesser extent, the frontal subcortical white matter is a common imaging feature of paediatric HIV infection. Calcification of the basal ganglia has been documented on CT scans in about 30-50% of children over age one year and in almost 90% of the autopsy studies [12, 13]. Pathologically, calcification is located in both small and medium-sized blood vessels and the surrounding parenchyma, with no histological changes of ischemia or infarction. However, movement disorders in the absence of toxoplasmosis or drug-related conditions are rare (3%) in adult patients with HIV infection [14, 15].

**Acute viral encephalitis** may be another cause of neuroimaging abnormalities of the basal ganglia in childhood, sometimes with persistent calcifications as sequelae of the acute insult. However, in most of the cases basal ganglia lesions take the form of MRI hypodensities, rarely calcified. *Varicella* has been associated with transient bilateral facial, jaw and arm chorea and dystonia, and less frequently, with hemichorea or generalised chorea [16] and parkinsonian manifestations have been reported in 3 children with post-varicella encephalitis and non-enhancing basal ganglia lesions on CT, giving on MRI a low signal intensity on T1-weighted images and high signal on T2 [17]. In *herpes simplex encephalitis*, although movement disorders may be present early in the course, they are more often due to a relapse [18-20]. Movement disorders have also been reported in other acute viral encephalites, such as *ECHO* virus [21], *Epstein-Barr* virus [22] and *West Nile* virus [23] infections. In West Nile Virus (WNV) infection movement disorders, including tremor (15 [94%]), myoclonus (5 [31%]), and Parkinsonism (11 [69%]) were present mainly during the acute phase of the disease. Movement disorders are also observed in a significant proportion of patients with *Japanese encephalitis* [24, 25]. Japanese encephalitis is endemic in several parts of the Indian subcontinent and in the Far East, birds are the natural reservoir for the causative virus and transmission to humans of an arbovirus is transmitted by mosquitoes [11]. Neuroimaging typically shows extensive bilateral thalamic lesions, but MRI reveals additional findings in lentiform nucleus in almost all cases and, less often, in midbrain and cerebellum. Movement disorders, in the form of Parkinsonism with bradykinesia, rigidity and masked facies, are present in about 70-80% of the patients who survive the acute encephalitic phase.

**Sydenham's chorea** is the classic infection-related movement disorder [26]. Neuroimaging studies may be normal or show reversible bilateral or contralateral basal ganglia involvement [27], in the form of hypodensities on CT scan and increased T2 signal on MRI. Positron emission tomography (PET) studies show reversible striatal hypermetabolism [28]. Bacterial meningitis caused by *Haemophilus influenzae*, *Streptococcus pneumoniae* and *Neisseria meningitidis* [29] have been related to movements disorders, probably because of the damage to the basal ganglia by infarcts consequent to vasculitis, sometimes detectable on neuroimaging. This mechanism, or more often an immunological one, may be the cause of the occasional movement disorders [30, 31].

**Tuberculosis** continues to be a major health problem in developing countries and, because of AIDS, is now an emergent disease in industrial countries. Movement disorders have been reported in a number of neurotuberculosis cases, including hemiballismus, tremor, myoclonus, chorea and dystonia [29, 32-34]. Neuroimaging studies may be normal, but more often show hydrocephalus and infarcts, and sometimes focal lesions in the basal ganglia or even tuberculomas that may be calcified. The correlation between the movement disorders and the neuroimaging findings is poorly established. Damage of the basal ganglia by infarcts consequent to vasculitis is probably the main mechanism for movement disorders in tuberculosis, although hydrocephalus [34] and tuberculomas [32, 34] may also play a role.

**Table I. Causes of calcification of the basal ganglia in infancy and childhood.**

1. **Inflammatory causes**
   - Cytomegalovirus infection
   - Toxoplasmosis
   - Congenital rubella
   - HIV infection and AIDS
   - Acute viral encephalitis
   - Polioencephalitis in immunodepressed patients
   - Bacterial meningoencephalitis
   - Tuberculosis
   - Neurocysticercosis
   - Parainfectious encephalomyelitis
   - Encephalitis in Cree Indians
   - Systemic lupus erythematosus

2. **Tumours and dysplasias**
   - Calcified astrocytoma of basal ganglia
   - Calcified cavernous hemangioma of basal ganglia
   - Calcified ganglioglioma of basal ganglia
   - Subependimal astrocytoma
   - Metastasis
   - Tuberous sclerose
   - Neurofibromatosis

3. **Vascular and hypoxic causes**
   - Perinatal hypoxic-ischaemic encephalopathy
   - Symmetrical thalamic degeneration in infancy
   - Calcified infarct
   - Arteriovenous malformations of basal ganglia

4. **Endocrine disorders**
   - Primary hypoparathyroidism
   - Pseudo- and pseudopseudohypoparathyroidism
   - Hyperparathyroidism
   - Hypothyroidism

5. **Toxic disorders**
   - CO poisoning
   - Lead poisoning
   - Chromium poisoning
   - X-ray therapy of leukaemia or tumours
   - Intrathecal methotrexate
   - Hypervitaminosis D
   - Nephrotic syndrome

6. **Genetic, metabolic and heredodegenerative diseases**
   - Mitochondrial encephalomyopathy
   - Cockayne syndrome and related syndromes
   - Down syndrome (Takashima and Becker, 1985)
   - Raine syndrome
   - MCA/MR syndrome
   - Krabbe leucodystrophy
   - CDG syndrome (diffuse calcification of white matter) (Stibler and Jaeken, 1990)
   - Calcification of basal ganglia with leukodystrophy and CSF lymphocytosis
   - Neuroaxonal dystrophy (Ramaekers et al., 1987)
   - Hallervorden-Spatz disease (may not be true calcification but rather iron storage) (Savoiardo et al., 1993)
   - Phenylketonuria (biopterin reductase deficiency) (Woody et al., 1989)
   - Biotinidase deficiency (Schulz et al., 1988)
   - Lipoid proteinosis (hyalinosis cutis)
   - Carbonic anhydrase II deficiency (Ohlsson et al., 1986; Strisciuglio et al., 1990; Venta et al., 1991)
   - Dystonia-basal ganglia calcification syndrome (Larsen et al., 1985)

**Table I continued.**

- Pycnodysostosis (hydrocephalus, growth retardation, mild facial dysmorphism)
- Microcephaly-intracranial calcification syndrome (congenital microcephaly, basal ganglia calcification, polymicrogyria, AR inheritance?) (Burn et al., 1986; Reardon et al., 1994)
- Microcephaly with calcification of basal ganglia (Baraitser et al., 1983)
- Craniosynostosis-basal banglia calcification-mild facial dysmorfism (autosomal recessive inheritance?) (Longman et al., 2003)
- Trichothiodystrophy (Happle et al., 1984)
- Retinopathy with calcification of basal ganglia (Hammerstein et al., 1982)
- Lethal arthrogryposis with calcification (Illune et al., 1988)
- renatal cerebral calcification, Coats disease, dysmorphism and movement disorder (Tolmie et al., 1988)
- Aicardi-Goutières syndrome

**7. Miscellaneous**
- Familial amentia with familial calcification of choroid plexus and raised CSF protein (calcification mainly in choroid plexuses) (Lott et al., 1979)
- Bilateral striato-pallido-dentate calcinosis (Boller et al., 1977; Ellie et al., 1989; Manyam et al., 1990, 1992)

**Table II. Pathological conditions resulting in neuroimaging abnormalities of the basal ganglia.**

**ACUTE**
- Hypoxia
- Hypoglycemia
- Toxins (carbon monoxide, cyanide)
- Hemolytic-uremic syndrome
- Osmotic myelinolysis
- Encephalitis
- Parainfectious encephalomyelitis
- Tegretol toxicity

**CHRONIC**
**1. Inborn errors of metabolism**
- Mitochondrial disorders
- Canavan's disease
- Glutaric aciduria types I and II
- Methylmalonic acidemia
- Ethylmalonic acidemia
- Propionic acidemia
- Molybdenum cofactor deficiency
- Mitochondrial adenosine triphosphate synthetase deficiency
- 3-Methylglutaconic aciduria
- β-Ketothiolase deficiency
- Malonic acidemia
- α-Ketoglutaric aciduria
- 3-Ketothiolase deficiency
- Biotinidase deficiencies
- L-2-hydroxyglutaric aciduria
- Maple syrup urine disease
- Wilson's disease
- Hallervorden-Spatz disease
- Dentatorubral and pallidoluysian atrophy

**2. Degenerative diseases**
- Juvenile Huntington's disease
- Sequelae of acute insults
- Basal ganglia calcification syndromes (i.e., Cockayne's syndrome)

**3. Other diseases**
- Neurofibromatosis type 1

**Parasitic infections** of the CNS, still frequent in tropical and subtropical countries, may also present as movement disorders or neuroimaging abnormalities of the basal ganglia. Movement disorders, especially tremor, are a common symptom in cerebral trypanosomiasis [35]. Contrariwise, although movement disorders have been described in several cases of *cerebral malaria* [36], they are not a frequent symptom of the disease. Likewise, they are rare in *neurocysticercosis*, although neuroimaging lesions in basal ganglia, sometimes calcified, may be found in about 30% of cases [37]. One case of *cat-scratch disease* with choreoathetosis and increased T2 signal in basal ganglia on MRI has been recently described [38].

Neuroimaging abnormalities of the basal ganglia may be found in *parainfectious encephalitis*. Acute *disseminated encephalomyelitis* (ADEM) is an autoimmune inflammatory disease, usually monophasic with gradual resolution, in relation to a virus, bacteria or immunization, but may also occur in the absence of any obvious cause. MRI shows demyelinating lesions in the form of hyperintensities in T2-weighted images and FLAIR, which are located mostly in white matter, but can extend to the grey matter. Basal ganglia involvement is found in about 15-30% of cases, although movement disorders are present in less than 5% [39, 40].

A rare condition, consisting in *acute neurological dysfunction associated with destructive lesions of the basal ganglia* in children, has been reported by Goutières and Aicardi [41]. Although the cause of this syndrome remains unknown, it has been related to some viral infections and an immunological mechanism could be involved. Main clinical features are acute disturbance of consciousness, motor rigidity, loss of spontaneous movements and language, axial hypotonia and a stereotyped response to any kind of stimulus. The cerebrospinal fluid shows a mononuclear cell reaction with negative bacterial and viral cultures. Neuroimaging studies disclose basal ganglia involvement compatible with vasculitis and necrosis. The acute onset is often followed by later spontaneous improvement associated with neuroimaging normalisation.

An immunological mechanism could be responsible for calcifications of the basal ganglia described in a rare neurological disorder among *Cree Indian* children in a northern Quebec village [42]. Other features are severe mental retardation, movement disorders, cerebral atrophy, white matter changes and systemic immunological abnormalities. The familial incidence of cases and the high degree of parental consanguinity suggest a genetic contribution, although the role of an unusual virus infection has also been proposed. The similarity of this disorder to the *Aicardi-Goutières syndrome* (AGS – see below) is striking. As described in AGS, a high level of interferon-α in the CSF has been found in one of the Cree children [43].

Movement disorders such as dystonia, athetosis and chorea have been described, correlating with atrophy of the caudate nucleus, in some cases of *Rasmussen syndrome* [44-47], a rare autoimmune disorder consisting in intractable epilepsy and progressive hemispheric dysfunction [48].

Movement disorders and neuroimaging abnormalities of the basal ganglia occasionally occur in other **autoimmune and collagen vascular diseases**. About 80-100% of cases of CNS *lupus* have abnormal findings on MRI, including brain atrophy, focal lesions in the white matter and changes in the basal ganglia, often with calcification [49]. Although movement disorders, mainly chorea, have been reported in a number of cases with neurolupus [50-52], they are only present in about 4% of cases and account for not more than 2% of all neurological symptoms. A correlation between them and the neuroimaging and pathological abnormalities of the basal ganglia has not been always established.

In patients without lupus, the primary antiphospholipid syndrome is characterized by the presence of antiphospholipid antibodies and thrombocytopenia resulting in a hypercoagulable state [53]. Patients may present movement disorders and neuroimaging abnormalities but, as for lupus, calcifications are rare and a correlation is not always noted. Hemidystonia in three paediatric cases of primary antiphospholipid syndrome related to a presumed immune-mediated thrombotic event involving the basal ganglia as shown by MRI has been reported [54].

Neuroimaging abnormalities of the basal ganglia have also been reported in cases of *haemolytic uremic syndrome* (HUS), sometimes associated with movement disorders [55-57], related to microangiopathy of cerebral vessels with microthrombosis resulting in infarction and coagulative necrosis.

## ■ Vascular and hypoxic causes

Movement disorders, accompanied by neuroimaging abnormalities, may result from hypoxic-ischemic injury to the basal ganglia in case of global cerebral hypoperfusion [58], particularly during the perinatal period. Symptoms appear after a variable interval of time, sometimes after decades, mainly in the form of focal or segmental dystonia [59-62]. Chorea and athetosis, may also appear. Despite the global insult, patients often have focal, less frequently unilateral, findings on neuroimaging studies, in the form of hyperintensity of basal ganglia on T2-weighted sequences of MRI *(Figure 1)*, and sometimes calcifications. Uncommonly, brain CT or MRI are normal or disclose mild diffuse atrophy or leukomalacia. Pathologically, the type of lesion most frequently found is status marmoratus of the striatum [63].

A rare distinct clinico-radiological entity is *symmetrical thalamic degeneration with calcifications* of infancy [64, 65]. Lesions follow pre- or intra-partum global cerebral hypoperfusion in premature infants and are clinically distinguished by prominent brain-stem dysfunction, particularly of lower cranial nerves. Neonatal thalamic calcifications in premature infants may serve as a radiological marker of an acute hypoxic-ischemic event and imply that injury was sustained to diencephalic and brain-stem structures at least 2 to 4 weeks prior to their appearance on CT scan.

In older children some cases of acute hypoxia related to asthma, anaesthesia or drowning developing progressive dystonia and lesions in the putamen have been reported [66]. Clinical and radiological features are different from those developed by some older patients after cardiac arrest, hypotension or anaesthesia, mainly consisting of a nonprogressive akinetic-rigid syndrome and imaging lesions in the globus pallidus.

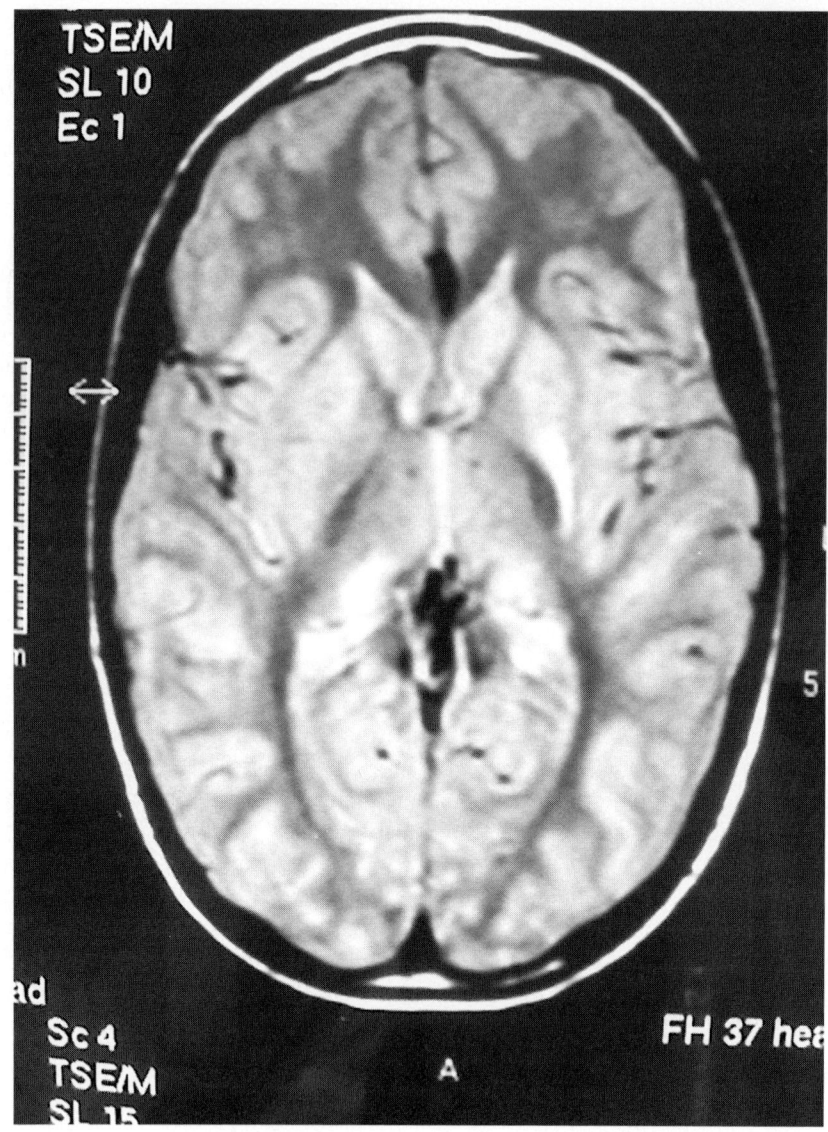

**Figure 1.** Hyperintense signal of the posterior part of the left putamen in a 14 years old girl with congenital right hemiplegia, later complicated by episodes of dystonic status.

A particular condition is *"post-pump chorea"* [67], a syndrome of chorea or ballismus, episodic eye deviation and hypotonia. It appears in 1-2% of infants and young children, after an asymptomatic period, within 12 days of cardiac surgery under hypothermia and cardiopulmonary bypass. It can be severe and irreversible, and has a significant death rate. Neuroimaging and pathological findings are mostly located in the external globus pallidus.

*Lacunar infarcts* in the basal ganglia are known to cause, particularly in adults, various movement disorders, such as chorea, focal dystonia, hemichorea-hemiballismus and Parkinsonism. Although lacunar infarcts in the basal ganglia are rare in children, they can occasionally occur in the clinical context of some autoimmune and collagen vascular diseases or conditions entailing a state of hypercoagulability, such a nephrotic syndrome (see above). Calcification is possible.

*Cerebral arteriovenous malformations* (AVMs) most frequently manifest by seizures or spontaneous intracranial haemorrhage. The bleeding risk in patients with AVMs of the basal ganglia or thalamus (9.8% per patient-year) is much higher than the risk in patients with AVMs in other locations (2-4%), so their risk of incurring a neurological deficit is higher [68-70]. Several cases of cerebral AVMs have been described in the literature to cause movement disorders, mainly dystonic syndromes such as cervical dystonia and hemidystonia, but also hemiathetosis, hemichorea, hemiballismus, tremor, action myoclonus and palatal myoclonus [71].

## ■ Endocrine Disorders

*Hypoparathyroidism* is probably the most frequent cause of secondary basal ganglia calcification. All types of hypoparathyroidism, including primary (idiopathic), post-thyroidectomy, pseudo-hypoparathyroidism and even pseudo-pseudohypoparathyroidism, have been reported to cause this abnormality.

*Primary hypoparathyroidism* is usually transmitted as an X-linked condition. Epileptic seizures and carpopedal and laryngeal spasm are major acute manifestations and can be precipitated by hyperpnea. Mental retardation or psychosis is present in 60% of cases, extrapyramidal signs in 30% and signs of intracranial hypertension in 25-30%. Cataracts and skin lesions are common. *Chovstek sign* is nonspecific, and the diagnosis rests on demonstration of low calcium and high phosphorus levels. Calcification in this condition, as well in post-surgical hypoparathyroidism, is often not limited to the globus pallidus, putamen and caudate, but also involves subcortical white matter and cerebral cortex (especially in the frontal lobes), internal capsule, dentate nucleus and cerebellar hemispheres [72-74].

In *pseudo-hypoparathyroidism*, similar manifestations are associated to short stature, obesity, moon-shaped facies, one or more shortened metacarpal (frequently 4$^{th}$ and 5$^{th}$ metacarpal) and metatarsal bones, mental retardation and impaired sense of taste and smell. Calcifications are present in one-third of the cases. This condition, more frequent in females, is also known as *Albright's hereditary osteodystrophy* and is dominantly inherited. The same morphological syndrome without abnormality of calcium/phosphorus metabolism is known as *pseudopseudohypo-parathyroidism*, but it seems to be a part of Albright's osteodystrophy as shown by the occurrence of cases both with and without calcium/phosphorus disturbances in the same kindred.

The clinical features of basal ganglia dysfunction in patients with these forms of intracranial calcifications vary considerably. Occasionally, completely asymptomatic patients in which basal ganglia calcification have been incidentally found on CT san, have been found to have laboratory evidence for hypoparathyroidism. In symptomatic patients, movement disorders are not always present despite calcification of the basal ganglia, and inversely, some cases presenting with movement disorders in the absence of basal ganglia calcification have been reported [75], evidencing the lack of correlation between clinical and radiological features.

Present in about 30% of the patients, movement disorders mostly demonstrate in the form of Parkinsonism with akinesia and rigidity, although some cases presenting with dystonia, choreoathetosis, hemiballismus, tremor and other features have been reported [72, 73, 76-82]. Treatment of the hypoparathyroidism has improved the movement disorder in some patients [79, 83-85]. However, many have failed to respond, although progression may be slowed or halted. Treatment with anti-parkinsonism drugs, such as L-dopa, often has little or no effect [83, 86, 87].

Basal ganglia calcification has also been reported in a few cases of congenital hypothyroidism [88].

## ■ Toxic Disorders

Poisoning by certain gases and heavy metals is a rare cause of movement disorders associated to neuroimaging abnormalities of the basal ganglia. They are even rarer in children, since most of the cases are related to a chronic, often occupational, exposure to the toxic agent. The physiopathological mechanism of neurological damage is cellular hypoxia due to mitochondrial dysfunction or generation of free radicals.

Survivors of *carbon monoxide (CO) poisoning* may show, after an initial improvement, delayed-onset Parkinsonism, sometimes with dystonia, often reversible with recovery within the first year [89]. Neuroimaging studies disclose generalised atrophy with focal injury particularly to the globus pallidus, but also in the striatum, hippocampus, cerebellum and substantia nigra. Calcification of the basal ganglia has been reported [90, 91]. A correlation between imaging findings and long-term clinical outcome has been noted [92].

Chronic exposure to *lead* has also been related to calcification of the basal ganglia in adults and, less frequently, of the subcortical area and the cerebellum [93]. MRI discloses high signal intensities on T2-weighted sequences in periventricular white matter, basal ganglia, insula, posterior thalamus and pons. Despite the basal ganglia lesions, movement disorders are not frequently observed. However, some cases of chronic lead exposure resulting in movement disorders, mainly tremor, have been reported [94, 95]. Acute exposure to organic lead may result in acute encephalopathy with vomiting and hallucinations and, in some cases, movement disorders [95, 96].

*Manganese* has been shown to increase free radical formation and inhibit antioxidant function. It also causes mitochondrial dysfunction and probably interferes with the striatal dopaminergic system. Chronic occupational exposure to manganese may result in progressive irreversible Parkinsonism and dystonia, associated with neuroimaging abnormalities of the basal ganglia, in the form of hyperintensity on T2-weighted MRI [94]. Similar neuroimaging findings have been described in regard to manganese intoxication in children receiving prolonged parenteral nutrition [97, 98].

*Cyanide* intoxication may also result in delayed reversible Parkinsonism and dystonia, associated with cerebral atrophy and hyperintensity of the basal ganglia on T2-weighted MRI [99].

*Methanol*, also by inhibition of cytochome oxidase, may cause Parkinsonism, dystonia and blindness, associated with injury to the retina and the optic nerve and necrosis of the putamen as well as the subcortical white matter, cerebellum, brainstem and spinal cord. Like methanol, other organic solvents such as toluene, n-hexane and carbon disulfide may cause tremor and Parkinsonism, besides cerebellar signs, by chronic occupational exposure [94, 100].

Neuroimaging abnormalities of the basal ganglia related to perivascular pallidal deposits containing *chromium*, phosphorus and calcium have been reported in the three cases, not associated with movement disorders [101]. Chromium, contrarily to calcium and phosphorus, has not been found before in CNS calcifications, and its presence in these three cases is thought to be related to chromium intoxication, which usually results in dermatological or pulmonary lesions without cerebral involvement.

Toxic effects of copper resulting in basal ganglia dysfunction and neuroimaging abnormalities are observed in Wilson's disease (see below).

Movement disorders may also be caused by a number of drugs, including neuroleptics, anticonvulsants [102] oral contraceptives [103], theophylline [104, 105], and amphetamines. Symptoms are often transient and resolve with discontinuation of the causal agent. Specific basal ganglia lesions are not reported.

Neuroimaging abnormalities of the basal ganglia, particularly calcifications, have been reported in children as a long-term complication of radiation treatment of tumours or leukaemia [106-110] and/or intrathecal methotraxate [111]. The exact pathogenesis of this condition is not well known. It appears, however, to be related to a vasculitis of the small vessels of the brain resulting in hyalinization and calcification. Patients are often asymptomatic, although some cases presenting with psychiatric symptoms [111] or movements disorders, mainly Parkinsonism [112, 113], have been reported.

Finally, neuroimaging abnormalities of the basal ganglia may be found in pathological conditions entailing hydroelectrolytic and metabolic disturbances. *Nephrotic syndrome* has been related to hypercoagulability and cerebral infarctions, sometimes involving the basal ganglia [114]. Hypervitaminosis D has been found a cause of pathological calcifications [115]. Severe hypoglycemia may be at the origin of neuroimaging abnormalities, in the form of high-signal lesions on T2-weighted MRI images, mainly involving the basal ganglia and hippocampus [116, 117].

## ■ Genetic, metabolic and heredodegenerative diseases

Lesions of the basal ganglia, frequently in the form of calcifications, are a common finding in several genetic, metabolic and heredodegenerative disorders of childhood. However, most of them do not present with movement disorders, at least as a main symptom. In this part of the chapter, we will mainly discuss those that combine basal ganglia lesions and a movement disorder.

*Mitochondrial encephalomyopathies* are a prominent cause of neuroimaging abnormalities of the basal ganglia [118-120] and should be systematically sought. Calcifications may be present, but most cases show hyperintensity on T2-weighted and FLAIR sequences on MRI. These signal abnormalities are present in more than 50% of reported cases. Consequently, in the presence of compatible clinical semeiology, they should be considered suggestive of a mitochondrial encephalomyopathy [120]. Movement disorders may be present, though they are not constant and not frequently the main symptom. The presence of such lesions should evoke a mitochondrial encephalo-myopathy, particularly in children presenting symptoms of cerebral palsy with no clear history of a pre- or perinatal acquired disorder [121].

*Pantothenate kinase-associated neurodegeneration* [122], also called Hallervorden-Spatz syndrome, is an autosomal recessive neuro-degenerative disease clinically characterized by a progressive movement disorder mainly consisting in dystonia or Parkinsonism. The main pathological feature is abundant iron deposition in the globus pallidus and areas of "loose" tissue with vacuolization and lesser amounts of iron in the anteromedial zone. Also called "eye-of-the-tiger", the MRI lesion corresponds to the low signal intensity in T2-weighted images due to iron deposits in a dense tissue associated to a high signal intensity of an area of loose tissue with vacuolization [123].

*Carbonic anhydrase II deficiency* is a rare autosomal recessive disease characterized by mental retardation, orteopetrosis, renal tubular acidosis and cerebral calcifications involving the basal ganglia [124]. Many other inborn errors of metabolism are at the origin of basal ganglia MRI abnormalities, including calcifications *(Table I)*.

*Familial progressive encephalopathy with calcification of the basal ganglia* (**Aicardi-Goutières syndrome**) is a rare autosomal recessive disorder described in 1984 [125]. True incidence is not known, to date about 70 cases have been reported in the literature [126-128]. The major neurological features of the syndrome are relatively common and nonspecific, despite some strinking characteristiques [127].

Aicardi-Goutières syndrome (AGS) is a progressive encephalopathy of early onset, almost always in the first year of life, often actually present from birth. Cerebral calcifications, mostly located in the basal ganglia, are one of the striking features *(Figure 2)* and they are usually associated to white matter disease. The presence of a cerebrospinal fluid lymphocytosis and a raised level of CSF interpheron-alpha (INF-α) are findings of high diagnostic value. The syndrome has superficial resemblance to the neurological sequelae of congenital infection. However, search for microbiological and serological evidence of embryopathic infections are negative.

Extraneurological features may also be part of the clinical picture. The most prominent of these are cutaneous lesions affecting fingers and toes, sometimes also ear lobes, in the form of scaly erythematous rash with swelling and acrocyanotic appearance reminiscent of chilblains. Some patients show a transient hepatomegaly, sometimes with slight hypertransaminasemia, and a mild thrombocytopenia has been found in some cases. In a recent publication [126], Lanzi *et al.* discussed the clinical, neuroradiological and biological characteristics of 21 new cases and compared them with the 48 cases reported in the literature.

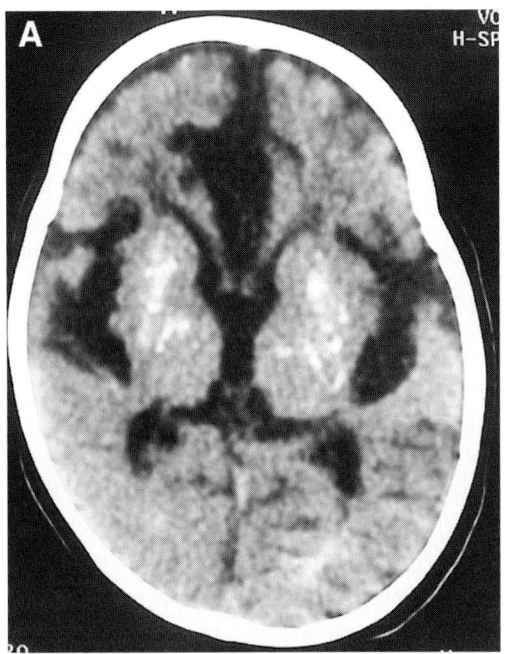

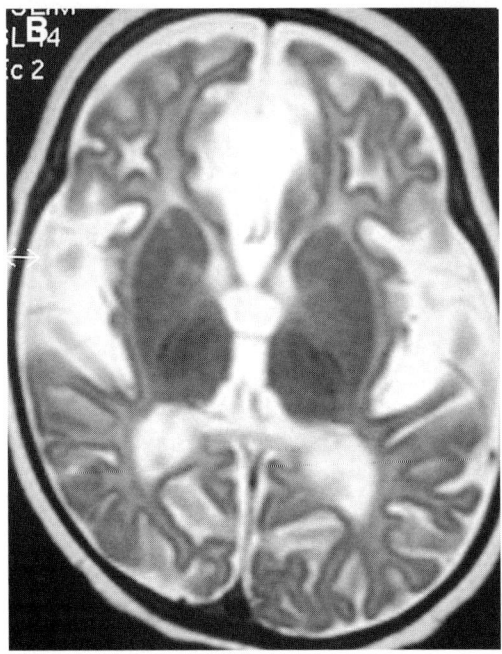

**Figure 2.** Aicardi-Goutières syndrome. CT scan (2A) is showing typical bilateral calcifications of the basal ganglia and Magnetic Resonance Imaging (2B) showing marked, diffuse atrophy.

The clinical picture in almost all of Lanzi's patients was characterized by severe neurodevelopmental delay and diffuse neurological signs, involving truncal hypotonia, generalized or peripheral hypertonia, pyramidal tract signs and reduced or absent vision with associated abnormal eye movements. Most patients developed microcephaly in the first months or years of life, a cardinal sign of the syndrome, which is usually not present at birth. Clear extrapyramidal signs, in the form of prominent dystonic movements and postures, and in some cases a very marked buccal-lingual dystonia, attacks of opisthotonos precipitated by minor external stimuli and persistence of asymmetrical tonic reflexes of the neck, were present in 50-85% of cases.

Calcifications were found in all cases, most often located in the basal ganglia. They could extend to the dentate nuclei, the white matter, in particular in the periventricular areas, and very occasionally the cortex. They have a punctuate appearance in the basal ganglia and are more widespread in the white matter. Cerebral atrophy, with ventricular and cortical sulci enlargement is also present in almost all cases. Leukodystrophy, localized prevalently around the ventricle horns, and cystic degeneration in cortical areas, are associated.

Chronic CSF lymphocytosis of variable degree is a consistent feature, particularly during the first year of life. However, the duration of this pleiocytosis is probably quite variable and remains to be defined more precisely. A relatively elevated level of protein in CSF, without oligoclonal banding or evidence of intrathecal synthesis, is associated in about half of the cases. Another major finding in laboratory investigations, demonstrated by Lebon et al. in 1988 [129], is the presence of high titres of interferon-$\alpha$ particularly in the CSF, but also in blood. It has become an essential diagnostic finding and is probably present in all cases, at least in the early stages of the syndrome. This finding has also been an important contribution to a better understanding of the physiopathology of the syndrome [130], whose main lesions appear to be a calcifying vasculitis involving both brain and systemis vessels [131]. This vasculitis is very similar to that induced in mice receiving astrocytes-targeted interferon [132, 133]. Although the cause of elevated INF-$\alpha$ levels remains unknown, recent investigations suggest that it may be due to a dysregulation by a mutated gene of the production of interferon [134-136].

The course of the syndrome is severe and prognosis, although not necessarily extremely bad in terms of survival during the first year of life, is really unfavourable in terms of neurological impairment. The symptoms are initially progressive, and seem to stabilize by the end of the second year of life. Serial laboratory measures, too, seem to support the hypothesis of a stabilisation of the syndrome. Pleocytosis and raised interferon-$\alpha$ in the CSF, can reach very high levels in the first months of life but tend to decrease over the years. Atypical forms of the syndrome exist. Mild clinical forms, with very mild neurological signs or no neurological signs at all, have been reported [137, 138]. Recently, three new cases with the classical clinical and neuroradiological characteristics have been reported, in which cerebrospinal fluid showed no lymphocytosis and no high levels of interferon-$\alpha$, but high levels of neopterin and biopterin combined with low levels of folates [139].

An autosomal recessive *congenital infection-like syndrome with microcephaly and intracranial calcification* (MICS, also called pseudo-TORCH syndrome or Baraitser-Reardon syndrome), sharing many features with Aicardi-Goutières syndrome, has also been described [65-68]. In MICS not only basal ganglia calcifications are present, but also microcephaly at birth, liver dysfunction and thrombocytopenia, signs that have also been reported in some cases of AGS. In MICS the presence of pleiocytosis in the CSF has been rarely found, while the presence of high levels of interferon-$\alpha$, though it has not been investigated, could be a point in favour of a diagnosis of Aicardi-Goutières syndrome. MICS is probably a heterogeneous group of diseases.

Other rare inherited congenital syndromes may evidence calcifications of the basal ganglia. A heredofamilial neurologic syndrome consisting in mental retardation associated with elevated CSF protein concentration and intracranial calcifications, mainly located in choroid plexuses, has been reported [140]. A probably autosomal dominant inherited syndrome consisting in symmetrical basal ganglia calcifications associated with retinal degeneration has been described in three members of a family [141]. *Raine syndrome* is a rare autosomal recessive inherited disorder characterised by generalised osteosclerosis with craniofacial anomalies and intracranial calcifications involving the basal ganglia [142]. A congenital recessively inherited syndrome, showing craniosynostosis, basal ganglia calcification and mild facial dysmorphism has also been described [143]. Basal ganglia calcifications have also been reported in some cases of *cerebro-oculo-facio-skeletal (COFS) syndrome*, of autosomal recessive inheritance [144, 145]. A familial syndrome associating Coat's disease, an idiopathic exudative retinopathy, with basal ganglia calcifications and other features has been reported [146-148]. Movement disorders have not been reported in any of these syndromes, despite the basal ganglia involvement.

*Cockayne syndrome* is an autosomal recessive inherited disorder of DNA repair. Main clinical features are dwarfism, microcephaly, mental retardation, ocular and hearing abnormalities, photosensitivity and progeroid appearance. Gait disturbances are frequent, and movement disorders, mainly dystonia, may be present. Neuroimaging studies typically disclose generalized atrophy, leukodystrophy and basal ganglia calcification [149-151]. In *congenital ichthyosis with trichothiodystrophy* (Tay syndrome), another autosomal recessive inherited disorder of DNA repair, basal ganglia calcification has been occasionally reported.

Neuroimaging abnormalities of the basal ganglia may also be found in patients with *infantile neuroaxonal dystrophy* (INAD), an early-onset autosomal recessive neurodegenerative disease clinically characterized by developmental regression leading to spastic tetraparesis, blindness, deafness and dementia. MRI evidences cerebellar atrophy and high-intensity-lesions on T2-weighted sequences mainly involving basal ganglia, cerebellum and deep white matter [152]. Cases with basal ganglia calcification have also been reported [153, 154].

Cerebral calcifications mainly involving temporal lobes, but sometimes extending to basal ganglia, have been described in *lipoid proteinosis*, an autosomal recessive inherited disorder characterized by widespread deposition of eosinophilic hyaline-like material in the skin, mucous membranes and some internal organs [155, 156].

*Huntington's disease* (HD) is an autosomal dominantly inherited disorder due to an intragenic expansion of a CAG trinucleotide repeat in the distal part of the short arm of chromosome 4 resulting in a wide expression of an abnormal protein named "huntingtin". Unlike the adult-onset form, juvenile HD is mostly characterized by a hypokinetic-rigid syndrome, while chorea is rare. Epileptic seizures, intellectual regression and behavioural disorders are other frequent features. Although it may be normal at the early stages of the illness, neuroimaging often discloses abnormalities of the basal ganglia. Atrophy of the caudate nucleus on CT scan has been largely reported, and recently related to the number of CAG trinucleotides and the severity of clinical expression [157, 158]. High-signal-lesions on T2-weighted MRI in the atrophic caudate nuclei and putamina are additional features [159].

*Dentatorubral-pallidoluysian atrophy* (DRPLA) is a rare, autosomal dominant neurodegenerative disorder, mainly diagnosed in Japan, attributed to CAG trinucleotide repeat expansion in the DRPLA gene on chromosome 12. Main clinical manifestations in the juvenile-onset form are myoclonic epilepsy and mental retardation or developmental regression, although cerebellar ataxia, choreoathetosis and dementia, more typical of adult-onset forms, may be present too. MRI discloses cortical, brain stem and cerebellar atrophy and high-signal lesions on T2-weighted sequences in white matter, globus pallidus, thalamus, midbrain and pons, showing a positive correlation with the patient's age and the size of the expanded CAG repeat [160, 161].

*Wilson's disease* (WD), or familial progressive hepatolenticular degeneration, is an autosomal recessive disorder, due to different mutations of WD gene mapped to chromosome 13, resulting in a defect of P-type ATPases involved in the cellular transport of copper and ensuing abnormal deposition of this metal in liver, brain, cornea and other tissues. Neurological involvement is present in 90% of cases, and usually manifests after the age of 10 years, mainly in the form of a dystonic syndrome, although chorea, tremor, asterixis and, less frequently, Parkinsonism may also be present. Epileptic seizures, mental deterioration and psychiatric disorders are frequent too. The Kayser-Fleischer ring surrounding the corneal limb and representing a granular deposit of copper in Descemet's membrane is practically pathognomonic for WD. CT scan shows brain atrophy and areas of hypodensity in putamen, caudate, dentate, red nucleus and cerebellar cortex [162]. MRI, more sensitive, discloses hypointensity in T1-weighted and hyperintensity in T2-weighted sequences in lenticular nuclei, thalami, brainstem, claustrum and white matter [163, 164], and sometimes cavitation in basal ganglia and thalami [165]. Hyperintensity in T1-weighted and hypointensity in T2-weighted sequences have been also reported, maybe related to a paramagnetic effect of copper deposition [166]. These neuroimaging abnormalities decrease and may disappear following chelating therapy.

Finally, in patients with *Down syndrome* a high incidence of calcification of the basal ganglia on CT scan, until 85% in some series, has been described [167]. Basal ganglia calcification are mainly located in the globus pallidus and become more prominent with increased age, so they may be considered as representing premature aging. Calcification and amyloid degeneration of the adjacent blood vessels are present, suggesting a physiopathogenic relationship. Despite the presence of basal ganglia lesions, clinical manifestations in the form of movement disorders are not present. In a report of a patient with Down syndrome who presented with movement disorders, CT scan disclosed bilateral calcification in the globus pallidus which resembled a sign of premature aging but the clinical course and MRI findings resembled those of Hallervorden-Spatz syndrome [168].

## ■ "Idiopathic" calcification of the basal ganglia

Calcification of the basal ganglia and other intracranial structures not associated with disorders of calcium metabolism, somatic abnormalities or a variety of other recognizable causes (*e.g.* "physiological" age-related calcification, birth anoxia, CO intoxication, lead poisoning, tuberous sclerosis, Cockayne's syndrome, Down's syndrome, postinfectious, AIDS, radiation therapy, methotrexate therapy, mitochondrial diseases, familial encephalopathies) has been observed, as either a familial – mostly inherited as an autosomal dominant trait – or a sporadic condition.

*Bilateral striato-pallido-dentate calcinosis* (BSPDC) is a rare disorder histologically characterized by calcification of small cerebral vessels which predominates in the basal ganglia but also involves the thalamus and dentate nuclei as well as the cerebral and cerebellar white matter [169-171].

Clinical distinction of BSPDC has been blurred by a variety of factors. There has been a lack of consistent terminology when reporting this "neuro-mineral" disease. A plethora of descriptive terms have been used, such as symmetric cerebral calcification, idiopathic calcification of cerebral capillaries, symmetrical calcification of the basal ganglia, idiopathic non-arteriosclerotic calcification of cerebral vessels, idiopathic familial cerebrovascular ferrocalcinosis, symmetrical intracranial advanced pseudocalcium, pallido-dentate calcifications, idiopathic basal ganglia calcification and others with a total of 35 names [170] resulting in considerable confusion as to what cases constitute BSPDC.

Pathological studies show that calcium is the major element present and it accounts for the radiological appearance of the disease. BSPDC is a very rare disorder, and less than one hundred cases have been described. Extremely rare in children, it is hard to diagnose BSPDC in the first or second decade of life without neuroimaging or an evident family history, because most of the patients, despite multiple calcifications, usually do not reveal any signs until the third decade of life. About 50% are asymptomatic even at late age. Symptoms mainly consist of mental deterioration, dysarthria and movement disorders, including Parkinsonism [172] and abnormal movements. One case of a 12-year-old girl with transient Parkinsonism has been reported [173]. In a recent review [174], clinical and radiological features of the 38 patients in the BSPDC Registry (including patients referred to this registry between 1985 and 1997) have been discussed and compared with the 61 patients with BSPDC reported in 20 other publications. Of the 99 patients, 73 belonged to 14 families with autosomal dominant inheritance, 12 from 5 families were grouped under "familial" without a clear pattern of inheritance and 14 were sporadic. Of the 99 patients, 67 were symptomatic and 32 were asymptomatic at the time of evaluation. The mean age of the symptomatic group (47 ± 15) was significantly higher than the mean age of the asymptomatic group (32 ± 20). Symptomatic patients had a substantially greater amount of calcifications in all regions, with statistically significant differences in dentate nucleus and centrum semiovale. The most common manifestation was a movement disorder (55%). Parkinsonism accounted for over half of all movement disorders (57%), while the hyperkinetic movement disorders accounted for the rest (chorea 19%, tremor

8%, dystonia 8% and athetosis 5%). Cognitive impairment was the second most common manifestation followed by cerebellar impairment and speech disorder. Seizures were present in 9%.

## Conclusions

Calcifications of the basal ganglia are rare in children. When present they are almost always suggestive of an underlying neurological disorder but not pathognomonic. Furthermore, no direct clinico-pathological correlation can be established between a movement disorder and basal ganglia calcification or other neuroimaging abnormalities, the underlying physiopathological mechanisms remaining largely obscure and subject to further research. In the presence of basal ganglia calcifications, or other MRI abnormalities, and movement disorders, the associated symptoms and findings must also be taken into account in order to achieve a diagnosis.

## References

1. Delacour A. Ossification des capillaires du cerveau. *Ann Med Psychol* 1850; 2: 486-61.
2. Fahr I. Idiopathische verkalking der hirume fasse. *Zbl Allf Path* 1930; 50: 129-33.
3. Klein C, Vieregge P. The confusing history of "Fahr's disease". *Neurology* 1998; 50 (Suppl 4): A59.
4. Koller WC, Cochran JW, Klawans HL. Calcification of the basal ganglia: computerized tomography and clinical correlation. *Neurology* 1979; 29 (3): 328-33.
5. Harrington MG, MacPherson P, McIntosh WB, *et al*. The significance of the incidental finding of basal ganglia calcification on computerized tomography. *J Neurol Neurosurg Psychiatry* 1981; 44: 1168-70.
6. Kendall B, Cavanagh N. Intracranial calcifications in paediatric computed tomography. *Neuroradiology* 1986; 28: 234-330.
7. Aicardi J. *Diseases of the nervous system in childhood*. 2nd ed. London: Mac Keith Press, 1998.
8. Barkovich AJ. "Toxic and metabolic brain disorders". In: Barkovich AJ. *Pediatric Neuroimaging*. 3rd ed. USA: Lippincott Williams & Wilkins, 2000, p. 71-156.
9. Fernández-Alvarez E, Aicardi J. "Diseases with several types of movement disorders". In: Fernandez-Alvarez E, Aicardi J. *Movement disorders in children*. 1st ed. London: Mac Keith Press, 2001, p. 130-51.
10. Janavs JL, Aminoff MJ. Dystonia and chorea in acquired systemic disorders. *J Neurol Neurosurg Psychiatry* 1998; 65 (4): 436-45.
11. Kumar A. Movement disorders in the tropics. *Parkinsonism Relat Disord* 2002; 9 (2): 69-75.
12. Dickson DW, Belman AI, Park YD, Wiley C, Horoupian DS, Llena J, Kure K, Lyman WD, Morecki R, Mitsudo S, *et al*. Central nervous system pathology in pediatric AIDS: an autopsy study. *APMIS Suppl* 1989; 8: 40-57.
13. Kauffman WM, Sivit CJ, Fitz CR, *et al*. CT and MR evaluation of intracranial involvement in paediatric HIV infection: A clinical-imaging correlation. *AJNR Am J Neuroradiol* 1992; 13: 949-57.
14. Iranzo A, Kulisevsky J, Cadafalch J, Serrano C, Grau JM. Movement disorders in AIDS. *Neurologia* 1996; 11 (2): 70-5.
15. Mattos JP, Rosso AL, Correa RB, Novis SA. Movement disorders in 28 HIV-infected patients. *Arq Neuropsiquatr* 2002; 60 (3-A): 525-30.
16. Gollomp SM, Fahn S. Transient dystonia as a complication of varicella. *J Neurol Neurosurg Psyquiatry* 1987; 50: 1228-9.

17. Darling CF, Larsen MB, Byrd SE, Radkowski MA, Palka PS, Allen ED. MRI and CT imaging patterns in post-varicella encephalitis *Pediatr Radiol.* 1995; 25 (4): 241-4.
18. Shanks DE, Blasco PA, Chason DP. Movement disorders following herpes simplex encephalitis. *Dev Med Chlid Neurol* 1991; 33: 343-55.
19. Barthez-Carpentier MA, Rozemberg F, Dussaix E, Lebon P, Goudeau A, Billard C, Tardieu M. Relapse of herpes simplex encephalitis. *J Child Neurol* 1995; 10 (5): 363-8.
20. Hargrave DR, Webb DW. Movement disorders in association with herpes simplex virus encephalitis in children: a review. *Dev Med Child Neurol* 1998; 40 (9): 640-2.
21. Peters AC, Vielvoye GJ, Versteeg J, et al. ECHO 25 focal encephalitis and subacute chorea. *Neurology* 1979; 29: 676-81.
22. Hsieh JC, Lue KH, Lee YL. Parkinson-like syndrome as the major presenting symptom of Epstein-Barr virus encephalitis. *Arch Dis Child* 2002; 87 (4): 358.
23. Sejvar JJ, Haddad MB, Tierney BC, Campbell GL, Marfin AA, Van Gerpen JA, Fleischauer A, Leis AA, Stokic DS, Petersen LR. Neurologic manifestations and outcome of West Nile virus infection. *JAMA* 2003; 290 (4): 511-5.
24. Misra UK, Kalita J. Movement disorders in Japanese encephalitis. *J Neurol* 1997; 244 (5): 299-303.
25. Murgod UA, Muthane UB, Ravi V, Radhesh S, Desai A. Persistent movement disorders following Japanese encephalitis. *Neurology* 2001; 57 (12): 2313-5.
26. Cardoso F, Eduardo C, Silva AP, et al. Chorea in 50 consecutive patients with rheumatic fever. *Mov Disord* 1997; 12: 701-3.
27. Giedd JN, Rapoport JL, Kruesi MJ, et al. Sydenham's chorea: magnetic resonance imaging of the basal ganglia. *Neurology* 1995; 45: 2199-202.
28. Goldman S, Amrom D, Szliwowski HB, et al. Reversible striatal hypermetabolism in a case of Sydenham's chorea. *Mov Disord* 1993; 8: 355-8.
29. Burstein L, Breningstall GN. Movement disorders in bacterial meningitis. *J Pediatr* 1986; 109 (2): 260-4.
30. Kim JS, Choi IS, Lee MC. Reversible Parkinsonism and dystonia following probable Mycoplasma pneumoniae infection. *Mov Disord* 1995; 10: 510-2.
31. Zambrino CA, Zorzi G, Lanzi G. Bilateral striatal necrosis associated with Mycoplasma pneumoniae infection in an adolestent: clinical and neuroradiologic follow-up. *Mov Disord* 2000; 15 (5): 1023-6.
32. Udani PM, Parekh UC, Dastur DK. Neurological and related syndromes in CNS tuberculosis. Clinical features and pathogenesis. *J Neurol Sci* 1971; 14 (3): 341-57.
33. Alarcon F, Duenas G, Cevallos N, Lees AJ. Movement disorders in 30 patients with tuberculous meningitis. *Mov Disord* 2001; 15 (3): 561-9.
34. Serrano-Duenas M. Tuberculous meningitis and dystonia. *Mov Disord* 2001; 16 (3): 582-3.
35. Duggan AJ, Hutchinson MP. Sleeping sickness in Europeans: a review of 109 cases. *J Trop Med Hyg* 1966; 69 (6): 124-31.
36. White RJ. "Malaria". In: Cook GC, editor. *Manson's Tropical Diseases.* London: W.B. Saunders, 1997, p. 1087-164.
37. Cosentino C, Velez M, Torres L, Garcia HH, Cysticercosis working group in Perú. Cysticercosis lesions in basal ganglia are common but clinically silent. *Clin Neurol Neurosurg* 2002; 104 (1): 57-60.
38. Anbu AT, Foulerton M, McMaster P, Bakalinova D. Basal ganglia involvement in a child with cat-scratch disease. *Pediatr Infect Dis J* 2003; 22 (10): 931-2.
39. Dale RC, de Sousa C, Chong WK, Cox TC, Harding B, Neville BG. Acute disseminated encephalomyelitis, multiphasic disseminated encephalomyelitis and multiple sclerosis in children. *Brain* 2000; 123 (Pt 12): 2407-22.
40. Tenembaum S, Chamoles N, Fejerman N. Acute disseminated encephalomyelitis: a long-term follow-up study of 84 pediatric patients. *Neurology* 2002; 59 (8): 1224-31.

41. Goutieres F, Aicardi J. Acute neurological dysfunction associated with destructive lesions of the basal ganglia in children. Ann Neurol 1982; 12 (4): 328-32.
42. Black DN, Watters GV, Andermann E, Dumont C, Kabay ME, Kaplan P, Meagher-Villemure K, Michaud J, O'Gorman G, Reece E, et al. Encephalitis among Cree children of northern Quebec. Ann Neurol 1988; 24 (4): 483-9.
43. Lebon P, Meritet JF, Krivine A, Rozenberg F. Interferon and Aicardi-Goutieres syndrome. Eur J Paediatr Neurol 2002; 6 (Suppl A): A47-53.
44. Bhatjiwale MG, Polkey C, Cox TC, Dean A, Deasy N. Rasmussen's encephalitis: neuroimaging findings in 21 patients with a closer look at the basal ganglia. Pediatr Neurosurg 1998; 29: 142-8.
45. Ben Zeev B, Nass D, Polack S, Manor Y, Duudevani P, Mendelson A, Goshen E, Zvas Z, et al. Progressive unilateral basal ganglia atrophy and hemidystonia: A new form of chronic focal viral encephalitis. Neurology 1999; 51 (Suppl 1).
46. Andermann F. Rasmussen Syndrome and movement disorder. Mov Disord 2002; 17 (3): 437-8.
47. Frucht S. Dystonia, athetosis and epilepsia partialis continua in a patient with late-onset Rasmussen's encephalitis. Mov Disord 2002; 17 (3): 609-12.
48. Hart Y. Rasmussen's encephalitis. Epileptic Disord. 2004; 6 (3): 133-44.
49. Nordstrom DM, West SG, Andersen PA. Basal ganglia calcifications in central nervous system lupus erythematosus. Arthritis Rheum 1985; 28 (12): 1412-6.
50. Bruyn GW, Padberg G. Chorea and systemic lupus erythematosus. A critical review. Eur Neurol 1984; 23 (6): 435-48.
51. Shahar E, Goshen E, Tauber Z, Lahat E. Parkinsonian syndrome complicating systemic lupus erythematosus. Pediatr Neurol 1998; 18 (5): 456-8.
52. Garcia-Moreno JM, Chacon J. Juvenile Parkinsonism as a manifestation of systemic lupus erythematosus: case report and review of the literature. Mov Disord 2002; 17 (6): 1329-35.
53. Asherson RA, Khamashta MA, Ordi-Ros J, et al. The primary antiphosholipid syndrome: major clinical and serological features. Medicine 1989; 68: 366-74.
54. Angelini L, Rumi V, Nardocci N, Combi ML, Bruzzone MG, Pellegrini G. Hemidystonia symptomatic of primary antiphospholipid syndrome in childhood. Mov Disord 1993; 8 (3): 383-6.
55. DiMario FJ Jr, Bronte-Stewart H, Sherbotie J, Turner ME. Lacunar infarction of the basal ganglia as a complication of hemolytic-uremic syndrome. MRI and clinical correlations. Clin Pediatr (Phila) 1987; 26 (11): 586-90.
56. Hue V, Leclerc F, Martinot A, Vallee L, Saunier P. Striatal involvement with abnormal movements in hemolytic-uremic syndrome. Arch Fr Pediatr 1992; 49 (4): 369-71.
57. Barnett ND, Kaplan AM, Bernes SM, Cohen ML. Hemolytic uremic syndrome with particular involvement of basal ganglia and favorable outcome. Pediatr Neurol 1995; 12 (2): 155-8.
58. Hawker K, Lang AE. Hypoxic ischemic damage of the basal ganglia: case report and review of the literature. Mov Disord 1990; 5: 219-24.
59. Scott BL, Jankovic J. Delayed-onset progressive movement disorders after static brain lesions. Neurology 1996; 46: 68-74.
60. Burke RE, Fahn S, Gold AP. Delayed-onset dystonia in patients with "static" encephalopathy. J Neurol Neurosurg Psychiatry 1980; 43: 789-97.
61. Saint Hilaire MH, Burke RE, Bressman SB, et al. Delayed-onset dystonia due to perinatal or early childhood asphyxia. Neurology 1991; 41: 216-22.
62. Rosenbloom L. Dyskinetic cerebral palsy and birth asphyxia. Dev Med Child Neurol 1994; 36 (4): 285-9.
63. Carpenter MB. Athetosis and the basal ganglia. Arch Neurol Psychiatry 1977; 63: 875-901.
64. Abuelo DN, Barsel-Bowers G, Tutschka BG, Ambler M, Singer DB. Symmetrical infantile thalamic degeneration in two sibs. J Med Genet 1981; 18 (6): 448-50.

65. DiMario FJ Jr, Clancy R. Symmetrical thalamic degeneration with calcifications of infancy. *Am J Dis Child* 1989; 143 (9): 1056-60.

66. Bhatt MH, Obeso JA, Marsden CD. Time course of postanoxic akinetic-rigid and dystonic syndromes. *Neurology* 1993; 43; 314-7.

67. Kupsky WJ, Drozd MA, Barlow CF. Selective injury of the glous pallidus in children with post-cardiac surgery choreic syndrome. *Dev Med Child Neurol* 1995; 37: 135-44.

68. Sasaki T, Kurita H, Saito I, Kawamoto S, Nemoto S, Terahara A, Kirino T, Takakura K. Arteriovenous malformations in the basal ganglia and thalamus: management and results in 101 cases. *J Neurosurg* 1998; 88 (2): 285-92.

69. Fleetwood IG, Marcellus ML, Levy RP, Marks MP, Steinberg GK. Deep arteriovenous malformations of the basal ganglia and thalamus: natural history. *J Neurosurg* 2003; 98 (4): 747-50.

70. Lehmann P, Toussaint P, Depriester C, Legars D, Deramond H. Lenticulostriate aneurysms. Radioclinical study. *J Neuroradiol* 2003; 30 (2): 115-20.

71. Krauss JK, Kiriyanthan GD, Borremans JJ. Cerebral arteriovenous malformations and movement disorders. *Clin Neurol Neurosurg* 1999; 101 (2): 92-9.

72. Barabas G, Tucker SM. Idiopathic hypoparathyroidism and paroxysmal dystonic choreoathetosis. *Ann Neurol* 1988; 24 (4): 585.

73. Cheek JC, Riggs JE, Lilly RL. Extensive brain calcification and progressive dysarthria and dysphagia associated with chronic hypoparathyroidism. *Arch Neurol* 1990; 47 (9): 1038-9.

74. Jorens PG, Appel BJ, Hilte FA, Mahler C, De Deyn PP. Basal ganglia calcifications in postoperative hypoparathyroidism: a case with unusual characteristics. *Acta Neurol Scand* 1991; 83 (2): 137-40.

75. Evans BK, Donley DK. Pseudohypoparathyroidism, Parkinsonism syndrome, with no basal ganglia calcification. *J Neurol Neurosurg Psychiatry* 1988; 51 (5): 709-13.

76. Tabaee-Zadeh MJ, Frame B, Kapphahn K. Kinesiogenic choreoathetosis and idiopathic hypoparathyroidism. *N Engl J Med* 1972; 286 (14): 762-3.

77. Goel A, Bhatnagar MK, Vashishta A, Verma NP. Hypoparathyroidism with extensive intracranial calcification: a case report. *Postgrad Med J* 1994; 70 (830): 913-5.

78. Hattori H, Yorifuji T. Infantile convulsions and paroxysmal kinesigenic choreoathetosis in a patient with idiopathic hypoparathyroidism. *Brain Dev* 2000; 22 (7): 449-50.

79. Kartin P, Zupevc M, Pogacnik T, Cerk M. Calcification of basal ganglia, postoperative hypoparathyroidism and extrapyramidal, cerebellar, pyramidal motor manifestations. *J Neurol* 1982; 227 (3): 171-6.

80. Siejka SJ, Knezevic WV, Pullan PT. Dystonia and intracerebral calcification: pseudohypoparathyroidism presenting in an eleven-year-old girl. *Aust NZJ Med* 1988; 18 (4): 607-9.

81. Blin O, Masson G, Serratrice G. Blepharospasm associated with pseudohypoparathyroidism and bilateral basal ganglia calcifications. *Mov Disord* 1991; 6 (4): 379.

82. Moriwaki Y, Matsui K, Yamamoto T, Hada T, Higashino K. Cerebral subcortical calcification and hypoparathyroidism – a case report and review of the literature. *Jpn J Med* 1985; 24 (1): 53-6.

83. Uncini A, Tartaro A, Di Stefano E, Gambi D. Parkinsonism, basal ganglia calcification and epilepsy as late complications of postoperative hypoparathyroidism. *J Neurol* 1985; 232 (2): 109-11.

84. Tambyah PA, Ong BK, Lee KO. Reversible Parkinsonism and asymptomatic hypocalcemia with basal ganglia calcification from hypoparathyroidism 26 years after thyroid surgery. *Am J Med* 1993; 94 (4): 444-5.

85. Pearson DW, Durward WF, Fogelman I, Boyle IT, Beastall G. Pseudohypoparathyroidism presenting as severe Parkinsonism. *Postgrad Med J* 1981; 57 (669): 445-7.

86. Klawans HL, Lupton M, Simon L. Calcification of the basal ganglia as a cause of levodopa-resistant Parkinsonism. *Neurology* 1976; 26 (3): 221-5.

87. Berendes K, Dorstelmann D. Unsuccessful treatment with levodopa of a parkinsonian patient with calcification of the basal ganglia. *J Neurol* 1978; 218 (1): 51-4.

88. Arii J, Tanabe Y, Makino M, Sato H, Kohno Y. Children with irreversible brain damage associated with hypothyroidism and multiple intracranial calcifications. *J Child Neurol* 2002; 17 (4): 309-13.
89. Choi IS. Delayed neurological sequelae in carbon monoxide intoxication. *Arch Neurol* 1983; 40: 433-5.
90. Illum F. Calcification of the basal ganglia following carbon monoxide poisoning. *Neuroradiology* 1980; 19 (4): 213-4.
91. Lugaresi A, Montagna P, Morreale A, Gallassi R. "Psychic akinesia" following carbon monoxide poisoning. *Eur Neurol* 1990; 30 (3): 167-9.
92. Sawada Y, Takahashi M, Ohashi N, Fusamoto H, Maemura K, Kobayashi H, Yoshioka T, Sugimoto T. Computerised tomography as an indication of long-term outcome after acute carbon monoxide poisoning. *Lancet* 1980; 1 (8172): 783-4.
93. Reyes PF, Gonzalez CF, Zalewska MK, Besarab A. Intracranial calcification in adults with chronic lead exposure. *AJR Am J Roentgenol* 1986; 146 (2): 267-70.
94. Louis ED. Etiology of essential tremor: should we be searching for environmental causes? *Mov Disord* 2001; 16 (5): 822-9.
95. Coulehan JL, Hirsch W, Brillman J, Sanadria J, Welty TK, Colaiaco P, Koros A, Lober A. Gasoline sniffing and lead toxicity in Navajo adolescents. *Pediatrics* 1983; 71: 113-7.
96. Goldings AS, Stewart RM. Organic lead encephalopathy: behavioral change and movement disorder following gasoline inhalation. *J Clin Psychiatry* 1982; 43 (2): 70-2.
97. Komaki H, Maisawa S, Sugai K, Kobayashi Y, Hashimoto T. Tremor and seizures associated with chronic manganese intoxication. *Brain Dev* 1999; 21: 122-4.
98. Mirowitz SA, Westrich TJ, Hirsch JD. Hyperintense basal ganglia on T1-weighted MR images in patients receiving parenteral nutrition. *Radiology* 1991; 181 (1): 117-20.
99. Valenzuela R, Court J, Godoy J. Delayed cyanide induced dystonia. *J Neurol Neurosurg Psychiatry* 1992; 55: 198-9.
100. Hormes JT, Filley CM, Rosemberg NL. Neurologic sequelae of chronic solvent abuse. *Neurology* 1986; 36: 698-702.
101. Duckett S. Abnormal deposits of chromium in the pathological human brain. *J Neurol Neurosurg Psychiatry* 1986; 49 (3): 296-301.
102. Zaccara G, Cincotta M, Borgheresi A, Balestrieri F. Adverse motor effects induced by antiepileptic drugs. *Epileptic Disord* 2004; 6 (3): 153-68.
103. Nausieda PA, Koller WC, Weiner WJ, et al. Chorea induced by oral contraceptives. *Neurology* 1979; 29: 1605-9.
104. Pranzatelli MR, Albin RL, Cohen BH. Acute dyskinesias in young asthmatics treated with theophylline. *Pediatr Neurol* 1991; 7: 216-9.
105. Stuart AM, Worley ML, Spillane J. Choreiform movements observed in an 8-year-old child following use of an oral theophylline preparation. *Clin Pediatr (Phila)* 1992; 31: 692-3.
106. Harwood-Nash DC, Reilly BJ. Calcification of the basal ganglia following radiation therapy. *Am J Roentgenol Radium Ther Nucl Med* 1970; 108 (2): 392-5.
107. Numaguchi Y, Hoffman JC Jr, Sones PJ Jr. Basal ganglia calcification as a late radiation effect. *Am J Roentgenol Radium Ther Nucl Med* 1975; 123 (1): 27-30.
108. Lee KF, Suh JH. CT evidence of grey matter calcification secondary to radiation therapy. *Comput Tomogr* 1977; 1(1): 103-10.
109. Smith D, Bloch S, Al-Rashid RA. Basal ganglia calcification on CT scanning in children with acute lymphocytic leukemia. *Neuroradiology* 1980; 20 (2): 91-3.
110. Lichtor T, Wollmann RL, Brown FD. Calcified basal ganglionic mass 12 years after radiation therapy for medulloblastoma. *Surg Neurol* 1984; 21 (4): 373-6.
111. Fernandez-Bouzas A, Ramirez Jimenez H, Vazquez Zamudio J, Alonso-Vanegas M, Mendizabal Guerra R. Brain calcifications and dementia in children treated with radiotherapy and intrathecal methotrexate. *J Neurosurg Sci* 1992; 36 (4): 211-4.

112. Wick W, Hochberg F, O'Sullivan J, Goessling A, Hughes A, Cher L. L-dopa-resistant Parkinsonism syndrome following cerebral radiation therapy for neoplasm. *Oncol Rep* 2000; 7 (6): 1367-70.

113. Skiming JA, McDowell HP, Wright N, May P. Secondary Parkinsonism: an unusual late complication of craniospinal radiotherapy given to a 16-month child. *Med Pediatr Oncol* 2003; 40 (2): 132-4.

114. Igarashi M, Roy S 3rd, Stapleton FB. Cerebrovascular complications in children with nephrotic syndrome. *Pediatr Neurol* 1988; 4 (6): 362-5.

115. Black AS, Kanat IO. A review of soft tissue calcifications. *J Foot Surg* 1985; 24 (4): 243-50.

116. Fujioka M, Okuchi K, Hiramatsu KI, Sakaki T, Sakaguchi S, Ishii Y. Specific changes in human brain after hypoglycemic injury. *Stroke* 1997; 28 (3): 584-7.

117. Cubo E, Andres MT, Rojo A, Guerrero A, Urra DG, Mendez R. Neuroimaging of hypoglycemia. *Rev Neurol* 1998; 26 (153): 774-6.

118. Valanne L, Ketonen L, Majander A, Soumalainen A, Pihko H. Neuroradiologic findings in children with mitochondrial disorders. *AJNR Am J Neuroradiol* 1998; 19 (2): 369-77.

119. Huang CC, Wai YY, Chu NS, Liou CW, Pang CY, Shih KD, Wei YH. Mitochondrial encephalomyopathies: CT and MRI findings and correlations with clinical features. *Eur Neurol* 1995; 35 (4): 199-205.

120. Barkovich AJ, Good WV, Koch TK, Berg BO. Mitochondrial disorders: analysis of their clinical and imaging characteristics. *AJNR Am J Neuroradiol* 1993; 14 (5): 1119-37.

121. Hoon AH Jr, Reinhardt EM, Kelley RI, Breiter SN, Morton H, Johnston MV. Brain magnetic resonance imaging in suspected extrapyramidal cerebral palsy: observations in distinguishing genetic-metabolic from acquired causes. *J Pediatr* 1997; 131 (2): 240-5.

122. Hayflick SJ. Unraveling the Hallervorden-Spatz syndrome: pantothenate kinase-associated neurodegeneration is the name. *Curr Opin Pediatr* 2003; 15 (6): 572-7.

123. Savoiardo M, Halliday WC, Nardocci N, Strada L, D'Incerti L, Angelini L, Rumi V, Tesoro-Tess JD. Hallervorden-Spatz disease: MR and pathologic findings. *AJNR Am J Neuroradiol* 1993; 14 (1): 155-62.

124. Ohlsson A, Cumming WA, Paul A, Sly WS. Carbonic anhydrase II deficiency syndrome: recessive osteopetrosis with renal tubular acidosis and cerebral calcification. *Pediatrics* 1986; 77 (3): 371-81.

125. Aicardi J, Goutières F. A progressive familial encephalopathy in infancy with calcifications of the basal ganglia and chronic cerebrospinal fluid lymphocytosis. *Ann Neurol* 1984; 15: 49-54.

126. Lanzi G, Fazzi E, D'Arrigo S. Aicardi-Goutières syndrome: a description of 21 new cases and a comparison with the literature. *Eur J Paediatr Neurol* 2002; 6 (Suppl A): A9-22.

127. Aicardi J. Aicardi-Goutieres syndrome: special type early-onset encephalopathy. *Eur J Paediatr Neurol* 2002; 6 (Suppl A): A1-7.

128. San Antonio V, Sachs P, Monier A, Aicardi J, Evrard P, Arzimanoglou A. Aicardi-Goutières syndrome: a familial, sometimes unrecognised, early-onset encephalopathy. *Rev Neurol* 2005; 161: 4, 445-50.

129. Lebon P, Badoual J, Ponsot G, Goutières F, Hemeury-Cukier F, Aicardi J. Intrathecal synthesis of interferon-alpha in infants with progressive familial encephalopathy. *J Neurol Sciences* 1988; 84: 201-8.

130. Lebon P, Meritet JF, Krivine A, Rozenberg F. Interferon and Aicardi-Goutieres syndrome. *Eur J Paediatr Neurol* 2002; 6 (Suppl A): A47-53.

131. Barth PG. The neuropathology of Aicardi-Goutieres syndrome. *Eur J Paediatr Neurol* 2002; 6 (Suppl A): A27-31.

132. Akwa Y, Hasset DE, Eloranta ML, et al. Transgenic expression of IFN-$\alpha$ in the central nervous system of mice protects against lethal neurotropic viral infection but induces inflammation and neurodegeneration. *J Immunol* 1998; 161: 5016-26.

133. Campbell IL, Krucker T, Steffensen S, et al. Structural and functional neuropathology in transgenic mice with CNS expression of IFN-$\alpha$. *Brain Res* 1999; 835: 46-61.

134. Fauré S, Bordelais I, Marquette C, et al. Aicardi-Goutières syndrome: monogenic recessive disease, genetically heterogeneous disease, or multifactorial disease? *Clin Genet* 1999; 56: 149-53.

135. Crow YJ, Jackson AP, Roberts E, van Beusekom E, Barth P, Corry P, et al. Aicardi-Goutières syndrome displays genetic heterogeneity with one locus (AGS1) on chromosome 3p21. Am J Hum Genet 2000; 67 (1): 213-21.
136. Crow Y. The genetics of Aicardi-Goutières syndrome. Eur J Paediatr Neurol 2002; 6 (Suppl A): A33-5.
137. Mehta L, Trounce JO, Moore JR, Young ID. Familial calcification of the basal ganglia with cerebrospinal fluid pleocytosis. J Medl Genet 1986; 23: 157-60.
138. McEntargart M, Kamel H, Lebon P, King MD. Aicardi-Goutières syndrome: an expanding phenotype. Neuropediatrics 1998; 29: 163-7.
139. Blau N, Bonafe L, Krageloh-Mann I, Thony B, Kierat L, Hausler M, Ramaekers V. Cerebrospinal fluid pterins and folates in Aicardi-Goutieres syndrome: a new phenotype. Neurology 2003; 61 (5): 642-7.
140. Lott IT, Williams RS, Schnur JA, Hier DB. Familial amentia, unusual ventricular calcifications, and increased cerebrospinal fluid protein. Neurology 1979; 29 (12): 1571-7.
141. Hammerstein W, Bischof G, Keck E. A tapetoretinal degeneration with symmetrical calcifications of the basal ganglia. A hereditary disease. Eur Neurol 1982; 21 (4): 249-55.
142. Rickert CH, Rieder H, Rehder H, Hulskamp G, Hornig-Franz I, Louwen F, Paulus W. Neuropathology of Raine syndrome. Acta Neuropathol (Berl) 2002; 103 (3): 281-7.
143. Longman C, Whiteford M, Koppel D, Donaldson M, Paterson W, Tolmie J. Craniosynostosis associated with intracranial calcification: a novel recessive syndrome. Clin Dysmorphol 2003; 12 (4): 215-20.
144. Linna SL, Finni K, Simila S, Kouvalainen K, Laitinen J. Intracranial calcifications in cerebro-oculo-facio-skeletal (COFS) syndrome. Pediatr Radiol 1982; 12 (1): 28-30.
145. Abdel-Salam GM, Svekus A, Pelle Z, Halasz AA, Czeizel AE. Microcephaly, microphthalmia, congenital cataract, with calcification of the basal ganglia: MCA/MR syndrome. Genet Couns 2000; 11 (4): 391-7.
146. Goutieres F, Dollfus H, Becquet F, Dufier JL. Extensive brain calcification in two children with bilateral Coats' disease. Neuropediatrics 1999; 30 (1): 19-21.
147. Tolmie JL, Browne BH, McGettrick PM, Stephenson JB. A familial syndrome with coats' reaction retinal angiomas, hair and nail defects and intracranial calcification. Eye 1988; 2 (Pt 3): 297-303.
148. Crow YJ, McMenamin J, Haenggeli CA, Hadley DM, Tirupathi S, Treacy EP, Zuberi SM, Browne BH, Tolmie JL, Stephenson JB. Coats' plus: a progressive familial syndrome of bilateral coats' disease, characteristic cerebral calcification, leukoencephalopathy, slow pre- and post-natal linear growth and defects of bone marrow and integument. Neuropediatrics 2004; 35 (1): 10-9.
149. Levinson ED, Zimmerman AW, Grunnet ML, Lewis RA, Spackman TJ. Cockayne syndrome. J Comput Assist Tomogr 1982; 6 (6): 1172-4.
150. Demaerel P, Kendall BE, Kingsley D. Cranial CT and MRI in diseases with DNA repair defects. Neuroradiology 1992; 34 (2): 117-21.
151. Ozdirim E, Topcu M, Ozon A, Cila A. Cockayne syndrome: review of 25 cases. Pediatr Neurol 1996; 15 (4): 312-6.
152. Farina L, Nardocci N, Bruzzone MG, D'Incerti L, Zorzi G, Verga L, et al. Infantile neuroaxonal dystrophy: neuroradiological studies in 11 patients. Neuroradiology 1999; 41: 376-80.
153. Ramaekers VT, Lake BD, Harding B, Boyd S, Harden A, Brett EM, Wilson J. Diagnostic difficulties in infantile neuroaxonal dystrophy. A clinicopathological study of eight cases. Neuropediatrics 1987; 18 (3): 170-5.
154. Venkatesh S, Coulter DL, Kemper TD. Neuroaxonal dystrophy at birth with hypertonicity and basal ganglia mineralization. J Child Neurol 1994; 9: 74-6.
155. Emsley RA, Paster L. Lipoid proteinosis presenting with neuropsychiatric manifestations. J Neurol Neurosurg Psychiatry 1985; 48 (12): 1290-2.

156. Nagasaka T, Tanaka M, Ito D, Tanaka K, Shimizu H. Protean manifestations of lipoid proteinosis in a 16-year-old boy. *Clin Exp Dermatol* 2000; 25 (1): 30-2.
157. Roth J, Zidovska J, Ruzickova S, Havrdova E, Preiss M, Uhrova T, Linek V, Doubek P, Volfova M, Jech R, Bauer J, Ruzicka E. Huntington's disease: the relationship between clinical signs, CAG repeats and the atrophy of the caudate nucleus in CT scans. *Sb Lek* 1999; 100 (1): 39-44.
158. Culjkovic B, Stojkovic O, Vojvodic N, Svetel M, Rakic L, Romac S, Kostic V. Correlation between triplet repeat expansion and computed tomography measures of caudate nuclei atrophy in Huntington's disease. *J Neurol* 1999; 246 (11): 1090-3.
159. Ho VB, Chuang HS, Rovira MJ, Koo B. Juvenile Huntington disease: CT and MR features. *AJNR Am J Neuroradiol* 1995; 16 (7): 1405-12.
160. Miyazaki M, Kato T, Hashimoto T, Harada M, Kondo I, Kuroda Y. MR of childhood-onset dentatorubral-pallidoluysian atrophy. *AJNR Am J Neuroradiol* 1995; 16 (9): 1834-6.
161. Koide R, Onodera O, Ikeuchi T, Kondo R, Tanaka H, Tokiguchi S, et al. Atrophy of the cerebellum and brainstem in dentatorubral pallidoluysian atrophy. Influence of CAG repeat size on MRI findings. *Neurology* 1997; 49 (6): 1605-12.
162. Williams FJ, Walshe JM. Wilson's disease. An analysis of the cranial computerized tomographic appearances found in 60 patients and the changes in response to treatment with chelating agents. *Brain* 1981; 104: 735-52.
163. King AD, Walshe JM, Kendall BE, Chinn RJ, Paley MN, Wilkinson ID, Halligan S, Hall-Craggs MA. Cranial MR imaging in Wilson's disease. *AJR Am J Roentgenol* 1996; 167 (6): 1579-84.
164. Saatci I, Topcu M, Baltaoglu FF, Kose G, Yalaz K, Renda Y, Besim A. Cranial MR findings in Wilson's disease. *Acta Radiol* 1997; 38 (2): 250-8.
165. Sener RN. Wilson's disease: MRI demonstration of cavitations in basal ganglia and thalami. *Pediatr Radiol* 1993; 23 (2): 157.
166. Mochizuki H, Kamakura K, Masaki T, Okano M, Nagata N, Inui A, Fujisawa T, Kaji T. Atypical MRI features of Wilson's disease: high signal in globus pallidus on T1-weighted images. *Neuroradiology* 1997; 39 (3): 171-4.
167. Takashima S, Becker LE. Basal ganglia calcification in Down's syndrome. *J Neurol Neurosurg Psychiatry* 1985; 48 (1): 61-4.
168. Okano S, Takeuchi Y, Kohmura E, Yoshioka H, Sawada T. Globus pallidus calcification in Down syndrome with progressive neurologic deficits. *Pediatr Neurol* 1992; 8 (1): 72-4.
169. Ellie E, Julien J, Ferrer X. Familial idiopathic striopallidodentate calcifications. *Neurology* 1989; 39: 381-5.
170. Manyam BV. Bilateral strio-pallido-dentate calcinosis: a proposed classification of genetic and secondary causes. *Mov Disord* 1990; 5 (suppl 1): 94.
171. Maynam BV, Bhatt MH, Moore WD, Devleschoward AB, Anderson DR, Calne DB. Bilateral striopallidodentate calcinosis: cerebrospinal fluid, imaging and electrophysiological studies. *Ann Neurol* 1992; 31: 379-84.
172. Maynam BV, Walters AS, Keller IA, Ghobrial M. Parkinsonism associated with autosomal dominant bilateral striopallidodentate calcinosis. *Parkinsonism and related disorders* 2001; 7: 289-95.
173. Yoshikawa H, Abe T. Transient Parkinsonism in bilateral striopallidodentate calcinosis. *Pediatr Neurol* 2003; 29: 75-7.
174. Maynam BV, Walters AS, Koteswara RN. Bilateral striopallidodentate calcinosis: clinical characteristics of patients seen in a registry. *Mov Disord* 2001; 16 (2): 258-64.

# Clinical, biochemical and molecular spectrum of aromatic L-Amino acid decarboxylase deficiency

Roser Pons MD[1], Blair Ford MD[1], Claudia A Chiriboga MD[1], Peter T Clayton MD[2], Veronica Hinton PhD[1], Keith Hyland PhD[3], Radhakant Sharma PhD[3], Darryl C De Vivo MD[1]

[1] Departments of Neurology and Pediatrics, College of Physicians and Surgeons of Columbia University, New York, NY
[2] Biochemistry Endocrinology and Metabolism Unit, Institute of Child Health at Great Ormond Street Hospital, University College London
[3] Institute of Metabolic Disease, Baylor University Medical Center, Dallas TX

Monoamine neurotransmitters include the catecholamines dopamine, norepinephrine and epinephrine and the indolamine serotonin. These compounds have numerous actions including modulation of psychomotor function, hormone secretion, cardiovascular, respiratory and gastrointestinal control, sleep mechanisms, body temperature and pain [1].

Aromatic L-amino acid decarboxylase (AADC) plays an important role in the synthesis of monoamines. It is a pyridoxal-phosphate dependent enzyme that converts L-dopa to dopamine and 5-hydroxytryptophan to serotonin respectively *(Figure 1)*. The catabolism of monoamines leads to the formation of homovanillic acid (HVA) from dopamine and 5-hydroxyindolacetic acid (5-HIAA) from serotonin *(Figure 1)*. The levels of these metabolites in CSF reflect the turnover of monoamine neurotransmitters within the brain [1].

In 1992, Hyland et al described the first patients with AADC deficiency [2]. These twin boys presented with motor, extrapyramidal and autonomic symptoms, decreased monoamine metabolites in CSF and severe reductions in AADC activity. This first description was the result of careful neurological observations, deductions regarding biochemical pathophysiology, and advances in laboratory technique [1, 2]. After the description of the first prototype cases, many other affected individuals came to attention. Based on the published cases to date [2-15], the spectrum of the disorder is well described, although it seems likely that patients with mild degrees of AADC activity have not yet come to light.

Deficiency in the activity of AADC leads to a generalized deficiency of monoamine neurotransmitters and has multiple effects on the CNS and on autonomic and endocrine function. This enzyme deficiency is the model of a biochemical disorder in which clinical aspects lead to predictable clinical consequences. While the main features of the disorder represent some of the expected consequences of dopaminergic and serotoninergic deficiency, the symptoms are not readily or completely reversed by dopaminergic or serotoninergic medication. In addition, the devastating and irreversible developmental abnormalities present in many patients with AADC deficiency, including disturbances of language, cognition, and motor function, suggest that neurological development is critically altered by catecholamine deficiencies in ways that are currently beyond our understanding.

## ■ Clinical Presentation

Approximately half of the patients present during the neonatal period with feeding difficulties, autonomic dysfunction and hypotonia as the most common findings [13, 14]. Recently two patients with neonatal hypoglycemia were reported [15].

During the first months of life all patients show evidence of motor symptoms and dystonic crises (Table I). Motor symptoms include axial hypotonia, decreased spontaneous movements and failure to make motor acquisitions. Although axial hypotonia is always present, appendicular tone may be increased, decreased or fluctuating [14].

Motor acquisitions are minimal in most patients. Patients usually lie in a frog-like position with minimal flickering of fingers and toes, unable to use their hands, hold their head or roll over. However, phenotypic variability exists and in 2 cases [5, 14] there has been development of axial control by the age of 2-to-3 years before treatment was started.

All patients develop paroxysmal events within the first months of life (Table I). These events are oculogyric crises (OGC), a form of paroxysmal dystonia. Patients show eye deviation upward, convergent, or to the side. The duration of these events, which occur several times a day to several times a week, ranges from few seconds to hours. When the events are prolonged they are associated with motor changes such as opisthotonic posturing and tonic or dystonic posturing of the limbs. Generally the patients appear conscious, the majority look upset, very distressed or cry inconsolably. EEG is usually normal or shows nonspecific findings (14). On video-EEG monitoring, no ictal correlate has been noted [14].

Approximately 2/3 of patients show other type of movement disorders in addition to OGC (Tables I, II). The most frequent movement disorder noted are other types of dystonia, including limb dystonia, stimulus provoked dystonia and cervical and facial dystonia. In order of frequency dystonia is followed by myoclonus, prominent startle, and distal chorea. Choreoathetosis, athetosis, non-epileptic flexor spasms, tremor and head drops are less often reported [4, 6, 7]. Two patients developed parkinsonism at 6 years of age with hypokinesia, shuffling gait and postural instability [14].

Drug-induced dyskinesias manifesting as chorea and/or dystonia are common in these patients and they can be provoked by dopamine agonist, MAO inhibitors, serotonin re-uptake inhibitors and serotonin agonists [13-14].

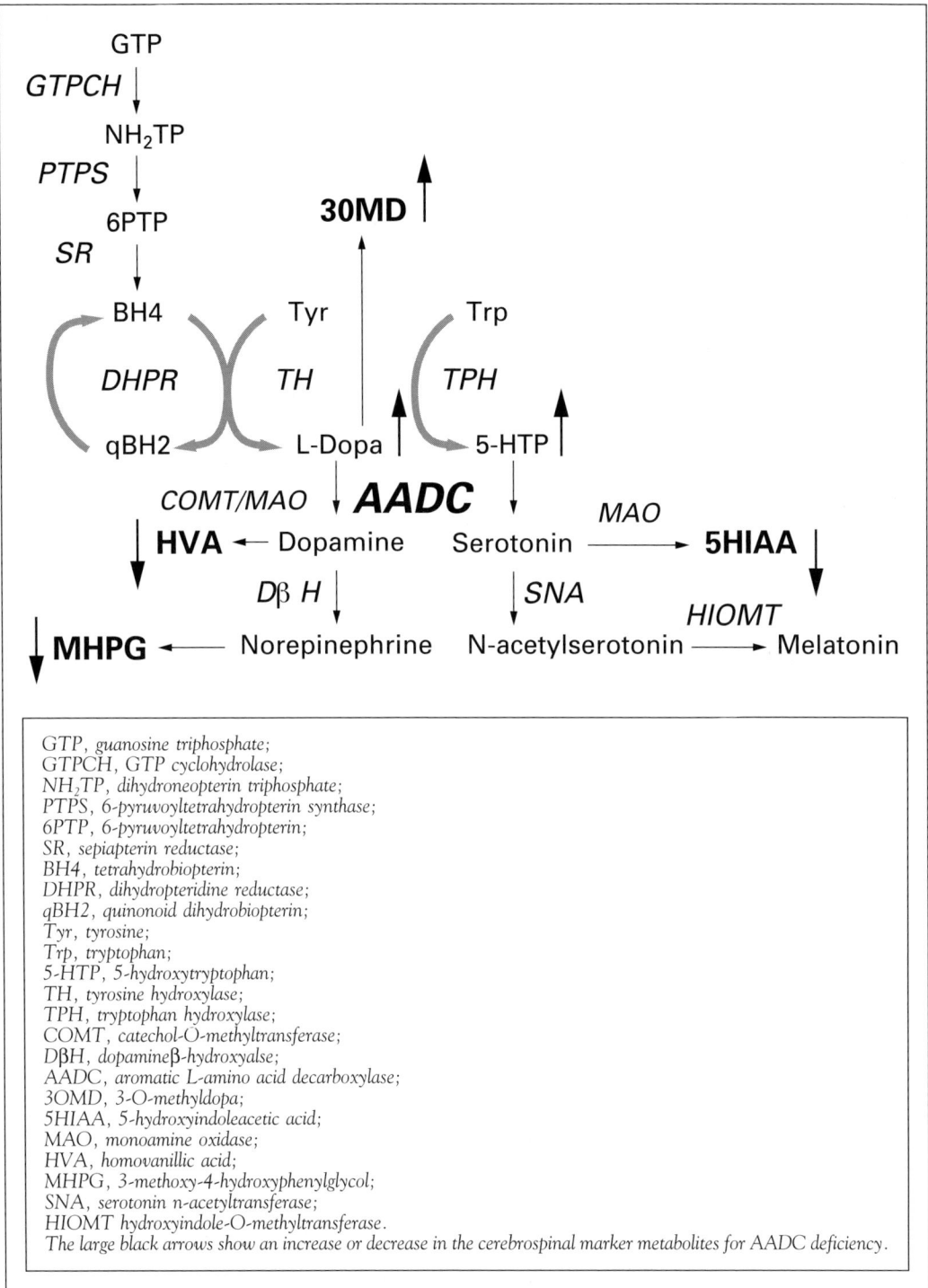

**Figure 1.** Central synthesis and catabolism of the catecholamines and serotonin.

Features of autonomic dysfunction are noted in most patients (Table I), most frequently excessive diaphoresis, temperature instability, nasal congestion, ptosis and miosis (Table III). Detailed testing of autonomic function has been reported in two patients, who showed severe impairment of sympathetic modulation in heart and blood vessels [13]. There was a tendency to suffer recurrent episodes of cardiorespiratory arrest provoked by painful stimuli in one patient, and this was attributed to the severe sympathetic dysfunction and the subsequent unopposed vagal tone [13].

Dysphoric mood is often noted (Table I). Parents may report inconsolable cry, irritability or moodiness. Sleep disturbances are also common (Table I) and they manifest as increased sleeping time or erratic sleep pattern with daytime sleepiness and/or frequent awakenings at night. These symptoms may be aggravated or precipitated by treatment.

Table I. AADC deficiency: main symptoms*.

| | |
|---|---|
| • Motor disturbance | 100% |
| • Oculogyric crises | 100% |
| • Autonomic dysfunction | 92% |
| • Other movement disorders | 69% |
| • Dysphoria | 69% |
| • Sleep disturbances | 62% |
| • Diurnal variation/improvement after sleep | 54% |

* Based on our series and the review of patients reported in the literature and described in sufficient detail [14].

Table II. AADC deficiency: movement disorders*.

- Dystonia:
    - Oculogyric Crises
    - Limb dystonia
    - Stimulus provoked dystonia
    - Cervicofacial dystonia
- Myoclonus/prominent startle
- Distal Chorea
- Parkinsonism
- Choreoathetosis/Athetosis
- Flexor spasms
- Tremor
- Head drops

* Shown in order of frequency.

Table III. AADC deficiency: autonomic dysfunction*.

- Diaphoresis
- Temperature instability
- Nasal congestion/hypersalivation
- Ptosis/pupilary changes
- Hypotension
- Bradyarrhytmia
- Poor distal perfusion
- GI dysmotility/Respiratory problems

* Shown in order of frequency.

Aggravation of neurologic symptoms late in the day and/or improvement by sleep is noted in half of the patients (Table I). This is reported as maximal motor activity in the morning or after a nap in the case of the more mobile patients; or by the occurrence of OGC mainly in the afternoon. The 2 patients with parkinsonism mentioned above showed this movement disorder in the afternoon, together with dysphoria and recurrent brief OGC. These symptoms resolved after a nap [14].

The cognitive function of these patients is very difficult to assess due to severe motor impairment. The majority are non-verbal, though they are often able to interact with the environment [13, 14]. Recently, a patient was reported who fulfilled DMS IV diagnostic criteria for autism [9]. The 3 more functional patients from our series made significant cognitive acquisitions. On testing, their cognitive functions placed them in the mild-to-moderate retardation range. They were cognisant of their surroundings, able to make their needs known, and responsive to educational interventions [14].

Neuroimaging studies are usually normal [2-4, 6, 7], though progressive brain atrophy has been reported in some patients [13]. F-18 Dopa PET scan in one patient revealed virtually absent uptake of tracer [13].

Endocrine dysfunction in these patients manifests as recurrent episodes of hypoglycemia [3, 13-15] and delayed bone maturation [3].

Other features include failure to thrive, hypersensitivity to light stimulation, tendency to breath-holding and apneic spells [13]. Recently one patient with generalized seizures at age 4 years was reported [13].

## ■ Diagnosis

All patients show the same pattern of CSF metabolites, pointing to a deficiency in the synthesis of monoamine neurotransmitters. This pattern includes reduced levels of HVA and 5-HIAA, indicating decreased synthesis of catecholamines and serotonin respectively, and increased levels of 3-O-methyldopa, which is the result of methylation of the accumulated precursor levodopa (Figure 1).

The diagnosis of AADC deficiency is confirmed by enzymatic analysis in plasma. Usually the residual activities range from undetectable to approximately 8% of normal values [2-7, 14].

AADC deficiency is an autosomal recessive condition, and the majority of the patients are compound heterozygotes [11, 14]. Screening of the AADC gene has led to the identification of a number of mutations, indicating that the mutational spectrum is highly heterogeneous [7, 11, 12, 14]. It is not known whether there is a correlation between specific mutations and the severity of the phenotype.

## ■ Pathophysiology

Deficiency in the activity of AADC leads to a generalized deficiency of the synthesis of catecholamines and serotonin. The clinical manifestations of AADC deficiency will derive from the deficiency of these neurotransmitters in the developing brain.

This is based on the similarity of some features of AADC deficiency with other known congenital and acquired states of deficient monoamine transmission [1] and on the development of animal models that affect the catecholamine system [16].

The motor symptoms in AADC deficient patients are thought to be secondary to dopamine deficiency, due to the known role of dopamine in coordination and regulation of movement [16]. In addition, similar motor manifestations were seen in a mouse model lacking tyrosine hydroxylase [16].

The phenomena of diurnal variation and sleep benefit are also thought to be related to dopamine deficiency, since these are known features of other dopamine deficiency states such as Segawa disease and juvenile Parkinson's disease. Diurnal fluctuation is thought to be related to circadian fluctuations in the regulation of monoamine metabolism in central serotoninergic and dopaminergic neurons [17, 18].

OGC are a feature of acquired or congenital states of dopamine deficiency and the pathophysiology is not fully understood. Neurotransmitter imbalance with deficient dopaminergic and increased cholinergic transmission is a postulated mechanism [19].

Levodopa induced dyskinesias which are commonly seen in Parkinson's disease, are attributed to hypersensitivity of dopamine receptors, abnormalities in non-dopamine transmitter systems, and alterations in the firing patterns that signal between the basal ganglia and the cortex [20]. The occurrence of drug-induced dyskinesias in AADC deficient patients may be due to similar pathophysiological mechanisms.

Features of autonomic dysfunction likely represent imbalance of the autonomic nervous system due to catecholamine deficiency. Temperature instability is thought to be secondary to serotoninergic and noradrenergic deficiency, given their role in thermoregulation [21].

Dysphoria and sleep disturbances are thought to be secondary to serotonin deficiency, since this neurotransmitter is implicated in anxiety disorders and pain mediation [22] and since serotonin is the precursor for the synthesis of melatonin and it is known to lower arousal and facilitate sleep [18]. Of note, a number of psychiatric and behavioral disorders have been noted in some families, including schizophrenia, anxiety disorders, mood disorders, phobias, panic attacks, attention deficit disorder and Tourette's syndrome [13]. This observation suggests that carriers of AADC deficiency may have a partially deficient monoamine transmission that in predisposed individuals may lead to psychiatric problems.

The cognitive deficits of these patients could be related to the early effects of monoamine deficiency in the developing brain. This is supported by animal models of prenatal manipulation of the monoaminergic system, which have shown structural abnormalities in brain development, particularly in the growth and laminar organization of the cerebral cortex [23].

In the area of endocrine dysfunction, the recurrent episodes of hypoglycemia are thought to reflect the relative lack of catecholamines as anti-insulinergic hormones [3]. Delayed bone maturation is thought to be associated with the lack of induction of growth hormone by catecholamines [3].

Failure to thrive is probably due to feeding difficulties, poor oral intake and gastrointestinal disturbances. Dopamine deficiency could also have a role, since stagnation of body length is a feature of dopa responsive dystonia due to GTP-cyclohydrolase deficiency, and improves by levodopa administration [17].

## ■ Differential Diagnosis

Early in infancy, due to profound hypotonia and hypokinesia, these patients may undergo diagnostic work up for a neuromuscular disorder. The presence of ptosis may raise the possibility of congenital myasthenia. Prolonged OGC, which are associated with dystonic posturing, are often though to be seizures. Features of autonomic dysfunction in the neonatal period, such as temperature instability or bradycardia, lead to the diagnostic work up of sepsis. The prominent startle response that some patients may suffer raised the possibility of hyperekplexia in one reported patient [6]. Finally, it is not rare for AADC deficient patients to carry the diagnosis of cerebral palsy at the time of diagnosis [13].

The clinical presentation of these patients is at times similar to other pediatric neurotransmitter disorders, such as tyrosine hydroxylase deficiency or disorders of pterin metabolism. CSF metabolite profiles together with enzymatic and molecular analysis will confirm the diagnosis [2].

## ■ Treatment

The main goal of treatment is to potentiate monoaminergic transmission. Since AADC is a vitamin B6 dependent enzyme, patients are supplemented with pyridoxine. However, up till now patients have not shown any significant clinical improvement [3, 4, 6, 13, 14], except for one case with a mutation in the pyridoxal phosphate binding site of the AADC gene who had a beneficial but transient response to high-dose vitamin B6 [7].

The main types of drugs used are dopamine agonists and MAO inhibitors. The majority of patients start on one type of drug and then a second type is added [3, 4, 6, 14]. A D2 receptor dopamine agonist (bromocriptine, pergolide) and a nonselective MAO inhibitor (tranylcypromine, phenelzine) have been the most frequent combination therapy used [3, 4, 6, 14]. The first patients described by Hyland et al [1] were started on treatment at 9 months of age and showed a favorable though slow developmental progress, suggesting that early treatment improves prognosis. However, with the report of further patients with AADC deficiency, this point is not clear, since other patients also started early on treatment have not shown such a favorable progress.

It is important to note that assessment of the response to treatment in these patients is difficult, since there is variability in the clinical status and age at the onset of treatment, in the period of follow up, and in the doses and combination of drugs used. Despite these difficulties, by reviewing the more detailed reported cases in the literature [3-7], together with our own experience [14], we detected 2 groups of patients based on their response to treatment. One group (Group I), comprising of

5 males [14], responded to a dopamine agonist and/or a nonselective MAO inhibitor. These patients showed improvement of tone and hypokinesia, decrease in frequency and/or duration of OGC, and improvement of autonomic dysfunction. Though variable, 4 patients had documented evidence of developmental progress [14]. It is unclear whether starting with an MAO inhibitor or with a dopamine agonist influences the clinical response.

The second group of patients (Group II), comprising 5 females and 1 male [3, 6, 7, 14], showed a transient or poor response to one drug and no further improvement when a second drug was added. This group of patients tended to suffer adverse effects from the medications, such as vomiting, dysphoria, insomnia and drug induced dyskinesias. It is unclear whether these patients would have shown a favorable response if they had been able to tolerate higher doses of medication, or whether they represent a subtype of AADC deficiency with a worse clinical phenotype.

It is interesting to note that the majority of AADC deficient patients with poor response to drugs (Group II) were females, while the majority of male patients had a positive response (Group I). Higher dependency on the dopamine system in females might contribute to clinical differences in deficiencies of monoamine synthesis and this could explain the worse phenotype and poorer response to treatment of the female patients with AADC deficiency [24].

Patients are generally not treated with dopamine or serotonin precursors, since deficient AADC activity would preclude monoamine production and would promote further accumulation of precursor metabolites. However, three reported siblings with AADC deficiency showed favorable response to levodopa [8, 12]. In these patients, molecular analysis demonstrated a mutation in the AADC gene that caused changes in the Km of the enzyme, suggesting that the mutation affected the enzyme-binding site for levodopa [12]. More recently, another patient treated with levodopa showed evidence of gradual improvement in his function that plateaued after 24 months of therapy [7]. These findings indicate that a trial of levodopa therapy could be attempted, although caution is recommended since levodopa administration may lead to decrease in methylation capacity [8].

A number of other therapeutic strategies have been used in AADC deficient patients [13, 14]. Anticholinergic therapy (trihexyphenidyl) produced a modest response in some patients [6, 7] but caused aggressive behavior in others [6, 7, 14]. Melatonin and chloral hydrate have helped to improve sleep in some patients [13, 14]. Buspirone, an anxiolytic with serotonergic and D2 agonist activity, improved rigidity and irritability but produced dyskinesias in 2 reported patients [6]. Serotonin reuptake inhibitors caused rigidity and drug induced dystonia in one patient [6]. Indirect catecholaminomimetics (dexamphetamine), amine re-uptake inhibitors (imipramine) and ergotamine have been of no benefit [2, 6]. Finally, local application of a sympathomimetic (oxymetazoline hydrochloride) has been useful for nasal congestion [6, 14].

Finally, one can speculate that AADC deficiency, like other enzymatic deficiency states, will be someday treatable using gene therapy. In AADC deficiency, as in other pediatric neurotransmitter diseases, the anatomical target of gene delivery will be of critical importance and may require delivery to multiple central and peripheral sites.

In addition, timing of gene therapy will be crucial, since replacement of missing neurotransmitters at later stages may not reverse developmental abnormalities that have already occurred [25].

## Concluding Remarks

AADC deficiency is a rare disorder, but should be suspected in infants with characteristic clinical findings, with or without family history. The diagnosis can be verified by biochemical and genetic analyses, but there may be marked variations in terms of severity and response to treatment. Although rationally developed, current therapeutic approaches are not optimal, and require careful selection and titration of medications that correct the underlying neurotransmitter deficits. Special attention needs to be paid to the potential of adverse side effects. The impact of the multiple neurotransmitter deficits on brain development is an intriguing subject that could be investigated further through creation of appropriate animal models and careful neuropsychological assessment of AADC patients, coupled with functional neuroimaging modalities.

## References

1. Hyland K. Presentation, diagnosis, and treatment of the disorders of monoamine neurotransmitter metabolism. *Sem Perinatol* 1999, 23: 194-203.
2. Hyland K, Surtees RA, Rodeck C, Clayton PT. Aromatic L-amino acid decarboxylase deficiency: clinical features, diagnosis, and treatment of a new inborn error of neurotransmitter amine synthesis. *Neurology* 1992, 42: 1980-8.
3. Korenke GC, Christen HJ, Hyland K, Hunneman DH, Hanefeld F. Aromatic L-amino acid decarboxylase deficiency: an extrapyramidal movement disorder with oculogyric crises. *Euro J Pediatr Neurol* 1997; 1: 67-71.
4. Maller A, Hyland K, Milstien S, Biaggioni I, Butler IJ. Aromatic L-amino acid decarboxylase deficiency: clinical features, diagnosis, and treatment of a second family. *J Child Neurol* 1997; 12: 349-54.
5. Abeling NG, van Gennip AH, Barth PG, van Cruchten A, Westra M, Wijburg FA. Aromatic L-amino acid decarboxylase deficiency: a new case with a mild clinical presentation and unexpected laboratory findings. *J Inherit Metab Dis* 1998; 21: 240-2.
6. Swoboda KJ, Hyland K, Goldstein DS, et al. Clinical and therapeutic observations in aromatic L-amino acid decarboxylase deficiency. Neurology. 1999; 12 (53): 1205-11.
7. Fiumara A, Brautigam C, Hyland K, et al. Aromatic L-amino acid decarboxylase deficiency with hyperdopaminuria. Clinical and laboratory findings in response to different therapies. *Neuropediatrics* 2002; 33: 203-8.
8. Brautigam C, Wevers RA, Hyland K, Sharma RK, Knust A, Hoffman GF. The influence of L-dopa on methylation capacity in aromatic L-amino acid decarboxylase deficiency: biochemical findings in two patients. *J Inher Metab Dis* 2000 23: 321-4.
9. Burlina AB, Burlina AP, Hyland K, Bonafe L, Blau N. Autistic syndrome and aromatic L-amino acid decarboxylase deficiency. *J Inher Metab Dis* 2001, 24 (Suppl 1): 34.
10. Sequeira S, Calado E, Wevers R. Aromatic L-amino acid decarboxylase deficiency. *J Inher Metab Dis* 2001, 24 (Suppl 1): 34.

11. Chang YT, Mues G, McPherson JD, Bedell J, Marsh JL, Hyland K. Mutations in the human aromatic L-amino acid decarboxylase gene. *J Inher Metab Dis* 1998, 21 (Suppl 2): 4.
12. Chang YT, Sharma R, Marsh JL, et al. Levodopa-responsive aromatic L-amino acid decarboxylase deficiency. *Ann Neurol* 2004; 55 (3): 435-8.
13. Swoboda KJ, Saul JP, McKenna CE, Speller NB, Hyland K. Aromatic L-amino acid decarboxylase deficiency. Overview of clinical features and outcomes. *Ann Neurol* 2003; 54 (suppl 6): S49-55.
14. Pons R, F Ford B, Chiriboga CA, et al. Aromatic L-amino acid decarboxylase deficiency: clinical features, treatment and prognosis. *Neurology* 2004; 62: 1058-65.
15. Menache CC, Haenggeli CA. Aromatic L-amino acid decarboxylase deficiency in two sibs. *Mov Disord* (abstract from the First international symposium on Paediatric Movement Disorders, Barcelona, 2004).
16. Chen L, Zhuang X. Transgenic mouse models of dopamine deficiency. *Ann Neurol* 2003; 54 (Suppl 6): S91-102.
17. Segawa M. Hereditary progressive dystonia with marked diurnal fluctuation. *Brain Dev* 2000; 22 (Suppl 1): S65-80.
18. Voog L, Eriksson T. Is rat brain content of large neutral amino acids (LNAAs) a reflection of plasma LNAA concentrations? *J Neural Transm Gen Sect* 1992; 87: 133-43.
19. Leigh RJ, Foley JM, Remler BF, Civil RH. Oculogyric crisis: a syndrome of thought disorder and ocular deviation. *Ann Neurol* 1987; 22: 13-7.
20. Bezard E, Brotchie JM, Gross CE. Pathophysiology of levodopa-induced dyskinesia: potential for new therapies. *Nat Rev Neurosci* 2001; 2: 577-88.
21. Lin MT. Effects of brain monoamine depletions on thermoregulation in rabbits. *Am J Physiol* 1980; 238: R364-71.
22. Saxena PR. Serotonin receptors: subtypes, functional responses and therapeutic relevance. *Pharmacol Ther* 1995; 66: 339-68.
23. Levitt P, Harvey JA, Friedman E, Simansky K, Murphy EH. New evidence for neurotransmitter influences on brain development. *Trends Neurosci* 1997 20: 269-74.
24. Reisert I, Pilgrim C. Sexual differentiation of monoaminergic neurons – genetic or epigenetic? *Trends Neurosci* 1991; 14: 468-73.
25. Kang UJ, Nakamura K. Potential of gene therapy for pediatric neurotransmitter diseases. Lessons from Parkinson's disease. *Ann Neurol* 2003; 54 (suppl 6): S103-9.

# Tyrosine hydroxylase deficiency: symptomatology, diagnosis, therapy and outlook

**Friederike Hörster, Georg F. Hoffmann**

*Division of Metabolic Diseases, Department of General Pediatrics, University Children's Hospital Heidelberg, Germany*

Tyrosine hydroxylase (TH, EC 1.14.16.2) catalyzes the hydroxylation of L-tyrosine to L-dihydroxyphenylalanine (L-dopa), the rate-limiting step in the biosynthesis of the catecholamines dopamine, norepinephrine and epinephrine *(Figure 1)*. The iron-containing mixed function oxidase requires molecular oxygen and the cofactor tetrahydrobiopterin ($BH_4$) for activity. TH is expressed in catecholaminergic neurons and the adrenal medulla.

TH deficiency (OMIM 191290) has recently become incorporated into concepts and classifications of dystonias as the cause of recessive L-dopa-responsive dystonia [1], but can also present as L-dopa-nonresponsive dystonia or progressive early-onset encephalopathy [2].

## ■ Genetics

The human TH gene contains 13 primary exons spanning ca. 8 kB. The gene map locus is 11p15.5. The single gene that encodes TH produces four different m-RNAs by alternative splicing. The first indication of primary genetic TH deficiency in humans was provided by Clayton and co-workers and confirmed by demonstrating a point mutation in exon 5 (L205P) of the TH gene [3]. Thereafter TH deficiency caused by a different mutation in exon 11 (Q381K) [4] with a relatively high residual enzyme activity of 15% [5] was identified in two siblings described as to suffer from recessive L-dopa-responsive dystonia. Recently, a different point mutation in exon 6 (R233H) could be identified in five patients with autosomal recessive L-dopa responsive infantile parkinsonism [6] and [7], as well as seven different novel mutations in children with the initial diagnoses of spastic paraplegia [8], recessive L-dopa-responsive dystonia [9] and L-dopa responsive progressive encephalopathy [2].

## ■ Clinical Features

A central role of TH in prenatal development, perinatal adaptation and postnatal survival is indicated by the non-viability of TH deficient knock-out mice [10]. In humans, impairment of TH was first studied in defects of $BH_4$ synthesis and recycling, mostly referred to as atypical phenylketonurias. Especially GTP cyclohydrolase I, the rate-limiting enzyme in the biosynthesis of $BH_4$, got into the focus of interest. Autosomal dominant L-dopa-responsive dystonia (Segawa's disease, OMIM 600225) is caused by haploinsufficiency of GTP cyclohydrolase I, and the autosomal recessive form of L-dopa-responsive dystonia was attributed to TH deficiency. So TH deficiency was integrated into concepts and classifications of primary dystonias and infantile parkinsonism [1, 4-6]. Later, the genetically and clinically rather homogenous group of patients with the R233H mutation in exon 6 [6] was characterised. The initial clinical symptoms motor retardation, hypokinesia, rigidity and truncal hypotonia were reported to develop between 3 and 7 months of age. All patients showed a substantial clinical improvement on low doses of L-dopa together with the decarboxylase inhibitor carbidopa although in contrast to L-dopa-responsive dystonia neither the neurological status nor the catecholamine levels in CSF could be normalized.

Recently the clinical picture of TH deficiency was further broadened. A child was described with TH deficiency and an even more severe clinical picture including prenatally impaired brain development and postnatal growth failure [12]. This extended concept of TH deficiency including the presentation as a progressive neurometabolic disorder in early childhood led to the recognition of additional patients [2]. These patients did not show dystonia as the presenting symptomatology but a progressive infantile encephalopathy characterized by abnormal extrapyramidal movements and affecting several cerebral and possibly cerebellar systems. It is important to stress that such patients also show symptoms of significant catecholamine deficiency, such as hypoglycemia and inadequate stress responses. There is an obvious tendency to pre-term birth with troublesome cardiorespiratory perinatal adaptation. It is reasonable to extrapolate that a number of patients can be assumed to die undiagnosed perinatally or even prenatally. Later on potentially life-threatening paroxysmal periods of general malaise with lethargy and vegetative symptoms of irritability, sweating and drooling can occur and are difficult to control. Growth can be compromised and bone age can be severely delayed, suggestive of an impaired secretion pattern and/or stimulation of growth hormone.

Surprisingly most infants with TH deficiency develop normally until an arrest of motor development with a characteristic combination of neurological symptoms around one year of age. Hypokinesia, marked truncal hypotonia, a mask face, oculogyric crises, myoclonic jerks and an extrapyramidal tremor can progressively develop. The latter three can be mistaken as epileptic phenomena. At the severe end of the spectrum virtually no movements are observed, including no dystonic movements. The first clinical impression of these infants in a frog-like position is that of a neuromuscular disorder. However, increased deep tendon reflexes and pyramidal tract signs point to cerebral dysfunction. Oculogyric crises are present, but as for the miosis, may stay undiagnosed because of prominent ptosis. In less severely affected patients progressive extrapyramidal symptoms, especially dystonia and rigidity are more

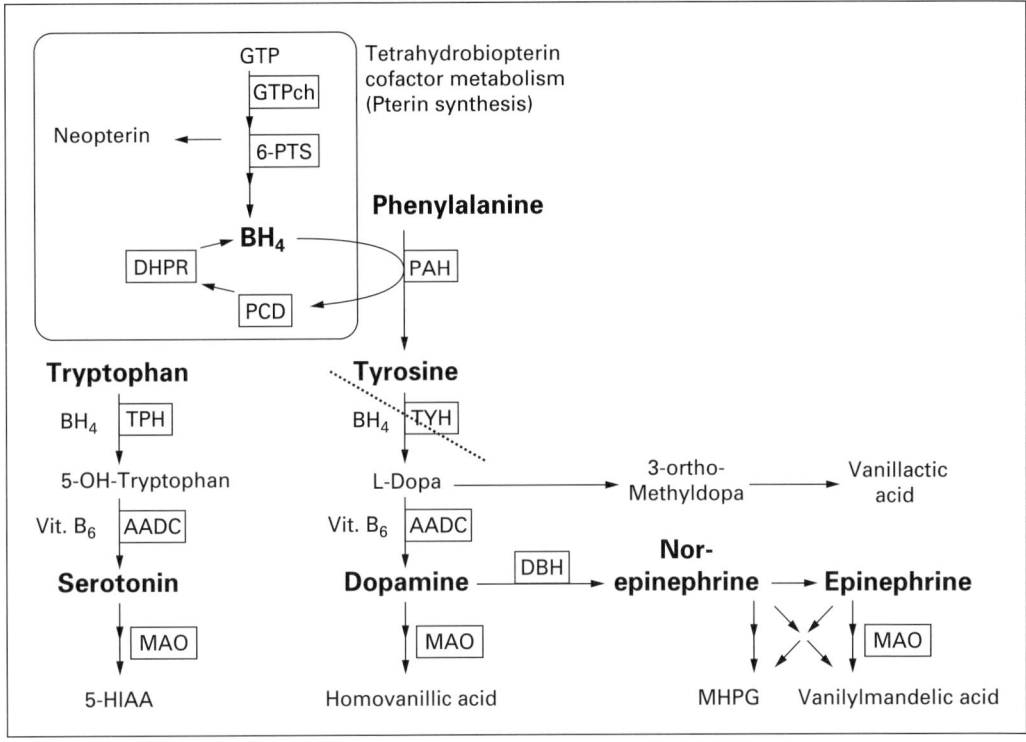

**Figure 1.** Phenylalanine hydroxylase (PAH) as well as tyrosine (TYH) and tryptophan (TPH) hydroxylases require tetrahydrobiopterin (BH$_4$) as cofactor. The synthesis and regeneration of this compound requires various enzymes. Aromatic L-amino acid decarboxylase (AADC) catalyses the formation of serotonin as well as dopamine; the latter may be converted by dopamine β-hydroxylase (DBH) into norepinephrine and epinerphrine. Breakdown of biogenic amines involves monoamine oxidase-A (MAO) and other enzymes. 5-HIAA = 5-hydroxyindoleacetic acid; MHPG = 3-methoxy-4-OH-phenylglycol; 6-PTS = 6-pyruvoyltetrahydropterin synthase; DHPR = dihydropteridine reductase; PCD = Pterin carbinolamine dehydratase; GTP = guanosine triphosphate; GTPch = guanosine triphosphate cyclohydrolase. The dotted line represents the enzymatic block at tyrosine hydroxylase.

obvious and point towards a dopamine deficiency syndrome. Such children may not develop pyramidal tract signs, and have no oculogyric crises or bouts of vegetative disturbance.

After infancy muscle tone increases progressively. Contractures, failure to thrive and immobilization may develop. Untreated adult patients with TH deficiency have not yet been diagnosed. It appears likely that life expectancy is significantly reduced; (dystonic) cerebral palsy is a likely descriptive (mis-)diagnosis. Some patients did not develop extrapyramidal symptoms in the first year of life, were able to walk independently and followed a clinical course best summarized as spastic paraplegia. Their symptoms fully resolved following L-dopa supplementation, and they are by now healthy and independently living adults [9].

Multiple therapeutic interventions with L-dopa together with the decarboxylase inhibitor carbidopa and selegilin were able to improve and to normalize the clinical picture in some patients but not in all. Despite of all therapeutic interventions disease course can be lethal [2].

Clear differences are obvious between the Segawa-like patients, who typically present in childhood with walking problems due to dystonia of the lower limbs or even much later with a Parkinson like disease and the majority of patients with TH deficiency, in whom several cerebral and possibly cerebellar systems are affected. Diurnal fluctuation, which is a hallmark of Segawa's syndrome, is mostly not prominent in TH deficiency.

## ■ Laboratory Findings and Diagnosis

The diagnosis of TH can only be made via cerebrospinal fluid investigations following a standardized lumbar puncture protocol [13]. In CSF a characteristic metabolite constellation is found: low concentrations of metabolites of dopaminergic neurotransmission homovanillic acid (HVA) and 3-methoxy-4-hydroxyphenylethylenglykol (MHPG) in the presence of normal concentrations for metabolites belonging to the serotonin neurotransmission system as 5-hydroxyindolacetic acid (HIAA) [14] (Figure 1). These compounds are mostly measured by high-performance liquid chromatography and have to be carefully compared with age-matched controls. Investigations of metabolites in peripheral fluids can lead to false-negative results. Urinary measurements of catecholamines, HVA and vanillylmandelic acid can be within the normal range in patients and are for this reason not informative. The only diagnostic helpful peripheral parameter is prolactin in serum. The secretion of serum prolactin is inversely regulated by feedback by dopaminergic $D_2$ receptors theoretically resulting in high prolactin, when dopamine is low.

A number of diseases and conditions such as mitochondrial encephalopathies, generalized hypoxia or severe epileptic encephalopathies can lead to secondary decrease of HVA, so before the diagnosis of TH can be suspected, others even more frequent causes of low CSF dopamine must be ruled out [15]. For this purpose a close communication between clinicians and diagnostic laboratories is mandatory.

Enzyme analysis is not possible in TH deficiency because tissues expressing enzyme activity, brain and adrenal medulla, are difficult to obtain. Thus mutation analysis is the only way to confirm the diagnosis.

## ■ Therapy

Substitution of L-dopa (1-10 mg/kg/day in two to six divided doses) is the principle of treatment. Some patients already respond to low-dose L-dopa treatment, some require higher doses and some don't respond at all or suffer from adverse effects such as dyskinesias, mainly hyperkinesia and ballism, or nausea.

For an successful therapeutic trial with L-dopa some points have to be taken into account:

- L-Dopa has to be administered in combination with an L-dopa-decarboxylase inhibitor (25% of L-dopa daily dosage, if L-dopa is below 400 mg/day, 10% of L-dopa daily dosage, if L-dopa is above 400 mg/day).

- L-Dopa treatment has to be started carefully and slowly with doses as low as 0.25 mg/kg/day in two to six divided doses to avoid dyskinesias due to hypersensitivity and up-regulation of dopamine receptors in dopamin-deficient patients. In such patients L-dopa can only be increased very slowly, sometimes over several years. Retarded preparations may be useful to ensure constant L-dopa levels. In general individual steps of increments L-dopa/carbidopa should not be more than 1 mg/kg/day.
- An L-dopa trial should last long (at least 3 month) with sufficient doses (10 mg/kg/day) before its effect is judged.
- L-dopa/carbidopa/5-hydroxytryptophan therapy may reduce CSF folates ($CH_3$-group trapping by L-dopa to 3-O-methyl-dopa) requiring folinic acid (5-formyltetrahydrofolate) substitution (15 mg/day).

Combination of L-dopa substitution with anticholinergic treatment (Trihexiphenidyl) or adjunctive treatment of L-dopa substitution with inhibitors of Monoaminoxidase B such as Selegelin, COMT inhibitors such as Entacapone, and dopamine agonists such as bromocriptine are therapeutic alternatives.

Monitoring of therapy requires repeated careful clinical evaluation by a (pediatric) neurologist including video documentation and follow-up of metabolite concentrations, including 5,10-metylenetetrahydrofolate by consecutive lumbar punctures. In some patients with high prolactin before L-dopa supplementation, prolactin levels can aid monitoring of therapy.

The long-term effects of life-long L-dopa treatment are not known and have to be investigated systematically [9].

## ■ Outlook

The clinical severity correlates with the biochemical phenotype, probably depending on the nature of the causative mutations. Children whose mutations are close to null mutations appear to be already compromised *in utero*: they are prone to fetal distress, are often born prematurely and barely survive the perinatal period. From the available data it appears that their levels of metabolites in the CSF are also very low [2]. They present the severe end of the spectrum of possible clinical phenotypes, but milder manifestations are no possible. In view of the broad spectrum of physiological functions, which are mediated by dopamine (*Table I*) a variety of complex clinical phenotypes can be expected.

Transgenic mouse models of dopamine deficiency are important to study the pathophysiologic mechanisms of dopamine deficiency and to perform therapeutic trials, but the generation of these animal models remains challenging [16]. It is particularly difficult to investigate the effects of isolated dopamine deficiency in TH knock-out animals, because the synthesis of epinephrine and norepinephrine is also affected and has clinical implications. A knock-out, which leads to a null mutation and zero enzyme activity is incompatible with life [10] due to cardiovascular failure in midgestation and survival can only be achieved, if TH activity is ensured in adrenergic cells by tissue-specific rescue of TH expression [17]. Thus the symptomatology in

**Table I. Dopamine mediated functions.**

| | |
|---|---|
| – Brain | Consciousness/emotion/Affect<br>Neuroendocrine secretion |
| – Retina | Dark adaption |
| – Pituitary Gland | Hormonal secretion<br>(prolactin and growth hormone) |
| – Kidney | Excretion of sodium and phosphate |
| – Vascular System | Tone of smooth muscles |
| – Gastrointestinal tract | Motility |
| Also heart, lung, vas deferens | |

men and in selective knock-out mice is different. These mice show parkinsonian motor dysfunction with symptoms only occurring in homozygotes. They respond to L-dopa treatment, but the life-limiting symptom is aphagia and starvation. The motivation of food-intake seems to be pertubated, which is not a major feature in human disease.

Therefore new animal models are required to study different degrees of enzyme deficiencies and their resulting phenotypes to achieve a better understanding of this new disease and help to develop new therapeutic opportunities to patients, who can not be treated sufficiently by L-dopa alone.

# References

1. Assmann B, Surtees R, Hoffmann GF. Approach to the diagnosis of Neurotransmitter Disease exemplified by the differential diagnosis of childhood-onset dystonia. Ann Neurol 2003; 54 (suppl 6): S18-S24.
2. Hoffmann GF, Assmann B, Bräutigam C, et al. Tyrosine Hydroxylase Deficiency causes progressive encephalopathy and dopa-nonresponsive Dystonia. Ann Neurol 2003; 54 (suppl 6): S56-S65.
3. Lüdecke B, Knappskog PM, Clayton PT, et al. Recessively inherited L-dopa-responsive parkinsonism in infancy caused by a point mutation (L205P) in the tyrosine hydroxylase gene. Hum Mol Genet 1996; 5: 1023-8.
4. Lüdecke B, Dworniczak B, Bartholomé K. A point mutation in the tyrosine hydroxylase gene associated with Segawa's syndrome. Hum Genet 1995; 95: 123-5.
5. Knappskog PM, Flatmark T, Mallet J, Lüdecke B, Bartholomé K. Recessively inherited L-dopa-responsive dystonia caused by a point mutation (Q381K) in the tyrosine hydroxylase gene. Hum Mol Genet 1995; 4: 1209-12.
6. van den Heuvel LPWJ, Luiten B, Smeitink JAM, de Rijk-van Andel JF, Steenbergen-Spanjers GCH, Jansen RJT, et al. A common point mutation in the tyrosine hydroxylase gene in autosomal recessive L-dopa responsive dystonia (DRD) in the Dutch population. Hum Genet 1998; 102: 644-6.
7. Grattan-Smith PJ, Wevers RA, Stennbergen-Spanjers, Fung VSC, Earl J, Wilcken B. Tyrosine Hydroxylase deficiency: clinical manifestations of catecholamine insufficiency in infancy. Movement Disorders 2002; 17: 354-9.

8. Furukawa Y, Graf WD, Wong H, Shimadzu M, Kish SJ. Dopa-responsive dystonia simulating spastic paraplegia due to tyrosine hydroxylase (TH) gene mutations. *Neurology* 2001; 56: 260-3.
9. Swaans RJM, Rondot P, Renier WO, van den Heuvel LP, Steenbergen-Spanjers GC, Wevers RA. Four novel mutations in the Tyrosine Hydroxylase Gene in patients with infantile parkinsonism. *Ann Hum Genet* 2000; 64: 25-31.
10. Zhou Q-Y, Qualfe CJ, Palmiter RD. Targeted disruption of the tyrosine hydroxylase gene reveals that catecholamines are required for mouse fetal development. *Nature* 1995; 374: 640-3.
11. de Rijk-van Andel JF, Gabreëls FJM, Geurtz, B, Steenbergen-Spanjers GCH, van den Heuvel LPWJ, Smeitink JAM, Wevers RA. L-dopa responsive infantile hypokinetic rigid parkinsonism due to tyrosine hydroxylase deficiency. *Neurology* 2000; 55: 1926-8.
12. Dionisi-Vici C, Hoffmann GF, Leuzzi V, *et al.* Tyrosine hydroxylase deficiency with severe clinical course: Clinical and biochemical investigations and optimization of therapy. *J. Pediatr.* 2000; 136: 560-2.
13. Hyland K. The Lumbar Puncture for Diagnosis of Pediatric Neurotransmitter Diseases. *Ann Neurol* 2003; 54 (suppl 6): S13-S17.
14. Bräutigam C, Wevers RA, Jansen RJT, *et al.* Biochemical hallmarks of tyrosine hydroxylase deficiency. *Clin Chem* 1998; 44 (9): 1897-904.
15. van der Heyden JC, Rotteveel JJ, Wevers RA. Decreased homovanillic acid concentrations in cerebrospinal fluid in children without a known defect in dopamine metabolism. *Eur J Ped Neurol* 2003; 31-7.
16. Chen L, Zhuang X. Transgenic mouse models of dopamine deficiency. *Ann Neurol* 2003; 54 (suppl 6): S91-S102.
17. Zhou QY, Palmiter RD. Dopamine-deficient mice are severely hypoactive, adipsic and aphagic. *Cell* 1995; 83: 1197-209.

# Dyskinetic features of succinate semialdehyde dehydrogenase deficiency, a GABA degradative defect

Phillip L. Pearl[1], Maria T. Acosta[1], Denise D. Wallis[1], Teodoro Bottiglieri[2], Karen Miotto[3], Cornelis Jakobs[4], K. Michael Gibson[5]

[1] Department of Neurology, Children's National Medical Center, George Washington University School of Medicine and Health Sciences, Washington, DC, USA
[2] Institute of Metabolic Disease, Baylor University Medical Center, Dallas, TX
[3] Department of Psychiatry and Biobehavioral Sciences, David Geffen School of Medicine at UCLA, University of California, Los Angeles, CA, USA
[4] Department of Clinical Chemistry, VU University Medical Center, Amsterdam, The Netherlands
[5] Department of Molecular and Medical Genetics, Oregon Health & Science University, Portland, OR, USA

---

Movement disorders represent some of the more common and heterogeneous abnormalities of neurological function. Classification is dependent upon detailed clinical investigation, with subgroups defined according to clinical presentation (acute, progressive, chronic), dyskinetic features (hyper-, hypo-, or akinetic), anatomical abnormalities (lesions of the *substantia nigra*, cerebellum, putamen, caudate, globus pallidus, subthalamic nucleus, or their pathways), and the predominant type of movement (ataxia, bradykinesia, rigidity, tremor, tic, dystonia, myoclonus, chorea, athetosis, ballismus) [1]. Underlying causes range from fixed anatomical lesions to degenerative, infectious, neoplastic, and metabolic diseases. In view of their role as a major computational center focusing input information regarding planned movements from the cortex, the basal ganglia have become a focus for investigation of pathology underlying movement disorders. Moreover, considerable biochemical attention has been devoted to the dopamine system since dopaminergic pathways emanating from the *substantia nigra* influence function of the basal ganglia and degenerate in Parkinson's disease [1].

Current research suggests that dopamine inhibits GABAergic pathways, with loss of that balance leading to pathological sequelae [1]. Our laboratory studies a rare, heritable disorder of GABA degradation, succinate semialdehyde dehydrogenase (SSADH) deficiency [2] (*Figure 1*). The clinical phenotype is nonspecific, involving developmental delay, mental retardation, delayed or absent speech, hypotonia, seizures, behavioral problems and ataxia as predominant features. Electroencephalography reveals predominantly diffuse slowing and generalized spike discharges [3], while neuroimaging shows cerebral atrophy and hyperintense signal in the white matter and globus pallidus.

The biochemical hallmark of SSADH deficiency is the accumulation of gamma-hydroxybutyric acid (GHB) in physiological fluids (*Figure 1*), a compound with unusual and varied pharmacological properties [4]. GHB inhibits pre-synaptic dopamine release [5], and appears to be associated with enhanced dopamine turnover, perhaps on a compensatory basis, in this disorder [6]. In support of this, brain concentrations of homovanillic acid (HVA; the end-product of dopamine metabolism) are significantly increased in SSADH-deficient knockout mice [6] in which GHB levels are increased. Further, the concentrations of HVA and 5-hydroxyindoleacetic acid (5-HIAA, the end-product of serotonin catabolism) demonstrate a significant linear correlation with GHB concentration in the cerebrospinal fluid of SSADH-deficient patients and mice [6, 7].

Enhanced catecholamine turnover may be implicated in many of the neuropsychological symptoms observed in these patients, including hyperactivity, aggression, hallucinations and sleep disturbances.

In addition to increases in GHB, SSADH deficiency is also associated with a significant elevation in brain GABA (*Figure 1*) [7]. The ability of GHB to freely inter-

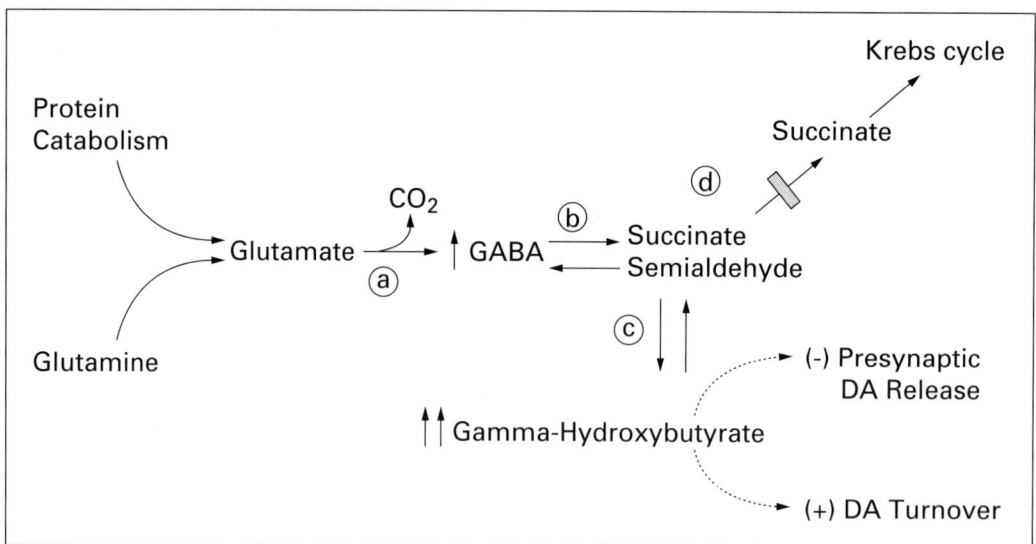

**Figure 1.** Mammalian synthesis and degradation of GABA (not all steps are shown). Enzymes include: a, glutamic acid decarboxylase; b, GABA-transaminase; c, an NAD(P)$^+$ dependent GHB oxidoreductase, perhaps consistent with so-called succinic semialdehyde reductase, or aldo-keto reductase 7A2 (*i.e.* AKR7A2); d, succinate semialdehyde dehydrogenase (SSADH), site of the inherited defect in human and murine SSADH deficiency. Metabolites increased in the latter are depicted by upward arrows. Regulatory properties of GHB are depicted by dashed lines, including decrease (-) of pre-synaptic DA release, and stimulation (+) of DA turnover. *GABA, gamma-aminobutyric acid; GHB, gamma-hydroxybutyric acid; DA, dopamine.*

convert to GABA, even in SSADH deficient patients and mice, leads to the hypothesis that much of the symptomatology in this disease is GABA-dependent. In support of this concept, the application of GABA agonists and neuroleptics, in humans and animals, can result in tardive dyskinesia and choreiform movements [8-10]. Intrathecal administration of GABA has been shown to elicit dyskinetic movements in mice [11]. Paradoxically, intervention with vigabatrin (an antiepileptic which increases GABA levels in CNS) was beneficial in reducing dyskinetic symptoms in a limited study of patients with tardive dyskinesia [12]. For its outflow pathways, the basal ganglia depend heavily on GABA as a neurotransmitter [13].

In the current review, we summarize our growing database of patients with SSADH deficiency, focusing attention on those dyskinetic features seen in this rare neurometabolic disorder. We review the results of applying GHB to rodent systems, and the ability of the monoamine oxidase inhibitor pargyline to block the effects of GHB on locomotion. Finally, we summarize the movement effects of illicitly consumed, high-dose GHB in human drug abusers [14].

## ■ Clinical Features of SSADH-Deficient Patients

Our current database includes a total of 92 patients, comprised of 50 patients from our own cohort and an additional 42 cases reported in the literature with clinical details. The majority of these patients have been previously reported [2, 3, 15]. The age at diagnosis varies from newborn to 25 years. Parental consanguinity is reported in 27 (29%) of cases. The clinical features from our cohort with systematically obtained questionnaire data are summarized in *Table I*. The most constant features are developmental delay, hypotonia, and mental retardation. Those patients not included as having mental retardation tend to be too young at the time of reporting to confirm this. Cognitive defects are particularly marked in expressive language. Other common features are ataxia, behavioral problems, seizures and hyporeflexia. Neonatal problems are uncommon but prematurity, lethargy, decreased sucking ability, respiratory difficulty, and hypoglycemia have been reported. Other occasional reported problems include decreased feeding and failure to thrive, strabismus, nystagmus, retinitis, disc pallor, and oculomotor apraxia.

Behavior problems have been notable in over half of patients, and have most commonly been characterized as sleep disturbances, inattention, and hyperactivity. Sleep disturbances have included both disrupted and excessive sleep. We have identified one patient with daytime hypersomnolence having typical polysomnographic features of narcolepsy, including sleep onset stage REM during diurnal naps. Medication management has focused on targeting behavioral symptomatology as well as seizures. Neuroimaging and EEG findings are presented in *Table II*.

The presence of movement disorders such as chorea, athetosis, dystonia, and myoclonus has been noted in only a limited number of patients. The actual incidence of these findings in the disorder is not accurately known, as the data is extracted from case reports and documents that have differing amounts of clinical detail. We discuss here in some clinical detail the cases reported with these movement disorders. The report by Rahbeeni *et al.* [16] is notable for signs of basal ganglia dysfunction reported in five patients from three families. The first patient presented at 2.5 years with developmental delay, choreoathetosis, slightly diminished deep tendon reflexes, and severe hypotonia. MRI revealed scattered bilateral T2-weighted high intensity focal lesions and mild atrophy. She was treated with vigabatrin and improved initially according to the parents. The patient later developed myoclonic seizures and regressed. An EEG demonstrated polyspike and wave activity, activated by sleep, which later progressed to a slow background and bilateral bifrontal paroxysmal sharp waves. At a repeat assessment, the child was found to be dystonic with autistic features.

The second patient, the brother of the index patient above, presented at age 13 months with choreoathetosis and developmental delay. His clinical course was milder than that of his sister. Neurological examination revealed hypotonia and hyporeflexia. He was treated with riboflavin, dextromethorphan and vigabatrin. His parents noted some improvement, but he began to demonstrate hyperactivity. At the age of 21 months, he developed seizures and EEG showed background slowing with paroxysms of spike, poly-spike and slow waves. Follow-up at 27 months revealed mild hyperkinetic behavior, severe hypotonia, and no verbal skills.

The third patient presented at the age of 4 days. He had a breech presentation and was noted to be severely hypotonic at birth with a poor sucking reflex. Physical findings included an anterior pole cataract and bilaterally undescended testicles. He was severely hypotonic and areflexic, with weak Moro, sucking and tonic neck reflexes. He also experienced myoclonus and suspected myoclonic seizures. An MRI suggested white matter oedema, and EEG indicated lack of differentiation between REM and non-REM sleep. This patient was treated with vigabatrin. His seizures, hypotonia, respiratory efforts and sucking improved.

The fourth patient presented at age 12 years with severe hypotonia, myoclonic seizures, dystonia, generalized tonic-clonic seizures and choreoathetosis. She is the paternal cousin of the patient above. Her deep tendon reflexes were decreased. An MRI revealed hypoplasia of the cerebellar vermis. EEG findings showed background slowing and frequent parietal and occipitotemporal paroxysmal activity. She was treated with vigabatrin, carbamazepine, thioridazine, and riboflavin. Follow-up revealed decreased severity of choreoathetosis.

The fifth patient presented at the age of 14 months with developmental delay and hypotonia. Evaluation revealed myoclonus and decreased deep tendon reflexes. EEG showed generalized background slowing, and MRI revealed scattered subcortical white matter lesions.

An additional report described the presence of chorea in a 3.5 year old patient presenting with a generalized tonic-clonic seizure associated with fever [15]. As an infant, she was weak and a poor feeder. Her development was delayed; she sat at 10 months, rolled at 11 months, and began to speak at 20 months. Upon examination, she was found to have ataxia, hypotonia, mental retardation, and choreiform movements. EEG was normal and MRI revealed atrophy. Her status at age 4 years 8 months revealed persistence of hypotonia, language delay, and frequent involuntary movements.

### Table I. Clinical features in SSADH deficiency (N = 50).

| | | |
|---|---|---|
| Developmental Delay | 50 | (100%) |
| Mental Retardation | 40 | (80%) |
| Behavior Problems | 35 | (70%) |
| Hypotonia | 32 | (64%) |
| Ataxia | 27 | (54%) |
| Seizures | 23 | (46%) |
| **Seizure types in SSADH deficiency (N = 22)** | | |
| Generalized Tonic-Clonic | 14 | (64%) |
| Absence | 10 | (45%) |
| Myoclonic | 5 | (23%) |
| Other | 8 | (36%) |
| **Behavior problems in SSADH deficiency (N = 35)** | | |
| Sleep Disturbances | 22 | (63%) |
| Inattention | 17 | (49%) |
| Hyperactivity | 14 | (40%) |
| Obsessive Compulsive | 11 | (31%) |
| Anxiety | 10 | (29%) |
| Aggression | 6 | (17%) |
| Hallucinations | 4 | (11%) |

### Table II. Diagnostic studies in SSADH deficiency.

| | | |
|---|---|---|
| **Neuroimaging findings (N = 60)** | | |
| Increased T2-weighted signal: | | |
|     Globus pallidus | 18 | (30%) |
|     White matter | 10 | (17%) |
|     Dentate nucleus | 6 | (10%) |
|     Brainstem | 4 | (7%) |
| Cerebral atrophy | 8 | (13%) |
| Cerebellar atrophy | 7 | (12%) |
| Delayed myelination | 2 | (3%) |
| Normal MRI | 20 | (33%) |
| **EEG findings (N = 54)** | | |
| Background abnormal/slowing | 20 | (37%) |
| Spike discharges | 17 | (31%) |
| ESES | 1 | (2%) |
| Photosensitivity | 2 | (4%) |
| Normal | 18 | (33%) |

ESES: electrographic status epilepticus during slow wave sleep.

A patient presenting at 11 months had severe choreoathetosis, lethargy, and nystagmus [17]. At age 2 years 9 months, the patient was begun on vigabatrin therapy, with initial improvement reported in crawling and pulling skills. At treatment day 71, however, there was significant deterioration and the patient became vegetative and dystonic. After some stabilization, later deterioration on day 79 was characterized by episodes of flailing movements and irritability. The medication was discontinued after 120 days without significant improvement.

An additional report describes a patient who presented at three months of age with hypotonia and delay in motor skills [18]. At eight months, he developed choreoathetosis and developmental regression following a febrile illness. CT and MRI scans showed an abnormality of the globus pallidus bilaterally, which progressed in later studies. Of interest, it was also found that this patient had a transient increase in his CSF glycine.

## Evaluation of GHB on Movement in Rodents and the Effect of Monamine Oxidase Inhibitors

The known capacity for GHB to alter dopaminergic function, and its accumulation in human and murine SSADH deficiency, would suggest a pivotal role for this metabolite in associated dyskinesia. Studies in rodents indicate that GHB inhibits locomotor function, when administered in relatively high doses [19]. These effects on motor activity appear to be mediated via depression of dopaminergic activity mediated via $GABA_B$ receptors, since 3-methoxytyramine, a marker of dopamine release, is depleted following GHB administration [20], and $GABA_B$ receptor antagonists blocked GHB-induced movement anomalies [19, 21].

We have taken the experimental approach of investigating drugs that increase dopaminergic activity as potential agents to either protect or rescue rodents from GHB-associated loss of locomotor function. Monoamine oxidase (MAO) inhibitors, such as pargyline and selegiline, have been used with some effectiveness, in the treatment of movement disorders such as Parkinson's disease. The inhibition of MAO results in increased concentrations of dopamine at the synaptic cleft, and prolonged stimulation of postsynaptic dopamine receptors [22]. Administration of the monoamine oxidase inhibitor pargyline (100 mg/kg), either 5 minutes before or 5 minutes after GHB was given to rodents, was effective in antagonizing the loss of motor activity [21] (Figure 2). These findings confirm that depression of neuronal dopaminergic activity is a primary mechanism involved in the loss of motor function induced by GHB, and that dopamine agonists may possess therapeutic potential to treat GHB toxicity when it is illicitly consumed, and potentially in the rare instances of dyskinesia associated with SSADH deficiency.

## Dyskinesia in GHB Abusers

Movement disorders have been reported with the medical use of GHB. Older anesthesia studies report seizure-like movements during induction with GHB [23]. In the 1980's and early 1990's, GHB was sold over-the-counter as a health supplement to enhance bodybuilding, and to aid dieting and sleep. Poison control center reports of nausea, confusion, seizure-like activity and agitation led to the FDA's ban of GHB use as a supplement [24]. GHB, also known as sodium oxybate, has emerged as a treatment of cataplexy. Clinical trials did not reveal any specific movement disturbance or abnormal EEG activity. However, confusion, amnesia and sleepwalking were noted as possible side effects [25].

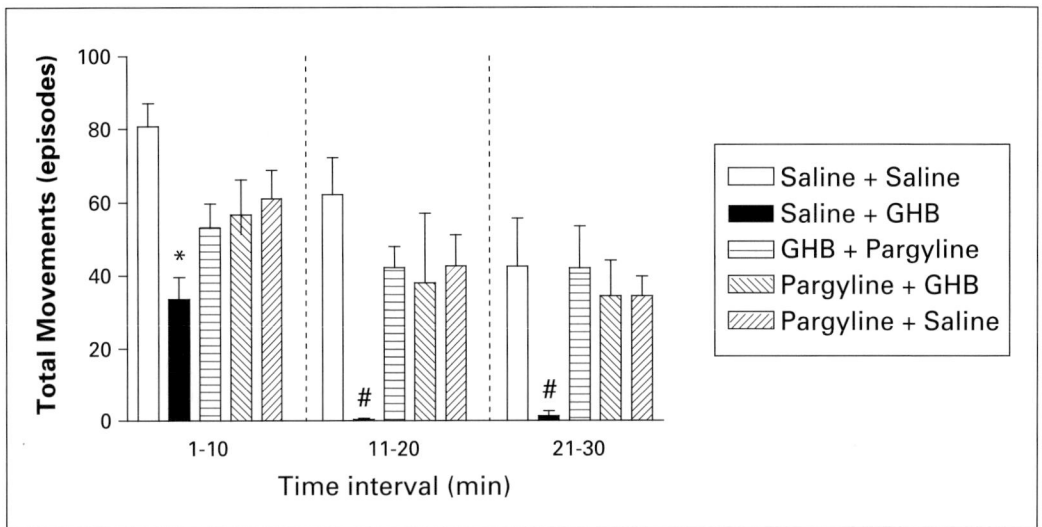

**Figure 2.** Total movement episodes in the rat monitored with the Truscan locomotion system [20, 21]. Movements were summed over three 10 minute epochs, and presented as means ± SEM. Treatment groups are depicted in the box, including vehicle (saline), GHB (500 mg/kg, intraperitoneal), or pargyline (100 mg/kg, intraperitoneal).
# $p < 0.01$; * $p < 0.05$, n = 6 animals per group.

GHB has become popular as a drug of abuse over the last 14 years. Since 1990, an increasing number of cases of both abuse and toxicity have been noted. GHB overdose is characterized by loss of consciousness, hypotonia, tremors, myoclonus, seizure-like activity, bradycardia, hypotension, respiratory depression, and possibly respiratory arrest. Resolution of symptoms can be spontaneous [26]. Unpredictable loss of consciousness, unusual clonic movements, and uncontrollable tremors have been associated with GHB abuse. Episodes of loss of consciousness can occur in new and dependent users. However, these appear to occur more frequently in tolerant users. Tolerance to the effects of GHB results in an increase in dosage, and a withdrawal syndrome on abrupt cessation of GHB use.

Illicit GHB preparations vary in concentrations, which can result in erratic dosing patterns. Users describe the loss of consciousness episodes as "drop-attacks" or even "cataplectic attacks". Morbidity and mortality associated with these episodes include motor vehicle accidents and head trauma. In severe cases of intoxication, users appear lost and unresponsive to verbal commands. Family members and friends have described users as engaging in repetitive sexual or alternatively purposeless behaviors. These episodes of GHB-induced delirium or encephalopathy are difficult to treat, as individuals are consistently amnestic of the events. GHB-induced delirium occurs more frequently at night when around-the-clock users increase their GHB dose to obtain hypnotic effects. To date, EEG and sleep studies are lacking in dependent users; therefore, it is not known whether high dose GHB actually causes cataplexy or seizure activity. Dependent GHB users and individuals with SSADH deficiency share some behavioral and motor disturbances, an observation which merits further investigation.

## ■ Discussion

SSADH deficiency, a disorder of GABA degradation, is associated with excessive GABA and GHB levels in physiologic fluids, and additionally invokes alterations in multiple other neurotransmitter systems. Data from both murine and human systems demonstrate changes involving glutamine, dopamine, and serotonin [6]. The disorder is heterogeneous with many neurologic symptoms, including developmental and cognitive effects, behavioral problems, sleep disorders, and epilepsy. Movement disorders, including chorea, athetosis, dystonia, and myoclonus, have been described in a limited number of patients [16].

Neuroimaging studies in SSADH deficiency have shown increased T2-weighted MR signal in the globus pallidus bilaterally and symmetrically [2]. Similar findings are seen in other organic acidopathies, including methylmalonic and propionic acidemia [27]. Other anatomical imaging abnormalities in SSADH deficiency have included increased signal in subcortical white matter, brainstem (including substantia nigra), and cerebellum. A pattern of dentate nucleus and globus pallidus involvement has been described [28]. MR spectroscopy has not demonstrated abnormalities of the neuronal markers N-acetylaspartate and choline or the presence of a lactate peak on single voxel imaging of the basal ganglia [3]. MR spectroscopy using special editing for neurotransmitters has shown elevation in GABA in human occipital lobe parenchyma [29]. The effects of elevated GABA, and GHB, on the dopaminergic system, particularly nigrostriatal connections, may result in abnormalities of basal ganglia function at an anatomical, biochemical, or clinical level.

Of our database of 92 patients with SSADH deficiency, eight have been reported as having notable abnormalities of movement apart from the more common ataxia. While longitudinal clinical or biochemical assessments are lacking in these patients, some trends may be identified. Relatively early clinical onset, typically in infancy and even in the neonatal period, is common in this patient subset. Their clinical phenotype appears relatively severe, although without markers on MRI or EEG testing that would appear specific or predictive of more basal ganglia or encephalopathic involvement, respectively. While SSADH deficiency is not typically a metabolic encephalopathy associated with intermittent decompensation in the face of systemic threats, there does appear to be a relative predisposition to episodic decompensation in those individuals exhibiting dyskinetic symptoms. In terms of movement disorders, the predominant features, apart from ataxia, suggest basal ganglia dysfunction, especially the abnormal MRI signal in the globus pallidus (probably gliosis). In one family with two affected sibs, both have shown worsening signal abnormality over time involving the globus pallidus plus substantia nigra [PL Pearl, KM Gibson, unpublished observations].

The effects of L-dopa in Parkinson's disease, and the ingestion of MPTP in drug abusers [30], laid the foundation for the investigation of neurochemical aspects of movement disorders. These observations provide a rationale for evaluating potential correlations between GHB and dyskinesia following acute administration in rodents and human drug abusers. Concentration effects may provide an explanation for the infrequency of dyskinesia in SSADH deficiency as opposed to the more common movement anomalies in high-dose GHB administration in rodents and humans. Brain GHB concentration approaches 0.25 mM in SSADH-deficient mice, comparable to patient cerebrospinal fluid levels of 0.2-1.2 mM [2, 6]. GHB is a weak $GABA_B$ receptor agonist, but the requisite concentrations approach 5 mM [31]. Although not evaluated, this concentration might be attained in high-dose application in rodents and in chronic GHB drug consumption.

In conclusion, human SSADH deficiency represents a rare heritable disorder of GABA metabolism with a wide spectrum of manifestations. The phenotype is heterogeneous, and appears to be expanding. Imaging studies indicate predominant involvement of the basal ganglia in this disorder. There appears to be a relative paucity of movement disorders other than ataxia as a prominent clinical manifestation, an interesting observation in view of the significant disturbances of GABA and GHB metabolism in this disease.

**Acknowledgements:** *Pediatric Neurotransmitter Disease Association, Delman Family Fund for Pediatric Neurology Research, members of the Partnership for Pediatric Epilepsy Research [including the American Epilepsy Society, the Epilepsy Foundation, Anna and Jim Fantaci, Fight Against Childhood Epilepsy and Seizures (FACES)], Neurotherapy Ventures Charitable Research Fund, and Parents Against Childhood Epilepsy (PACE), and NIH NS 40270.*

# References

1. Clarke M, McKinlay I. *Disorders of movement*. In McIntosh N, Helms P, Smyth R, eds. *Forfeil & Arneil's Textbook of Pediatrics*, 6$^{th}$ ed. New York: Churchill Livingstone, 2003: 957-68.
2. Pearl PL, Novotny EJ, Acosta MT, Jakobs C, Gibson KM. Succinic semialdehyde dehydrogenase deficiency in children and adults. *Ann Neurol* 2003; 54 (suppl 6): S73-S80.
3. Pearl PL, Acosta MT, Gibson KM, et al. Clinical spectrum of succinic semialdehyde dehydrogenase deficiency. *Neurology* 2003; 60: 1413-7.
4. Snead OC. Evidence for a pre-synaptic G protein coupled gamma hydroxybutyric acid receptor. *J Neurochem* 2000; 75: 1986-96.
5. Maitre M. The gamma-hydroxybutyrate signalling system in brain: organization and functional implications. *Progr Neurobiol* 1997; 51: 337-61.
6. Gupta M, Hogema BM, Grompe M, et al. Murine succinate semialdehyde dehydrogenase deficiency. *Ann Neurol* 2003; 54 (suppl 6): S81-S90.
7. Gibson KM, Gupta M, Pearl PL, et al. Significant behavioral disturbances in succinic semialdehyde dehydrogenase (SSADH) deficiency (Gamma-hydroxybutyric aciduria). *Biol Psych* 2003; 54: 763-8.
8. Soares KV, McGrath JJ, Deeks JJ Gamma-aminobutyric acid agonists for neuroleptic-induced tardive dyskinesia. *Cochrane Database Syst Rev* 2001; CD000203.
9. Burbaud P, Bonnet B, Guehl D. Lagueny A, Bioulac B. Movement disorders induced by gamma-aminobutyric agonist and antagonist injections into the internal globus pallidus and *substantia nigra* pars reticulata of the monkey. *Brain Res* 1998; 780: 102-7.
10. Bartholini G. GABA system, GABA receptor agonists and dyskinesia. *Mod Prob Pharmacopsychiat* 1983; 21: 143-54.
11. Larson AA. Intrathecal GABA, glycine, taurine or beta-alanine elicits dyskinetic movements in mice. *Pharmacol Biochem Behav* 1989; 32: 505-9.

12. Stahl SM, Thornton JE, Simpson ML, Berger PA, Napoliello MJ. Gamma-vinyl-GABA treatment of tardive dyskinesia and other movement disorders. *Biol Psych* 1985; 20: 888-93.
13. Marsden CD, Sheehy MP. GABA and movement disorders. *Adv Biochem Psychopharmacol* 1981; 30: 225-34.
14. Nicholson KL, Balster RL. GHB: a new and novel drug of abuse. *Drug Alcohol Depend* 2001; 63: 1-22.
15. Gibson KM, Christensen E, Jakobs C, et al. The clinical phenotype of succinic semialdehyde dehydrogenase deficiency (4-hydroxybutyric aciduria): case reports of 23 new patients. *Pediatrics* 1997; 99: 567-74.
16. Rahbeeni Z, Ozand PT, Rashed M, et al. 4-Hydroxybutyric aciduria. *Brain Develop* 1994; 16 (suppl): 64-71.
17. Gibson K, DeVivo DC, Jakobs C. Vigabatrin therapy in patient with succinic semialdehyde dehydrogenase deficiency. *Lancet* 1989; ii: 1105-6.
18. Shih VE, Younes MC, Gotoff JM, Dooling EC, Gibson K. Transient increase in CSF glycine in a patient with succinic semialdehyde dehydrogenase deficiency. *Am J Hum Genet* 1990; 47: A166.
19. Carai MAM, Colombo G, Brunetti G, et al. Role of $GABA_B$ receptors in the sedative/hypnotic effect of γ-hydroxybutyric acid. *Eur J Pharmacol* 2001; 428: 315-21.
20. Bottiglieri T, Anderson D, Gibson KM, Froestl W, Diaz-Arrastia R. Effect of gamma-hydroxybutyrate and GABAb receptor antagonist on locomotor activity and brain dopamine metabolism in the rat. *Neurosci Abst* 2001; 27: 971-7.
21. Anderson D, Bottiglieri T, Gibson KM. Pargyline antagonizes the effect of gamma-hydroxybutyrate (GHB) on locomotor activity in the rat. Program No. 749.15. Abstract Viewer/Itinerary Planner. Washington, DC: *Society for Neuroscience*, 2002. Online.
22. Culver KE, Rosenfeld JM, Szechtman H. Monoamine oxidase inhibitor-induced blockade of locomotor sensitization of quinpirole; role of striatal dopamine uptake inhibition. *Neuropharmacol* 2002; 43: 385-93.
23. Solway J, Sadove MS. 4-Hydroxybutyrate: a clinical study. *Anesth Analg* 1965; 44: 532-9.
24. Dyer JE. Gamma-hydroxybutyrate: A health-food product producing coma and seizure-like activity. *Am J Emerg Med* 1991; 9: 321-4.
25. US Xyrem Multicenter Study Group. A randomized, double blind, placebo-controlled multicenter trial comparing the effects of three doses of orally administered sodium oxybate with placebo for the treatment of narcolepsy. *Sleep* 2002; 25: 42-9.
26. Chin RL, Sporer KA, Cullison B, Dyer JE, Wu TD. Clinical course of gamma-hydroxybutyrate overdose. *Ann Emerg Med* 1998; 31: 716-22.
27. Brismar J, Ozand PT. CT and MR of the brain in disorders of propionate and methylmalonate metabolism. *Am J Neuroradiol* 1994; 15: 1459-73.
28. Ziyeh S, Berlis A, Korinthenberg R, Spreer J, Schumacher M. Selective involvement of the globus pallidus and dentate nucleus in succinic semialdehyde dehydrogenase activity. *Pediatr Radiol* 2002; 32: 598-600.
29. Novotny EJ, Fulbright RK, Pearl PL, Gibson KM, Rothman DL. Magnetic resonance spectroscopy of neurotransmitters in human brain. *Ann Neurol* 2003; 54 (suppl 6): S25-S31.
30. Grondin R, Doan VD, Gregoire L, Bedard PJ. D1 receptor blockade improves L-dopa-induced dyskinesia but worsens parkinsonism in MPTP monkeys. *Neurology* 1999; 52: 771-6.
31. Lingenhoehl K, Brom R, Heid J, et al. Gamma-hydroxybutyrate is a weak agonist at recombinant $GABA_B$ receptors. *Neuropharmacol* 1999; 38: 1667-73.

# Tetrahydrobiopterin deficiencies and movement disorders

**Nenad Blau**

*Division of Clinical Chemistry and Biochemistry, University Children's Hospital, Zurich, Switzerland*

Tetrahydrobiopterin ($BH_4$) cofactor is essential for various processes and is present in probably every cell or tissue of higher organisms. $BH_4$ is required for various enzyme activities, and for less defined functions on the cellular level. The *de novo* biosynthesis pathway of $BH_4$ from GTP involves GTP cyclohydrolase I (GTPCH), 6-pyruvoyl-tetrahydropterin synthase (PTPS), and sepiapterin reductase (SR). Cofactor regeneration requires pterin-4a-carbinolamine dehydratase (PCD) and dihydropteridine reductase (DHPR) [1, 2]. The enzymes that depend on $BH_4$ are the phenylalanine, tyrosine, and tryptophan hydroxylases, all NO synthase (NOS) isoforms, and glyceryl-ether monooxygenase *(Figure 1)*.

With regard to human disease, $BH_4$ deficiency due to autosomal recessive mutations in all enzymes (except sepiapterin reductase) has been described as a cause of hyperphenylalaninemia. Under normal conditions the intracellular $BH_4$ level is thought to play a pivotal role in the regulation of tyrosine and tryptophan hydroxylase, the initial and rate-limiting steps in the biosynthesis of the catecholamines and serotonin. Disturbance of biogenic amine metabolism has been implicated as an etiological factor in a variety of neurological disorders. Alterations in $BH_4$ metabolism have been observed in several neuropsychiatric diseases, such as Parkinson's disease, familial dystonia, Alzheimer's disease, and endogenous depression [3]. Mutations in the gene for GTPCH are closely related to Dopa-responsive dystonia (DRD; hereditary progressive dystonia) [4]. This evidence strongly supports the importance of $BH_4$ and dopaminergic transmission in dystonia.

## ■ Tetrahydrobiopterin Deficiencies

Tetrahydrobiopterin ($BH_4$) deficiencies, a group of rare inherited neurological diseases with monoamine neurotransmitters deficiency, may present phenotypically with or without hyperphenylalaninemia (HPA)[5]. It is a heterogenous group of diseases affecting either all organs, including the central nervous system, or only the peripheral hepatic phenylalanine hydroxylating system [5, 6]. $BH_4$ deficiency can be caused by mutations in genes encoding the enzymes involved in its biosynthesis [7, 8] (GTPCH and PTPS) or regeneration [9-11] (PCD/DCoH and DHPR). The mutations are all inherited autosomal recessively. Biochemical, clinical and DNA data of patients with $BH_4$ deficiencies are tabulated in the BIODEF and BIOMDB databases and are available on the internet (www.bh4.org) [12]. Depending on the enzyme defect and the mode of inheritance patients are diagnosed by different analytical and biochemical approaches.

Two forms of $BH_4$ deficiency may occur without hyperphenylalaninemia. The autosomal dominantly inherited form of GTPCH deficiency (Dopa-responsive dystonia), initially described as Segawa disease) [13], together with the Sepiapterin reductase deficiency [14] have recently been described, none of which have been associated with elevated plasma phenylalanine levels in infancy.

Patients presenting *with* HPA are usually detected through the neonatal screening programs for PKU, while those presenting *without* HPA are recognized either by the typical clinical signs and symptoms or by analysis of neurotransmitter metabolites and pterins in CSF and by investigations of cultured skin fibroblasts [15] (see below).

## ■ Dopa-responsive Dystonias

DRD as a syndrome may have different causes and should be divided into three groups:

1) *autosomal dominant GTPCH deficiency* (adGTPCH) [16] (few patients are reported with autosomal recessive mutations (arGTPCH), but without hyperphenylalaninemia [17 18]); 2) *tyrosine hydroxylase (TH) deficiency* [19, 20]; 3) *other forms of $BH_4$ deficiency* (arGTPCH, PTPS, DHPR, SR) [14, 21, 22]. *Tables I-IV* summarize the most important clinical features of these three groups. In the following, this paper will deal only with some disorders included in groups 1 and 3.

In adGPCH deficiency, typically, dystonic posture or movement of one limb (there is a preference for the left side) appear insidiously between the ages of 1 and 9 years and all limbs are involved within 5 years of onset *(Table I)*. The DRD phenotype may be encompassed by a number of atypical presentations, including Parkinsonism (postural instability, cogwheel rigidity, hypomimia, bradykinesia and/or rest tremor), spastic paraplegia, and a presentation mimicking athetoid cerebral palsy. No axial torsion and no action dystonia or oculogyric crises are noted, as well as no mental retardation. Symptoms are remarkably alleviated after sleep and aggravate gradually toward evening. Diurnal fluctuation is present in about 70% of all cases reported and attenuates with age. There is a marked and sustained response to low doses of L-Dopa/Carbidopa without any unfavourable side effects.

Common but variable symptoms, found in other autosomal recessive variants of $BH_4$ deficiency, are mental retardation, convulsions, disturbance of tone and posture, abnormal movements, hypersalivation and swallowing difficulties. Onset of symptoms is in the first months of life.

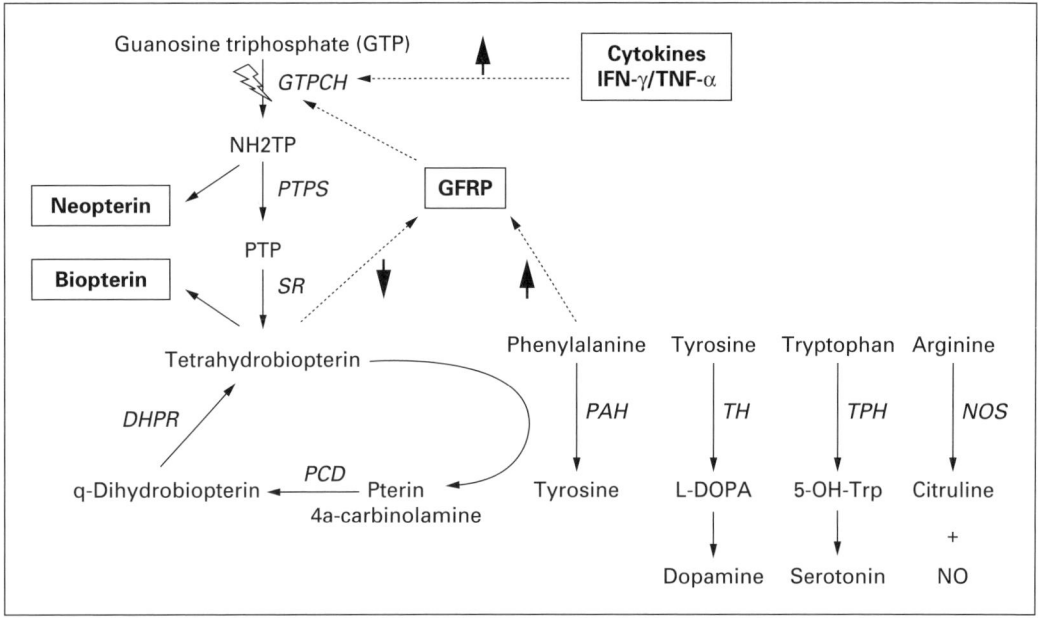

**Figure 1.** Biosynthesis, regeneration, and functions of BH4. Neopterin and biopterin are the two main metabolites in CSF and stimulated fibroblasts. GTPCH: GTP cyclohydrolase I; PTPS, 6-pyruvoyl-tetrahydropterin synthase; SR: sepiapterin reductase; PCD: pterin-4a-dehydratase; DHPR: dihydropteridine reductase; PAH: phenylalanine-4-hydroxylase; TH: tyrosine-3-hydroxylase; THP: tryptophan-5-hydroxylase; NOS: nitric oxide synthase; GFRP: GTPCH feed-back regulatory protein.

The clinical features of patients with SR deficiency are summarized in *Table IV*. The first two patients were diagnosed at the age of 5 and 10 years and were initially classified as having a "central" form of dihydropteridine reductase deficiency [23, 24]. They both presented with progressive psychomotor retardation, spasticity, and dystonia. Both subjects responded to administration of L-Dopa/Carbidopa (1-2 mg/kg/d), however, attempts to introduce 5-hydroxytryptophan resulted in severe vomiting and/or leucopenia [14]. Due to the late diagnosis and thus probably irreversible brain damage a trial with BH$_4$ in one patient was not successful. The third patient was diagnosed as SR-deficient at the age of 25 years, however, the diagnosis at the age of two years had been cerebral palsy presenting with diurnal dystonia and hypersomnolence [25]. Although this patient improved on L-Dopa and 5-hydroxytryptophan, initially she also did not tolerate the therapy. Further patients with cerebral palsy initially classified as DRD were found to be SR-deficient. Thus, SR deficiency may be more common than initially assumed.

## ■ Laboratory Diagnosis of BH4 Deficiency

Classical BH$_4$ deficiencies present with hyperphenylalaninemia and laboratory diagnosis starts with the newborn screening for PKU. A few simple tests (urinary pterins, DHPR activity in blood, and BH$_4$ loading test) discriminate between classical PKU and cofactor defects and additional investigations on neurotransmitter metabolites in CSF define the severity of the disease.

**Table I. Signs and symptoms in patients with Dopa-Responsive-Dystonia due to GTPCH deficiency (Group 1).**

|  | Symptoms | Frequency (%) | Neonatal <30 days | Infancy <18 m | Childhood <10 y | Adolescence >11 y | Adulthood |
|---|---|---|---|---|---|---|---|
| Characteristic features | Dystonia (lower limbs, trunk, arms, neck) | 98 | | + | ++ | ++ | ++ |
| | Diurnal fluctuations of symptoms | 70 | | ± | + | + | ± |
| | Parkinsonism (association of tremor, rigidity, bradykinesia) | 14 | | | ± | ± | + |
| Other extrapyramidal signs | Tremor | 23 | | | | + | + |
| | Rigidity | 16 | ± | + | + | + | + |
| | Neck tilting/poor head control | 7 | | ± | ± | ± | ± |
| | Bradykinesia | 5 | | ± | ± | ± | ± |
| | Hypo/akinesia | 4 | | ± | ± | ± | ± |
| | Oromandibular-orofacial dyskinesia | 4 | | | | ± | ± |
| | Dysphasia | 2 | | ± | ± | ± | ± |
| Other neurological signs | Hyperreflexia | 5 | ± | ± | ± | ± | ± |
| | Hypotonia (at onset) | 5 | | ± | ± | ± | ± |
| | Hypertonia | 5 | ± | ± | ± | ± | ± |
| | Spasticity | 2 | ± | ± | ± | ± | ± |
| Postural and orthopedic complications | Scoliosis | 5 | | | ± | ± | |
| | Wry neck | 5 | | | | ± | |
| | Pes equinovarus | 2 | | | ± | ± | |

From Ref. 29.
GTPCH: Gruanosine TriPhosphate CycloHydrolase.

The most informative biochemical investigations in patients with DRD are the measurement of pterins (neopterin and biopterin) and neurotransmitter metabolites HVA and 5HIAA in CSF. Both neopterin and biopterin have been found to be significantly reduced in CSF of patients with DRD (*Figure 2*). Although CSF levels of neopterin and biopterin are higher in DRD than in autosomal recessive GTPCH deficiency, both groups of patients can be clearly differentiated from other forms of $BH_4$ deficiency and from controls. CSF neopterin may be non-specifically elevated due to viral infections. A decrease in the levels of 5HIAA is a frequent but not invariable finding, while HVA levels are mostly reduced. Again, reduction of 5HIAA and HVA is less pronounced in DRD patients than in autosomal recessive GTPCH deficiency.

**Table II. Signs and symptoms in patients with Tyrosine Hydroxylase deficiency (Group 2).**

| System | Symptoms | Infancy < 18 m | Childhood < 10 y |
|---|---|---|---|
| Characteristic features | Truncal hypotonia | + | + |
| | Chorea/athetosis | + | + |
| | Ptosis of eyelids | + | + |
| | Parkinsonian symptoms | + | + |
| | Tremor | + | + |
| | Hypokinesia | + | + |
| Other neurological signs and symptoms | Oculogyric crises | ± | ± |
| | Ptosis | + | + |
| | Chorea/athetosis | ± | ± |
| | Irritability | + | + |
| | MR/DD | ± | ± |
| | Truncal hypotonia | + | + |
| | Developmental delay | + | + |
| | Dystonia | ± | ± |
| | Tremor | ± | ± |
| | Hypokinesia | ± | ± |
| | Limb hypertonia | + | + |
| | Seizures | ± | ± |

From Ref. 29.

**Table III. Signs and symptoms in patients with autosomal recessive GTPCH deficiency (Group 3).**

| System | Symptoms | Neonatal < 30 days | Infancy < 18 m | Childhood < 10 y |
|---|---|---|---|---|
| Characteristic features | Progressive psychomotor retardation despite treatment for PKU | ± | + | + |
| Other neurological signs and symptoms | Hypotonia/hypertonia/dystonia | + | + | + |
| | Temperature instability | + | + | + |
| | Seizures – myoclonic | | + | + |
| | Microcephaly | + | + | + |
| | Hypersalivation | + | + | + |
| | Mental retardation | | + | + |
| | Feeding difficulties | + | + | + |

From Ref. 29.

Table IV. Signs and symptoms in patients with PTPS and DHPR deficiency (Group 3).

| System | Symptoms | Neonatal < 30 days | Infancy < 18 m | Childhood < 10 y | Adolescence > 11 y |
|---|---|---|---|---|---|
| Characteristic features | Progressive mental and physical retardation despite dietary phenylalanine restriction | ± | + | + | + |
| Other neurological signs and symptoms | Myoclonic or tonic clonic seizures | | + | + | + |
| | Temperature instability | + | + | + | |
| | Hypersalivation | + | + | + | + |
| | Lethargy and irritability | | + | + | |
| | Hypotonia/hypertonia/ dystonia | + | + | + | + |
| | Retardation and regression | + | + | + | + |
| | Choreoathetosis | | + | + | |
| | Feeding difficulties | + | + | + | |

From Ref. 29.
PTPS: 6-pyruvoyl-tetrahydropterin synthase.
DHPR: Dihydroptetidine reductase.

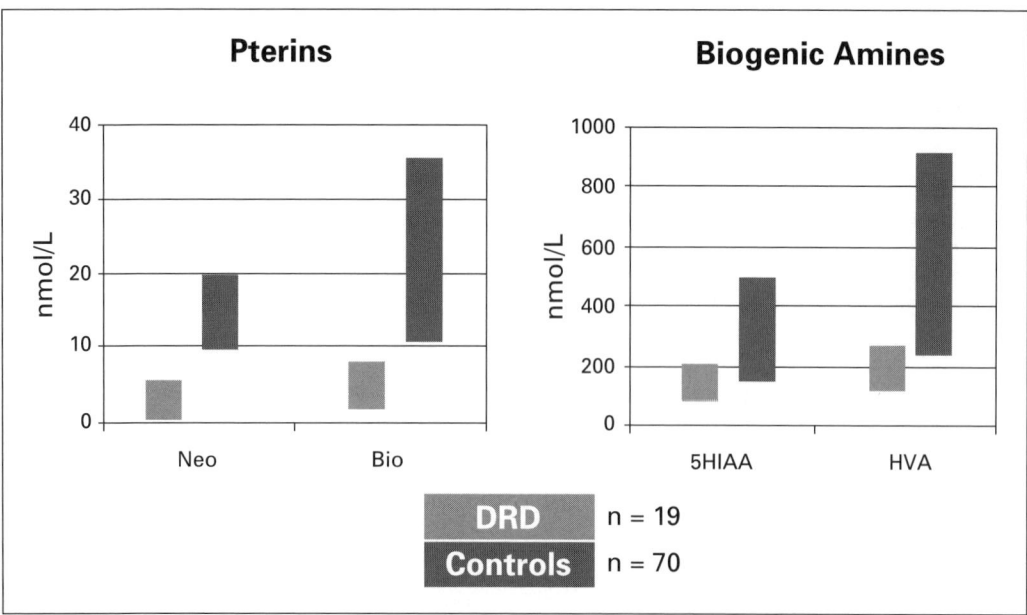

**Figure 2.** Pterins (neopterin and biopterin) and biogenic amine metabolites (5HIAA and HVA) in CSF from patients with Dopa-responsive dystonia (adGTPCH deficiency) and control persons.

Table V. Signs and symptoms in patients with Sepiapterin reductase deficiency (Group 3).

| System | Symptoms | Neonatal < 30 days | Infancy < 18 m | Childhood < 10 y Adolescence > 11 y |
|---|---|---|---|---|
| Characteristic features | Progressive psychomotor retardation | ++ | ++ | ++ |
| | Dystonia | + | + | + |
| | Spasticity | + | + | + |
| Other neurological signs and symptoms | Microcephaly | + | + | + |
| | Hypersalivation | + | + | + |
| | Hypotonia of the trunk | + | + | + |
| | Hypertonia of the limbs | + | + | + |
| | Tremor | | + | + |
| | Extrapyramidal signs | | + | + |
| | Seizures | | ± | ± |
| | Hypersomnolence | | | |
| | Oculogyric crises | | ± | ± |
| | Diurnal fluctuations of dystonia | | | ± |
| | Cortical atrophy | | | + |

An oral loading test with phenylalanine (100 mg/kg) is frequently used when CSF is not available [26]. This test is based on the fact that, due to the partial $BH_4$ deficiency in the liver, under loading conditions phenylalanine hydroxylase is not able to convert phenylalanine to tyrosine at a normal rate. Profiles of plasma phenylalanine and tyrosine and phenylalanine/tyrosine ratios are abnormal at 1, 2, and 4 hours after challenge (Figure 3). Although this test can differentiate between asymptomatic and symptomatic gene carriers, false-positive results are possible. In fact, heterozygote carriers for phenylketonuria (PKU) show the same abnormal phenylalanine/tyrosine profiles, whereas a small number of genetically confirmed DRD subjects showed no abnormalities with this test [27]. Additional measurement of plasma total biopterin improves the sensitivity, and blood sampling at 0, 1, 2, and 4 hours seems to be sufficient.

Enzymatic diagnosis of DRD is limited by the fact that the enzyme GTPCH is not expressed in various cell types, including blood cells and fibroblasts. We showed recently that cytokine-stimulated fibroblasts are highly useful to measure neopterin and biopterin production patterns and GTPCH activity [28]. After stimulation for 24 hours with interferon-γ and tumour necrosis factor-α the concentrations of neopterin and biopterin were extremely low compared with the normal fibroblasts. GTPCH activity in cytokine-stimulated fibroblasts from patients with DRD was significantly reduced (Figure 4). Thus, the skin fibroblast assay is confirmatory for GTPCH

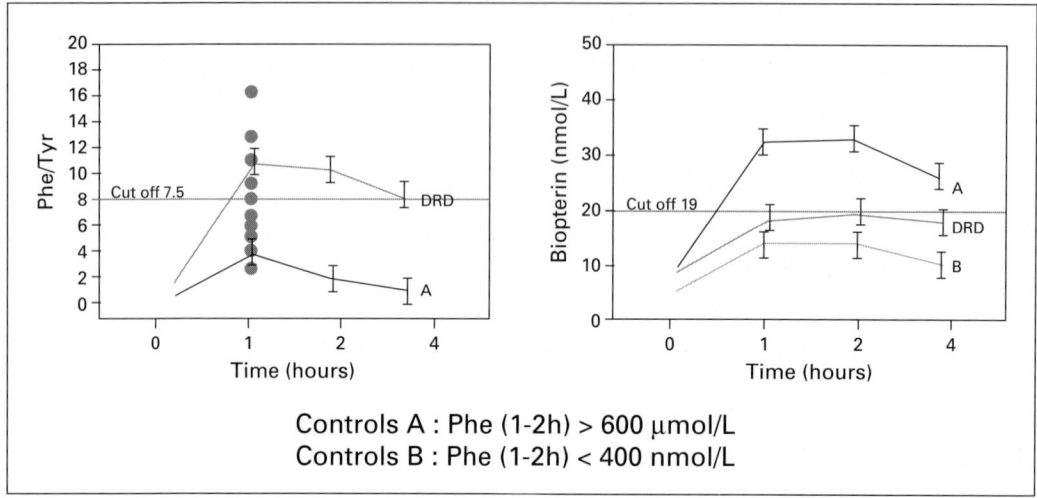

**Figure 3**. Plasma Phe/tyr ratio (A) and biopterin concentrations (B) during loading test with phenylalanine (100 mg/kg) in patients with DRD (adGTPCH deficiency) and control persons. Dots in graph A show a group of genetically proven DRD patients with Phe/Tyr ratios below the cut-off of 7.5 (for details see Saunders-Pullman et al. [27]).

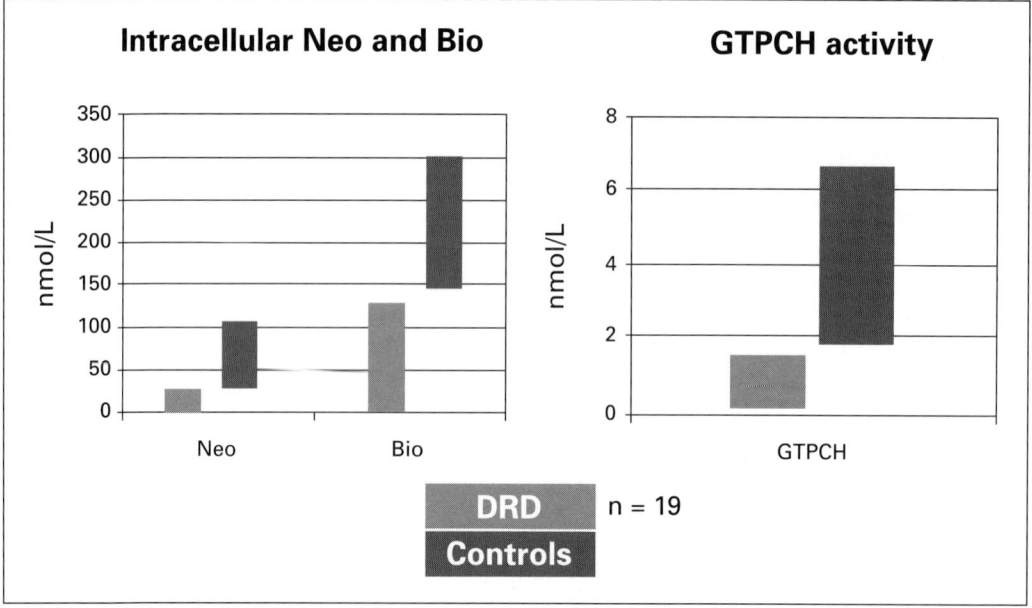

**Figure 4**. Intracellular neopterin and biopterin concentrations and GTPCH activity in cytokine-stimulated fibroblasts from patients with DRD (adGTPCH deficiency) and control persons. For details see Bonafé et al. [28].

deficiency and allows differential diagnosis from other forms of $BH_4$ deficiency. Patients with suspicion of DRD can be first screened by the neopterin and biopterin production assay in fibroblasts and positive cases can be further assayed for GTPCH activity in the same cultured cells.

## ■ Diagnostic procedures

The following sequence of clinical and laboratory investigations is recommended in the diagnosis of DRD due to adGTPCH deficiency:

1. Clinical signs and symptoms,
2. Clinical response to low-dosage L-Dopa/Carbidopa administration,
3. CSF investigation for pterins and biogenic amines,
4. Phenylalanine loading test,
5. Mutations analysis,
6. GTPCH activity in fibroblasts.

The first two tests are highly specific for DRD due to adGTPCH deficiency, but may interfere with disorders such as tyrosine hydroxylase deficiency or others. The pattern of CSF pterins and biogenic amine metabolites 5HIAA and HVA is also specific, but may be seen also in some neurodegenerative diseases. Radiological investigations (MRI and CT) should be included. The phenylalanine loading test may be difficult to interpret in patients with poor intestinal absorption and low phenylalanine blood levels after 1-2 hours. Mutation analysis is not always positive ($< 60\%$) and additional search for small deletions should be included. The enzyme activity measurement is in our hands most useful, but it is time-consuming and rather expensive.

**Acknowledgements:** *This work was supported by the Swiss National Science Foundation grant no. 3100-066953.01*

## References

1. Thöny B, Auerbach G, Blau N. Tetrahydrobiopterin biosynthesis, regeneration and functions. *Biochem J* 2000; 347: 1-26.
2. Werner-Felmayer G, Golderer G, Werner ER. Tetrahydrobiopterin biosynthesis, utilization and pharmacological effects. *Curr Drug Metab* 2002; 3: 159-73.
3. Levine RA. Tetrahydrobiopterin and biogenic amine metabolism in neuropsychiatry, immunology, and aging. *Ann N Y Acad Sci* 1988: 129-39.
4. Ichinose H, Ohye T, Takahashi E, et al. Hereditary progressive dystonia with marked diurnal fluctuation caused by mutation in the GTP cyclohydrolase I gene. *Nature Genet* 1994; 8: 236-41.
5. Blau N, Thöny B, Cotton RGH, Hyland K. *Disorders of tetrahydrobiopterin and related biogenic amines*. In: Scriver CR, Beaudet AL, Sly WS, et al., eds. *The Metabolic and Molecular Bases of Inherited Disease*. 8th ed. New York: McGraw-Hill, 2001: 1725-76.
6. Blau N. Inborn errors of pterin metabolism. *Ann Rev Nutr* 1988; 9: 185-209.
7. Blau N, Ichinose H, Nagatsu T, et al. A missense mutation in a patient with guanosine triphosphate cyclohydrolase I deficiency missed in the newborn screening program. *J Pediatr* 1995; 126: 401-5.

8. Thöny B, Blau N. Mutations in the GTP cyclohydrolase I and 6-pyruvoyl-tetrahydropterin synthase genes. Hum Mutat 1997; 10: 11-20.
9. Thöny B, Neuheiser F, Kierat L, et al. Mutations in the pterin-4a-carbinolamine dehydratase gene cause a benign form of hyperphenylalaninemia. Hum Genet 1998; 103: 162-7.
10. Smooker PM, Cotton RGH. Molecular basis of dihydropteridine reductase deficiency. Hum Mutat 1995; 5: 279-84.
11. Ponzone A, Spada M, Ferraris S, et al. Dihydropteridine reductase deficiency in man: From biology to treatment. Med Res Rev 2004; 24: 127-50.
12. Blau N, Barnes I, Dhondt JL. International database of tetrahydrobiopterin deficiencies. J Inherit Metab Dis 1996; 19: 8-14.
13. Furukawa Y. Update on dopa-responsive dystonia: locus heterogeneity and biochemical features. Adv Neurol 2004; 94: 127-38.
14. Bonafé L, Thöny B, Penzien JM, et al. Mutations in the sepiapterin reductase gene cause a novel tetrahydrobiopterin-dependent monoamine neurotransmitter deficiency without hyperphenylalaninemia. Am J Hum Genet 2001; 69: 269-77.
15. Blau N, Bonafé L, Thöny B. Tetrahydrobiopterin deficiencies without hyperphenylalaninemia: Diagnosis and genetics of Dopa-responsive dystonia and sepiapterin reductase deficiency. Mol Genet Metab 2001; 74: 172-85.
16. Steinberger D, Korinthenberg R, Topka H, et al. Dopa-responsive dystonia: mutation analysis of GCH1 and analysis of therapeutic doses of L-dopa. Neurology 2000; 55: 1735-7.
17. Hirano M, Ueno S. Mutant GTP cyclohydrolase I in autosomal dominant dystonia and recessive hyperphenylalaninemia. Neurology 1999; 52: 182-4.
18. Nardocci N, Zorzi G, Blau N, et al. Neonatal Dopa-responsive extrapyramidal syndrome in twins with recessive GTPCH deficiency. Neurology 2003; 60: 335-7.
19. Knappskog PM, Flatmark T, Mallet J, et al. Recessively inherited L-DOPA-responsive dystonia caused by point mutation (Q381K) in the tyrosine hydroxylase gene. Human Mol Genetics 1995; 4: 1209.
20. Grattan-Smith PJ, Wevers RA, Steenbergen-Spanjers GC, et al. Tyrosine hydroxylase deficiency: Clinical manifestations of catecholamine insufficiency in infancy. Mov Disord 2002; 17: 354-9.
21. Hanihara T, Inoue K, Kawanishi C, et al. 6-Pyruvoyl-tetrahydropterin synthase deficiency with generalized dystonia and diurnal fluctuation of symptoms – a clinical and molecular study. Movement Dis 1997; 12: 408-11.
22. Blau N, Thöny B, Spada M, Ponzone A. Tetrahydrobiopterin and inherited hyperphenylalaninemias. Turk J Pediatr 1996; 38: 19-35.
23. Blau N, Thöny B, Renneberg A, et al. Variant of dihydropteridine reductase deficiency without hyperphenylalaninemia: Effect of oral phenylalanine loading. J Inher Metab Dis 1999; 22: 216-20.
24. Blau N, Thöny B, Renneberg A, et al. Dihydropteridine reductase deficiency localized to the central nervous system. J Inherit Metab Dis 1998; 21: 433-4.
25. Friedman J, Hyland K, Blau N, et al. CNS dihydropteridine reductase deficiency associated with diurnal dystonia and hypersomnolence. AAN Abstract Book 1999.
26. Hyland K, Fryburg JS, Wilson WG, et al. Oral phenylalanine loading in Dopa-responsive dystonia – a possible diagnostic test. Neurology 1997; 48: 1290-7.
27. Saunders-Pullman R, Blau N, Hyland K, et al. Phenylalanine loading as a diagnostic test for Dopa-responsive dystonia: Interpreting the utility of the test. Mol Genet Metab 2004: in press.
28. Bonafé L, Thöny B, Leimbacher W, et al. Diagnosis of Dopa-responsive dystonia and other tetrahydrobiopterin disorders by the study of biopterin metabolism in fibroblasts. Clin Chem 2004; 83: 207-12.
29. Blau N, Duran M, Blaskovics M, Gibson KM. Physician's Guide to the laboratory Diagnosis of Metabolic Diseases. Heidelberg: Springer, 2003.

# Cerebral creatine deficiency and movement disorders

### Saadet Mercimek-Mahmutoglu, Sylvia Stöckler-Ipsiroglu

*Department of Pediatrics, and National Newborn Screening Laboratory, University Hospital and General Hospital of Vienna, Austria*

Creatine deficiency syndromes represent a newly described group of inborn errors of creatine synthesis (arginine: glycine amidinotransferase [AGAT] deficiency and guanidinoaceteate methyltransferase [GAMT] deficiency) and of creatine transport (creatine transporter [CRTR] deficiency). The common clinical feature of creatine deficiency syndromes is mental retardation and epilepsy suggesting main involvement of cerebral gray matter. The typical biochemical abnormality of creatine deficiency syndromes is cerebral creatine deficiency, which is demonstrated by *in vivo* proton magnetic resonance spectroscopy. Measurement of guanidinoacetate in body fluids may discriminate GAMT (high concentration), AGAT (low concentration) and CRTR (normal concentration) deficiency. Specific neurologic symptoms and signs including pathologic signal intensities in globus pallidus and hyperkinetic extrapyramidal movement disorder are mainly observed in GAMT deficiency. GAMT and AGAT deficiency are treatable by oral creatine supplementation, while patients with CRTR deficiency do not respond to this type of treatment.

## ■ Introduction

Creatine is synthesized mainly in liver and pancreas by the action of arginine: glycine amidinotransferase (AGAT) and guanidinoacetate methyltransferase (GAMT). Creatine reaches muscle and brain via an active transmembrane creatine transport system (CRTR). Creatine is then utilized in the cellular pool of creatine/creatine-phosphate, which together with creatine kinase and ATP/ADP, provides a high energy phosphate buffering system. Intracellular creatine and creatine-phosphate are non-enzymatically converted to creatinine, with a constant daily turnover of 1.5% of body creatine. Creatinine is excreted in urine and the daily urinary creatinine excretion is directly proportional to total body creatine *(Figure 1)*.

According to the metabolic pathway of creatine, creatine deficiency syndromes may be due to disorders of creatine synthesis including AGAT (MIM 602360) and GAMT (MIM 601240) deficiency and disorders of creatine transport including the transmembrane creatine transporter (CRTR, MIM 300036) deficiency. GAMT deficiency was recognized as the first inborn error of creatine metabolism in 1994 [1], and a few years later, AGAT deficiency [2] and CRTR (SLC6A8) deficiency [3] were described. Inheritance of GAMT and AGAT deficiency is autosomal recessive, while CRTR deficiency is X-linked. So far, about 20 patients with GAMT deficiency, 4 patients with AGAT deficiency, and more than 20 patients with CRTR deficiency have been diagnosed.

## ■ Clinical Characteristics

The main clinical symptoms observed in all three creatine deficiency syndromes (GAMT, AGAT, CRTR) are: mental retardation, seizures and speech delay.

Patients with GAMT deficiency exhibit a more complex clinical phenotype with severe to mild presentation. The severe GAMT phenotype includes intractable epilepsy, early global developmental delay, extrapyramidal movement disorder and abnormal signal intensities of the basal ganglia. Patients with the intermediate GAMT type exhibit a moderate to severe mental retardation, speech delay, behavioural changes (autistic, hyperkinetic behaviour), and epilepsy (treatable with common anticonvulsive drugs) with minor or unspecific EEG changes. The few patients described so far with the mild phenotype presented with mental retardation, autistic behavior, and speech delay.

The spectrum of movement disorders spans from ataxia to ballismus and chorea with hypotonia and hyperkinesia as common denominator *(Table I)*. In most cases, clinical evidence of movement disorder is associated with pathological signal intensities in the basal ganglia (globus pallidus mainly). The characteristic involvement of basal ganglia and the pattern of clinical manifestation including mental retardation and epilepsy point to main involvement of grey cerebral matter in GAMT deficiency.

Table I. Extrapyramidal movement disorders in 17 patients with GAMT deficiency.

| Type of EPMD | Patient number (total: n = 17) | % |
|---|---|---|
| Atactic/dyskinetic/dystonic | 4/17 | 23 |
| Choreic-ballistic | 1/17 | 6 |
| Hemiballistic-dystonic | 1/17 | 6 |
| Dystonic-ballistic-choreic | 1/17 | 6 |
| EPMD (all together) | 7/17 | 41 |

EPMD = extrapyramidal movement disorder.

## ■ Biochemical and Molecular Diagnostics

### Extra- and intracellular creatine pool

Patients with disorders of creatine synthesis have systemic depletion of creatine and creatine-phosphate due to impairment of *de novo* creatine biosynthesis. Patients with CRTR deficiency – due to impairment of cellular creatine transport – have intracellular depletion of creatine and creatine-phosphate, while extracellular (urinary) creatine concentrations are normal or even elevated.

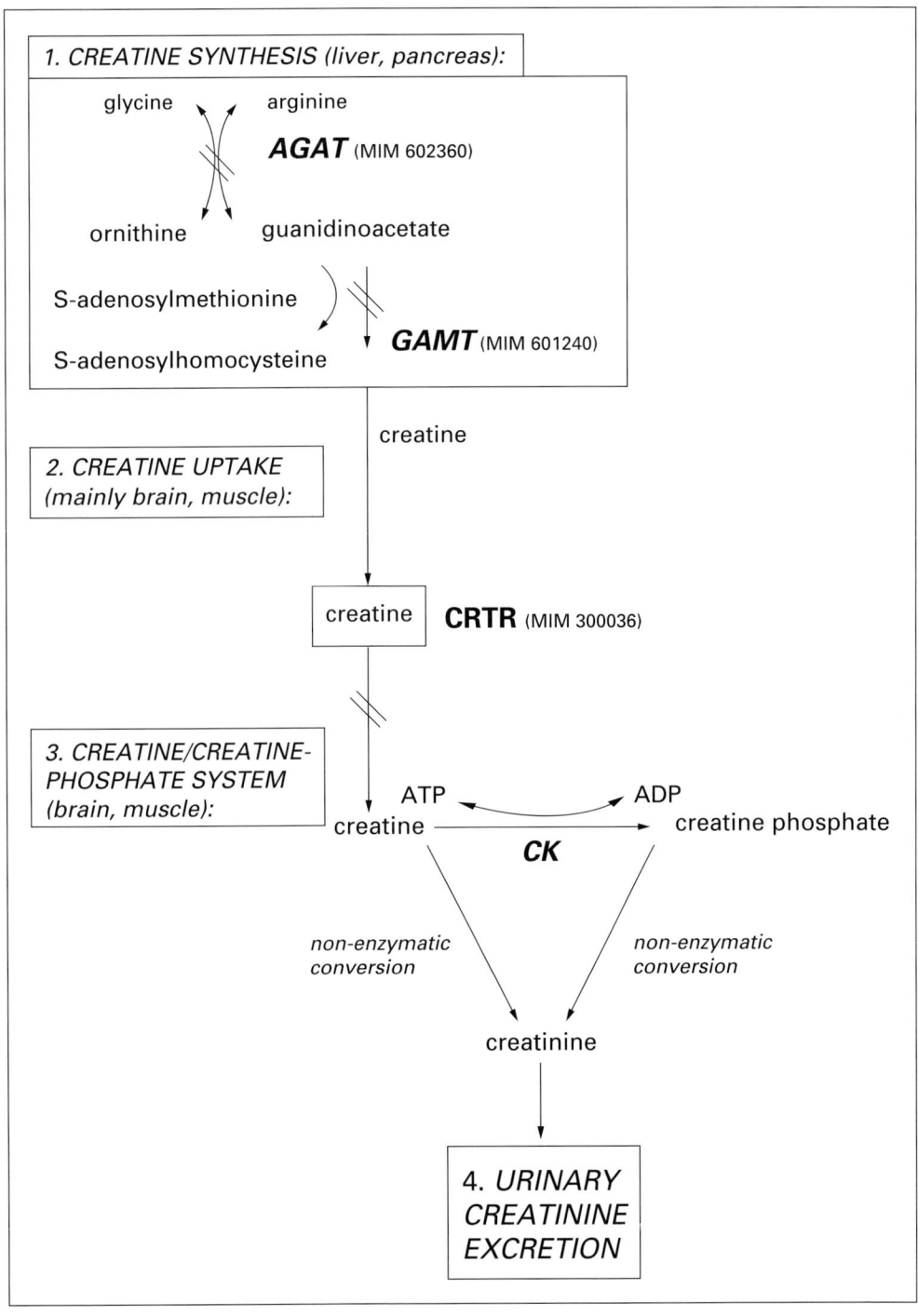

**Figure 1.** Metabolic pathway of creatine/creatine-phosphate.
AGAT = arginine: glycine amidinotransferase; GAMT = guanidinoacetate methyltransferase; CRTR = creatine transporter; CK = creatine kinase.

## Creatine in brain

Common denominator of GAMT, AGAT and CRTR deficiency is depletion of the cerebral creatine pool. Direct measurement of total creatine levels in the brain is possible by *in vivo* proton magnetic resonance spectroscopy: Complete lack of creatine, in the presence of a normal spectral pattern of the remaining metabolites, is a striking and unique pattern. Creatine has a prominent proton magnetic spectrum in the brain, and its deficiency cannot be overlooked *(Figure 2)*.

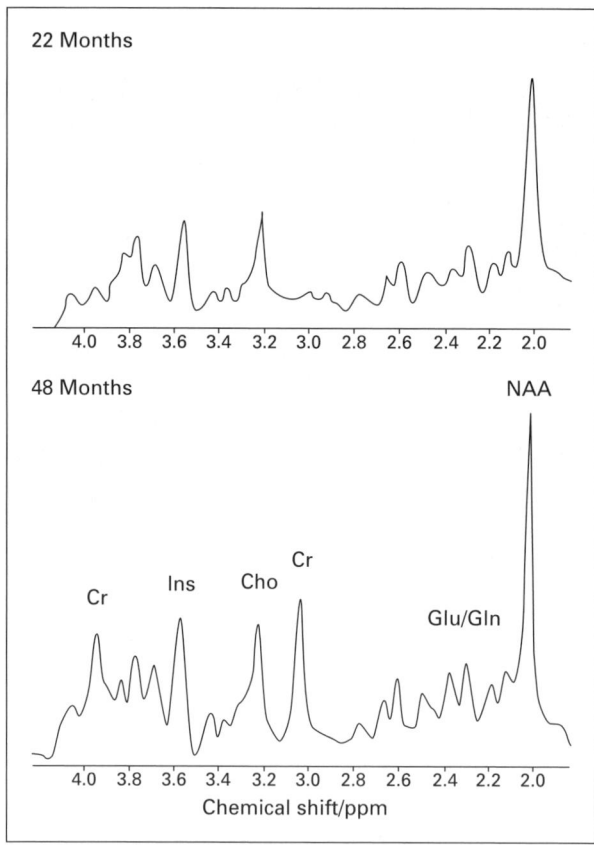

**Figure 2.** *In vivo* proton magnetic resonance spectroscopy (1H MRS) of the brain of a patient with cerebral creatine deficiency due to GAMT deficiency. A) complete lack of creatine resonance. B) Normalisation of creatine spectrum after 6 months of treatment with oral creatine monohydrate.

## Creatine in body fluids

In patients with GAMT deficiency, plasma, urinary and CSF creatine concentrations are low, but in patients with AGAT deficiency, plasma creatine was found to be within normal range, and urinary creatine concentration was only moderately reduced [4]. Therefore, determination of creatine in body fluids seems to be a specific marker

### Table II. Clinical characteristics of GAMT, AGAT and CRTR deficiency.

| Disorder | Mental retardation | Epilepsy | EPMS |
|---|---|---|---|
| GAMT (20 patients) | +++/++/+ | +++/++/+ | +/- |
| AGAT (4 patients) | ++/+ | +/- | - |
| CRTR (> 20 patients) | + | - | - |

Mental retardation: +++ = severe; ++ = moderate; + = mild.
Epilepsy: +++ = drug resistant; ++ = drug responsive; + = occasional fever-induced seizures; - = no seizures.
EPMS = extrapyramidal movement disorder; + = yes; - = no.

### Table III. Biochemical characteristics of GAMT, AGAT and CRTR deficiency & diagnostic tests.

| Disorder | Brain creatine Proton MRS | Guac U/P/CSF | Creatinine 24 h Urine | Creatine/creatinine Urine |
|---|---|---|---|---|
| GAMT | low – absent | high | low | normal |
| AGAT | low – absent | low | (low) | normal |
| CRTR | low – absent | normal | (low) | high |

( ) = expected but insufficient data in patients diagnosed so far.
Guac = guanidinoacetate; U = Urine; P = Plasma; CSF = spinal fluid.

### Table IV. Principles of treatment of Creatine Deficiency Syndroms.
Note that CRTR cannot be treated by any of the given principles.

| Disorder | Correction of creatine deficiency | Correction of guac accumulation | Additional |
|---|---|---|---|
| GAMT | oral creatine supplementation | arginine restriction | ornithine supplementation |
| AGAT | oral creatine supplementation | not required | not available |
| CRTR | no correction by oral creatine supplementation | not required | not available |

Guac = guanidinoacetate.

of GAMT deficiency, but not for AGAT deficiency. In the patients with CRTR deficiency, the urinary creatine excretion relative to the creatinine excretion is elevated, and the ratio creatine/creatinine can be used as a first biochemical diagnostic marker for this disease.

## Guanidinoacetate

The accumulation of guanidinoacetate in tissues and body fluids is pathognomonic for GAMT deficiency, while levels below normal are characteristic for AGAT deficiency. Guanidinoacetate is not altered in CRTR deficiency.

## Creatinine

Urinary creatinine excretion is directly related to the intracellular creatine pool. As the cellular creatine pool is diminished both in disorders of creatine synthesis and in disorders of creatine transport, assessment of the daily creatinine excretion in 24-hour urine samples may be helpful in the diagnosis of GAMT, AGAT, and CRTR deficiency. However in various conditions with reduced muscle mass (*e.g.* in newborns and very young infants and in patients with muscle disease) this test may not be reliable as it merely reflects an unspecific reduction of the body creatine pool.

Plasma creatinine concentrations have been found both below and within (the lower) normal range in patients with creatine deficiency syndromes. Therefore, determination of plasma creatinine concentrations alone is not a sensitive tool for the recognition of these disorders.

## Enzymatic diagnosis

GAMT and AGAT deficiency are confirmed enzymatically by determination of the respective enzyme activities. Highest activities are measured in liver biopsy samples [5]. For less invasive diagnosis, sensitive assays for the measurement of GAMT and AGAT activities have been developed in fibroblasts and virus (EBV) transformed lymphoblasts [6-8]. CRTR deficiency may be diagnosed by creatine uptake studies in cultured fibroblasts [9].

## Mutation analysis

Molecular analysis of GAMT, AGAT and CRTR gene is available. Thirteen different mutations located on various exons of the GAMT gene have been found in the patients with GAMT deficiency [10, 11]. Three patients with AGAT deficiency (all of them from the same pedigree) were homozygous for a T149X nonsense mutation [11, 12]. Different mutations have been identified in the CRTR deficient families [3, 13, 14].

For review of diagnostic procedures see reference [15].

For overview of clinical and biochemical characteristics see *table I* and reference [16].

# ■ Treatment and Outcome

Systemic creatine deficiency as caused by disorders of creatine synthesis (GAMT and AGAT deficiency), can be corrected by oral supplementation of creatine-monohydrate. Dosages from 350 mg to 2 g/kg BW/day have been used in patients with GAMT and AGAT deficiency. The dose level of 350 mg/kg BW/day is about 20 times the daily creatine requirement and has been reported not to induce side effects in healthy volunteers [17].

## GAMT deficiency

Clinical response to oral creatine supplementation as demonstrated in the first described patient with GAMT deficiency [18] includes resolution of extrapyramidal signs and symptoms, substantial developmental progress, improvement of epilepsy and of general condition [18, 19, 20]. During a 25-month period of treatment, almost complete recovery of brain creatine was achieved. Although creatine supplementation leads to substantial clinical benefit, none of the patients has achieved normal development.

The accumulation of guanidinoacetate cannot be sufficiently corrected by creatine monohydrate supplementation alone. Therefore dietary restriction of arginine, which is the rate limiting substrate to the synthesis of guanidinoacetate, and substitution of ornithine, which competitively inhibits the synthesis of guanidinoacetate, is an additional therapeutic approach. Reduction of guanidinoacetate concentrations via competitive inhibition of AGAT activity by additional substitution with high dose ornithine failed [21]. Restriction of dietary arginine, which is the immediate precursor of guanidinoacetate and substrate to AGAT activity, has failed to lower guanidinoacetate levels either [22]. Combined arginine restriction and ornithine supplementation is able to decrease elevated guanidinoacetate concentrations permanently. As shown in one patient, the correction of the metabolite pattern is also associated with a significant improvement of the clinical outcome [22, 23].

## AGAT deficiency

In the three published patients with AGAT deficiency, upon oral creatine supplementation (300 mg/kg) almost complete restoration of extremely low pre-treatment cerebral creatine levels was obtained. Correction of cerebral creatine was accompanied by a favourable clinical response as shown by significant improvement of highly abnormal developmental scores [4, 12]. As guanidinoacetate concentration is low in AGAT deficiency, creatine substitution alone might effectively prevent neurological sequelae in early treated patients.

## CRTR deficiency

Unlike in the patients with GAMT and AGAT deficiency, in CRTR deficiency oral creatine substitution does not result in an increase of brain creatine levels.

For review of treatment see reference [24].

# Conclusion

Up to now creatine deficiency syndromes are underdiagnosed. An alertness of clinicians is necessary to identify new patients. Therefore it is important to establish laboratories offering selective screening for specific analytes (quantitative methods for guanidinoacetate and creatine), as well as combined MRI/MRS investigations in the patients at clinical risk. For interpretation of MRS results it is important to know that in creatine deficiency syndromes almost complete lack of cerebral creatine is a striking feature.

## References

1. Stockler S, Holzbach U, Hanefeld F, et al. Creatine deficiency in the brain: A new treatable inborn error of metabolism. *Pediatr Res* 1994; 36: 409-13.
2. Item CB, Stockler-Ipsiroglu S, Stromberger C, et al. Arginine: Glycine amindinotransferase (AGAT) deficiency: The third inborn error of creatine metabolism in humans. *Am J Hum Genet* 2001; 69: 1127-33.
3. Salomons GS, van Dooren SJ, Verhoeven NM, et al. X-linked creatine-transporter gene (SLC6A8) defect: A new creatine-deficiency syndrome. *Am J Hum Genet* 2001; 68 (6): 1497-500.

4. Bianchi MC, Tosetti M, Fornai F, Cipriani P, De Vito G, Canapicchi R. Reversible brain creatine deficiency in two sisters with normal blood creatine level. *Ann Neurol* 2000; 47: 511-3.
5. Stockler S, Isbrandt D, Hanefeld F, Schmidt B, Figura von K. Guanidinoacetate methyltransferase deficiency: the first inborn error of creatine metabolism in man. *Am J Hum Genet* 1996; 58: 914-22.
6. Ilas J, Mühl A, Stockler-Ipsiroglu S. Guanidinoacetate methyltransferase (GAMT) deficiency: non-invasive enzymatic diagnosis of a newly recognized inborn error of metabolism. *Clin Chim Acta* 2000; 290: 179-88.
7. Verhoeven NM, Roos B, Struys EA, Salomons GS, van der Kmaap MS, Jakobs C. Enzyme assay for diagnosis of guanidinoacetate methyltransferase deficiency. *Clin Chem* 2004; 50: 441-3.
8. Verhoeven NM, Schor DS, Roos B, et al. Diagnostic enzyme assay that uses stable-isotope-labeled substrates to detect L-arginine: glycine amidinotransferase deficiency. *Clin Chem* 2003; 49: 803-5.
9. Salomons GS, van Dooren SJM, Bunea D, Verhoeven NM, Degrauw TJ, Jakobs C. Creatine transporter deficiency: Development of a new functional test for creatine uptake in cultured cells. *J Inher Metab Dis* 2001; 24 (suppl 1): 119.
10. Item CB, Stromberger C, Muhl A, et al. Denaturing gradient gel electrophoresis for the molecular characterization of six patients with guanidinoacetate methyltransferase deficiency. *Clin Chem* 2002; 48: 767-69.
11. Item CB, Mercimek-Mahmutoglu S, Battini R, et al. Characterization of seven novel mutations in seven patients with GAMT deficiency. *Hum Mutat* 2004; 23 (5): 524.
12. Battini R, Leuzzi V, Carducci C, et al. Creatine depletion in a new case with AGAT deficiency: clinical and genetic study in a large pedigree. *Mol Genet Metab* 2002; 77: 326-31.
13. Bizzi A, Bugiani M, Salomons GS, et al. X-Linked creatine deficiency syndrome: A novel mutation in creatine transporter gene SLC6A8. *Ann Neurol* 2002; 52: 227-31.
14. Hahn KA, Salomons GS, Tackels-Horne D, et al. X-linked mental retardation with seizures and carrier manifestations is caused by a mutation in the creatine-transporter gene (SLC6A8) located in Xq28. *Am J Hum Genet* 2002; 70: 1349-56.
15. Stockler-Ipsiroglu S, Stromberger C, Item CB, Mühl A. *Disorders of creatine metabolism*. In: Blau N, Duran M, Blaskovics ME, Gibson KM, eds. *Physician's guide to the laboratory diagnosis of metabolic diseases*. Heidelberg (Germany): Springer Verlag, 2003: 467-80.
16. Stromberger C, Bodamer O, Stockler-Ipsiroglu S. Clinical characteristics and diagnostic clues in inborn errors of creatine metabolism. *J Inher Metab Dis* 2003; 26: 299-308.
17. Greenhaff PL, Casey A, Short AH, Harris R, Soderlund D, Hultman E. Influence of oral creatine supplementation on muscle torque during repeated bouts of maximal voluntary exercise in man. *Clin Sci* 1993; 187: 219-27.
18. Stockler S, Hanefeld F, Frahm J. Creatine replacement therapy in guanidinoacetate methyltransferase deficiency, a novel inborn error of metabolism. *Lancet* 1996; 348: 789-90.
19. Ganesan V, Johnson A, Connelly A, Eckhardt S, Surtees RA. Guanidinoacetate methyltransferase deficiency: New clinical features. *Pediatr Neurol* 1997; 17: 155-7.
20. Schulze A, Hess T, Wevers R, Echhardt S, Surtees RA. Creatine deficiency syndrome caused by guanidinoacetate methyltransferase deficiency: diagnostic tools or a new inborn error of metabolism. *J Pediatr* 1997; 131: 626-31.
21. Stockler S, Marescau B, De Deyn PP, Trijbels JMF, Hanefeld F. Guanidino compounds in guanidinoacetate methyltransferase deficiency, a new inborn error of creatine synthesis. *Metabolism* 1997; 46: 1189-93.
22. Schulze A, Mayatepek E, Bachert P, Marescau B, De Deyn PP, Rating D. Therapeutic trial of arginine restriction in creatine deficiency syndrome. *Eur J Pediatr* 1998; 157: 606-7.
23. Schulze A, Bachert P, Schlemmer H, et al. Lack of creatine in muscle and brain in an adult with GAMT deficiency. *Ann Neurol* 2003; 53 (2): 248-51.
24. Stockler-Ipsiroglu S, Battini R, de Grauw T, Schulze A. *Disorders of creatine metabolism*. In: Blau N, Hoffmann GF, Leonard J, Clarke JTR, eds. *Physician's guide to the treatment and follow up of metabolic diseases*. Heidelberg (Germany): Springer Verlag, 2005, in press.

# Tourette syndrome: autoimmune mechanisms

Francisco Cardoso

*Neurology Service, The Federal University of Minas Gerais, Belo Horizonte, Brazil*

---

Sydenham's chorea (SC) is the first described neuropsychiatric disorder associated with streptococcus. Despite the emphasis on its motor aspects, older descriptions already emphasize the coexistence of behavioral disturbances. In 1860, Marcé mentioned that 2/3 of his patients with chorea also had mental symptoms. Fifty one years later Diefendorf found that mood changes, restlessness, emotional lability, nocturnal terror and attention deficit were common features of patients with acute chorea. In the middle of the XXth century the relationship between chorea and behavioral disorders became so much appreciated that authors submitted that schizophrenia and other psychiatric conditions were caused by SC [1] or even that chorea resulted from behavioral disorders [2]. In a controlled study undertaken in 1965, Freeman and colleagues described that "personality disturbances" were present in 26 of 40 patients with previous history of CS in contrast with just 8 of 30 controls.

However, up to the late 1980s there was no description of neuropsychiatric syndromes distinct from SC associated with streptococcus infection. The only possible exception was a single case report from Japan, where Kondo and Kabasawa in 1978 described one 11-year-old boy who developed Tourette's syndrome (TS) a few days after a febrile illness associated with elevated antistreptolysin O titer [3]. This situation changed in 1989 with Kiessling's description of 8 patients with tic disorder and evidence of recent infection with group A beta-hemolytic streptococcus (GABHS) at its onset or symptom worsening [4]. In this same year, Swedo's group at the National Institutes of Mental Health in Washington, DC, EUA, published a systematic assessment of 23 patients with previous history of SC and 13 subjects with rheumatic fever without chorea [5]. In this study the authors found obsessive-compulsive behavior (OCB) in five subjects of the SC group, of whom three met criteria for obsessive-compulsive disorder (OCD) whereas no patient of the rheumatic fever group presented with OCB. These findings led Swedo and her group [6, 7] to propose that SC is a model for childhood autoimmune neuropsychiatric disorders. According to this theory, infection with GABHS leads to formation of antibodies which cross-react with basal ganglia epitopes, leading to movement disorders (chorea, tics and others) as well as behavioral disturbances (*e.g.*, OCD). Following this speculation, these authors published several case reports and uncontrolled case series of patients with variable combination of OCB, OCD and tic disorder presumably associated with GABHS infection [8-13]. The authors initially proposed the term PITANDS (pediatric infection-triggered autoimmune neuropsychiatric disorders) [8] which was replaced by PANDAS (pediatric autoimmune neuropsychiatric disorders associated with streptococcus) in the next year [9].

Since the first articles implying a casual relationship between streptococcal infections and neuropsychiatric conditions other than SC, there have been many publications related to the issue. For instance, an electronic search on PubMed using PANDAS as the keyword results in 55 studies published since 1996. Many of these studies enthusiastically and noncritically accept the notion that GABHS infection of the oropharynx can lead to neuropsychiatric disorders as diverse as tics, myoclonus, parkinsonism, dystonia, abdominal contractions, OCD, OCB, attention deficit and hyperactivity disorder, anorexia nervosa, body dysmorphic disorder, aggressiveness, autism, and adult PANDAS. On the other hand, there are articles expressing scepticism of the existence of a casual relationship between streptococcal infection and many of these syndromes [14]. In summary, despite the flurry of articles, the literature remains far from a consensual view of the relationship between streptococcus and neuropsychiatric disorders. The aim of the present chapter is to provide a review of this topic. As the concept of PANDAS is based on the idea of events similar to those present in CS leading to different clinical profiles, I will first review the pathogenesis of rheumatic chorea. Subsequently, the discussion will be focused on PANDAS, emphasizing proposed diagnostic criteria, epidemiology, clinical and laboratory features, immune mechanism and therapeutic implications.

## ■ Pathogenesis of Sydenham's Chorea

Taranta and Stollerman established the casual relationship between GABHS infection and occurrence of SC [15]. Using indirect immunofluorescence, Husby et al. [16] were the first to identify antibodies against basal ganglia (ABGA) in SC. In their study, antibodies against cytoplasm of caudate and subthalamic neurons were detected in the serum of 46% of 30 patients with SC and 14% of 50 subjects with rheumatic carditis without chorea whereas the positivity in normal controls and patients with other conditions did not exceed 4%. Exposure of the positive sera to GABHS cell wall preparations resulted in significant reduction of the fluorescence. These results led to the hypothesis that infection with GABHS leads to formation of cross-reactive antibodies that disrupt the basal ganglia function. A specific epitope of streptococcal M proteins that cross-reacts with basal ganglia has been identified [17]. To account for the finding that just a minority of subjects infected with GABHS develop rheumatic fever (RF), it has been proposed that these complications occur in individuals genetically predisposed. The genetic marker for RF and related conditions would be either human leukocyte antigen-linked antigen expression (HLA) [18] or the B-cell alloantigen D8/17 [19]. Other findings suggesting the autoimmune nature of SC is the observation that immunosuppressive doses of steroids are effective in controlling the movement disorder and other manifestations of patients refractory to conventional therapies [20]. It must be emphasized that despite the popularity of the molecular mimicry theory, there remain many unsolved points which will be reviewed in the next paragraphs.

Firstly, it is necessary to reflect about the techniques used to demonstrate ABGA and how the results are presented. The advantage of indirect immunofluorescence technique is the demonstration of binding to an area of interest. On the other hand, it is a qualitative method whose reading (the intensity of fluorescence) can be quite subjective. Ideally, the observer must remain blinded to the clinical status of the subject donor of the serum. Unfortunately, in most instances this has not been done. Enzyme-linked immunosorbent assay (ELISA) lacks the morphologic precision of the previous method but allows quantification of the results. Using this technique, we have demonstrated that virtually all patients with acute SC are "positive" for ABGA [21]. The reason for the quotation marks is to remind the reader that all subjects tested do have some degree of absorbance, ie, antibodies against basal ganglia are present in all of them. What differentiates patients from controls is the degree of reactivity: positivity has been defined as an absorbance value greater than the mean plus two standard deviations of the optical density of controls. Others, however, prefer to present the data without employing this stratagem, just reporting the optical density values of each group [22]. Western blot (WB) techniques have also been used by us and others to study circulating antibodies in SC. Although more sensitive, it clearly lacks the specificity of ELISA since the material used as substrate to react with the antibodies is made up of denatured proteins. In fact, WB is more useful to trace targets of the immune response because of its capability to detect the molecular weight of the epitopes. Positivity on WB studies is usually presented in a nonquantitative manner (reactivity against targets not present in controls) or, less often, quantitatively with more sophisticated statistical techniques such as discriminant analysis [23].

Regardless of the methodology employed, essentially all studies of antibodies in SC agree that IgG ABGA are more seen in 50 to 90% of patients with chorea [16, 21]. In a study of patients from the Movement Disorders Clinic of the Federal University of Minas Gerais (MDC-UFMG), Church et al. [21] demonstrated that ABGA ELISA had a sensitivity of 95% and specificity of 93% in 20 patients with acute SC whereas these values on both immunofluorescent method (IF) and WB were, respectively, 100% and 93%. The sensitivity of WB and IF were, respectively, 69% and 63% in 16 subjects with persistent SC. The latter was defined as chorea lasting at least two years despite best treatment. Singer et al. [22], however, failed to find a statistical significant difference between SC patients and controls on ELISA for ABGA. However, rather than implying that the concentration of ABGA in SC is not raised, this study may reflect a small (nine patients) and clinically heterogeneous cohort. The WB studies point out to numerous antigens as important targets in SC: 40 kDa, 45 kDa, 60 kDa, 126 kDa and 131 kDa.

Another problem of the theory of molecular mimicry in SC is the target of the antibodies. Based on the circuitry of the basal ganglia [24], one can assume that ABGA directed against subthalamic nucleus could lead to interruption of its outflow, causing disinhibition of the ventrolateral thalamus and subsequent excessive activation of the motor cortex which would result in hyperkinesia. However, although not impossible to conceptualize, it is less clear how disruption of the caudate nucleus function could cause chorea. The possible explanation would be binding to medium spiny neurons belonging to the indirect pathway. The cessation of its function could release the lateral pallidum which, by its turn, would inhibit the subthalamic nucleus. It remains to be determined, however, if the anticaudate antibodies do bind to this specific subpopulation of neurons.

More crucial, however, is the question of how the ABGA reach the central nervous system. Under normal conditions, the blood-brain barrier (BBB) is impermeable to IgGs. This situation could change, however, if there is inflammation in the central nervous system. RF is unequivocally an inflammatory disease. In the heart, for instance, there can be severe inflammation of the endocardium. There is lack of evidence, however, of existence of a similar process in the brain of SC patients. The old autopsy studies do not support such theory since the findings reported by these authors are just consistent with nonspecific post-mortem diffuse abnormalities (for review, see [25]). More recently, most of the imaging studies have failed to find abnormalities in SC. Just one investigation, employing volumetric technique, identified increase in the size of the caudate, putamen and globus pallidus in 24 SC patients [26]. One possible interpretation for this finding is inflammation of the basal ganglia although this hypothesis is weakened by the lack of change in the signal. Similarly, we did not find evidence of inflammation in our recent CSF study [21]. In summary, there is no evidence of rupture of the BBB in CS which could explain how large molecules, such as IgG ABGA, could have access to the central nervous system. One alternative hypothesis that remains to be determined is the traffic of lymphocytes through the BBB. Inside the brain these cells would produce antibodies.

The most fundamental of all points pertaining to the hypothesis of cross-reactive antibodies is the demonstration of their biological activity. In many conditions, antibodies are merely epiphenomena: destruction of neurons by nonimmune mechanisms may lead to exposure of antigens which trigger formation of immunoglobulins which lack any pathogenic role. So far, no one has reported the passive transfer of ABGA of SC patients inducing meaningful biological response *in vivo* models. Classically, this type of experiment consists of injection of antibodies in experimental animals, causing an anatomical and/or physiological change. In SC, it is expected that infusion of ABGA in the basal ganglia (subthalamus, for instance) of an animal would cause dyskinesias or some other abnormality. Another approach was recently pursued by Kirvan et al. [27]. These authors demonstrated that IgM of SC induces expression of calcium-dependent calmodulin in culture of neuroblastoma cells. Although an interesting finding, this study has several limitations: it is an *in vitro* investigation, employing an artificial paradigm which does not necessarily reflect the situation observed in human patients; the antibody was obtained from one single patient; and, finally, the authors studied IgM whereas all investigations of ABGA in SC have detected IgG. In conclusion, although SC patients do have GABHS-induced antibodies which cross-react with basal ganglia antigens, it remains unknown whether they have any pathogenic value.

Because of the difficulties with the molecular mimicry hypothesis to account for the pathogenesis of SC, recently there have been studies addressing the role of immune cellular mechanisms in this condition. Investigating sera and CSF samples of CSF patients of the MDC-UFMG, Church and colleagues [28] in London found elevation of cytokines which take part in the Th2 (antibody-mediated) response, interleukins 4 (IL-4) and 10 (IL-10), in the serum of acute SC in comparison to persistent SC. They also described increase of IL-4 in 31% of the CSF of acute SC whereas just IL-4 was raised in the CSF of persistent SC. The authors concluded that SC is characterized by a Th2 response. However, as they have found elevation of IL-12 in acute SC and, more recently, we described increased concentration of chemokines CXCL9 and CXCL10 in the serum of patients with acute SC [29], it can be concluded that Th1 (cell-mediated) mechanisms may also be involved in the pathogenesis of SC.

One additional limitation of the autoimmune theory of the pathogenesis of SC is the finding that the proposed markers of genetic susceptibility, HLA loci as well as the D8/17 alloantigen, are nonspecific. A more recent study, for instance, failed to identify any relationship between SC and human leukocyte antigen class I and II alleles [30]. Despite repeated reports of the group which developed the essay claiming its high specificity and sensitivity [31, 32], findings of other authors suggest that the D8/17 marker lacks specificity and sensitivity. For instance, Kaur et al. [33] demonstrated that the discriminating power of monoclonal antibody against D8/17 was relatively low among patients of North Indian ethnic origin with rheumatic fever. Studying Caucasians in the USA, Murphy et al. [34] showed that 65.6% of their patients with OCD and/or chronic tic disorder and 8.3% of controls tested positive for D8/17. In Netherlands, Jansen and colleagues [35] found that just a minority of their patients with post-GABHS arthritis have elevation of D8/17-positive lymphocytes.

The above-mentioned shortcomings have led authors to even question the autoimmune theory of the pathogenesis of SC [36]. Other mechanisms have been proposed to explain the basal ganglia dysfunction in SC: streptococcal infection inducing vasculitis of medium-sized vessels; vascular lesions produced by antiphospholipid antibodies. Both theories do not seem tenable, however. There are no imaging or CSF investigations that lend support to existence of vasculitis in SC. Moreover, with one exception, all studies have failed to detect antiphospholipid antibodies in this condition.

Nevertheless, in conclusion, despite many obscure points, the current weight of evidence is in favor of the hypothesis that immune mechanisms induced by infection with GABHS interferes with the function of the basal ganglia leading to a constellation of signs and symptoms which characterize SC.

## ■ Clinical Features and Diagnostic Criteria of Streptococcus Related Neuropsychiatric Disorders

The usual age at onset of Sydenham's chorea (SC) is 8 to 9 years, although there are reports on patients developing chorea in the third decade of life, and in most series there is a female preponderance [37]. Typically, patients develop this disease 4 to

8 weeks after an episode of GABHS pharyngitis. It does not occur after streptococcal infection of the skin. The chorea, characterized by a random and continuous flow of contractions, rapidly spreads, becoming generalized but 20% of patients remain with hemichorea [37, 38]. Patients display motor impersistence, particularly noticeable during tongue protrusion and ocular fixation. The muscle tone is usually decreased; in severe and rare cases (1.5% of all patients seen at the MDC-UFMG) this is so pronounced that the patient may become bedridden (*chorea paralytica*).

Patients often display other neurologic and non-neurologic symptoms and signs. There are reports of common occurrence of tics in SC. We found it virtually impossible to distinguish simple tics from fragments of chorea. Even vocal tics, found in 70% or more of patients with SC in one study [39], are not of simple diagnosis in patients with hyperkinesias. Physicians experienced with movement disorders patients are well aware that involuntary vocalizations may result from dystonia or chorea of the pharynx and larynx. This has been reported in subjects with, for instance, oromandibular dystonia or Huntington's disease [40]. Under these circumstances the vocalization lacks the subjective feeling (premonitory urge or sensory tic) so characteristic of idiopathic tic disorders such as Tourette's syndrome. Investigation of premonitory feeling of tics as well as of complex tics (another feature also more specific of tic disorders) in SC will help solve this controversy. In the cohort of 120 SC patients followed up at the MDC-UFMG, we have identified complex tics in less than 4% of subjects.

There is evidence that many patients with active chorea have hypometric saccades, and a few of them also show oculogyric crisis. Dysarthria is common, and Gowers had already recognized in the XIXth century that SC patients present with a "disinclination to speak". In fact, a recent case-control study of patients at the MDC-UFMG described a pattern of decreased verbal fluency reflecting reduced phonetic, but not semantic, output [41]. This finding is suggestive of dysfunction of the dorsolateral pre-frontal-basal ganglia circuit. In a recent survey of 110 patients with rheumatic fever, half of whom had chorea, we found that migraine is more frequent in SC (21.8%) than normal controls (8.1%, $p = 0.02$) [42]. This is similar to what has been described in Tourette syndrome although in this study the authors have compared their results with data of the literature rather than their own controls [43]. In the older literature, there are also references to papilledema, central retinal artery occlusion, and seizures in a few patients with SC.

Lately, attention has been drawn to behavioral abnormalities. Previously in this chapter, it has already been mentioned that Swedo and her colleagues [5] found obsessive-compulsive behavior in five of 13 SC patients, of whom three met criteria for OCD, whereas no patient of the rheumatic fever (FR) group presented with OCB. In another study of 30 patients with SC, Asbahr et al. [44] demonstrated that 70% of the subjects presented with obsessions and compulsions, whereas 16.7% of them met criteria for OCD. None of 20 patients with RF without chorea had obsessions or compulsions [44]. These results were roughly replicated by a more recent study that, however, found that patients with RF without chorea had more obsessions and compulsions than healthy controls [45]. The text of this study, however, is not clear about the actual percentage of SC patients who had OCD. It is stated that 11.9% of the patients with RF (with or without chorea) met criteria for this disorder but in no point of the article are the two groups presented separately. As the authors write that there was no difference in the frequency of OCD in patients with and without RF, one can presume that about 12% of the 22 SC patients met criteria for this condition.

Mercadante and colleagues [45] also tackled the issue of hyperactivity and attention deficit disorder (ADHD) in SC and found that 45% of their 22 patients met criteria for this condition. In a recent survey of 156 subjects at the MDC-UFMG, Maia et al. [46] found that the score on the Leyton inventory was 14.8 ± 8.6 and 25.8 ± 22.5 in, respectively, 50 patients with RF without chorea and 56 subjects with SC. In this study the authors demonstrated that OCB displays little degree of interference in the performance of the activities of daily living. Comparing patients with acute and persistent Sydenham's chorea, ADHD was significantly more common in the latter (50% *versus* 16%) whereas there was a trend towards more OCB/OCD among subjects with more prolonged forms of SC but the difference failed to reach statistical significance. ADHD was also more common in the SC group in comparison with normal controls and subjects with RF without chorea. One note of caution must be made regarding the interpretation of data of hyperactivity in SC. As there is no biological marker used in the current diagnostic criteria (DSM-IV), it is not always easy to differentiate restlessness associated with chorea from true hyperactivity of ADHD.

Finally, it must be kept in mind that SC is a major manifestation of RF: 60% to 80% of patients display cardiac involvement, particularly mitral valve dysfunction, in SC, whereas the association with arthritis is less common, seen in 30% of subjects, although in approximately 20% of the patients chorea is the sole finding [37]. The current diagnostic criteria of SC are a modification of the Jones criteria: chorea with acute or subacute onset and lack of clinical and laboratory evidence of alternative cause are mandatory findings; the diagnosis is further supported by the presence of additional major or minor manifestations of rheumatic fever [37, 47, 48].

Outside the context of SC, there have been descriptions of numerous neuropsychiatric syndromes presumably in causal association with GABHS infection. The latter has been diagnosed usually using the classical laboratory findings anti-streptolysin-O (ASTO) and anti-DNAse B antibodies. It is also relevant to mention that all investigations of PANDAS are noncontrolled studies of which the majority corresponds to single case reports or series of few patients. The largest cohort so far reported is 50 patients [13]. In a more recent study, the authors searched for ABGA in 100 patients who met the TS diagnostic criteria. Positivity for the antibodies was found in 20 of the enrolled patients [49]. Tic disorder, meeting criteria of TS, and related conditions are the movement disorders most often described as part of PANDAS. The most commonly reported behavioral disorders related to GABHS are OCB and OCD. With three exceptions, the phenomenology presented by these patients does not differ substantially from their usual, presumably non-autoimmune, counterparts. The distinguishing features are the positivity of markers of GABHS infection; sudden, explosive onset; and presence of choreiform movements. There are, however, problems related to the former. First, streptococcal infection not leading to RF or any related complication remains a quite common problem in the first two decades of life regardless of the considered geographic region. For instance, in a recent survey of school children in the US, Morita et al. [50] found colonization of the oropharynx by streptococcus in 50% of them. In other words, this means that positivity of these markers lacks any meaningful specificity. Second, these very markers are usually negative in SC because of the long latency between the streptococcal infection and onset of chorea. As to sudden onset, it would reflect the abrupt beginning of a biological response triggered by infection. It is not unusual, however, that patients with idiopathic TS develop tics in a sudden manner. Moreover, because of the lack of controlled studies it remains to be determined whether this feature is indeed characteristic or even more common among patients with neuropsychiatric syndromes related to streptococcus. As to the other supposedly distinguishing feature, choreiform movements, it is a troublesome concept: they lack definition and, if one considers them as chorea, the patient would meet criteria of SC and not other condition such as PANDAS. Other movement disorders described in association with streptococcal infection have been myoclonus, dystonia, paroxysmal dyskinesia, abdominal contractions, and parkinsonism [51-57].

In some instances, the clinical picture of movement disorders emerges in the context of acute disseminated encephalomyelitis or encephalitis lethargica-like syndrome [52, 57]. As to the latter, recently the authors reported on 20 patients with a combination of sleep disorder, lethargy, movement disorders (parkinsonism and dyskinesias) and behavioral changes which were preceded by pharingitis in 55% of cases. Neuroimaging studies showed inflammatory changes in the basal ganglia in 40% of patients, elevated anti-ASTO in 65% of cases and antibodies against basal ganglia (ABGA) on Western blot (WB) studies in 95%. Although interesting, these cases should be viewed with great caution since it has been well demonstrated that the clinical findings of encephalitis lethargica are quite nonspecific [25]. Numerous agents, particularly viruses, have the potential to cause such phenomenology. One good example of this possibility is Japanese encephalitis, an endemic condition in south Asia. Up to 66% of patients with this illness, particularly children, present with a movement disorder [58]. From a laboratory point of view, WB studies have high sensitivity but low specificity. In situations of extensive and severe inflammation such as encephalitis, a nonspecific process may lead to exposure of antigens resulting in formation of antibodies which lack pathogenic value (epiphenomenon). Therefore, until more experience of assay of ABGA in encephalitis is gathered, these results must be viewed with skepticism.

The behavioral disorders often reported in association with GABHS infection are OCB/OCD and ADHD. Church et al. [49] have been the only ones to compare the behavioral findings of patients with and without evidence of streptococcal infection. They failed to find difference in the frequency of OCD between the two groups but ADHD was less common among the ABGA positive patients. To my knowledge, there is no comparative study of the content of OCB between idiopathic and streptococcus related forms of OCD. OCD, however, is more common in idiopathic TS than in SC: 50% *versus* 19% in patients seen at the MDC-UFMG [59, 46]. Moreover, based on our clinical experience with a large cohort of patients with these disorders, it can be suggested that OCD is more disabling in TS than in SC. This hypothesis is supported by the finding that interference is low in patients with the latter condition. In the recent study of the MDC-UFMG, the resistance and interference score on the Leyton inventory were, respectively, 9.6 ± 9.1 e 6.7 ± 7.5 [46]. Other behavioral disorders described as part of PANDAS or related to ABGA are encephalitis lethargica, anorexia nervosa, body dysmorphic disorder, aggressiveness, and autism [57, 60-62].

It is also necessary to draw the attention of the reader to the lack of reports describing non-neurologic findings of RF among patients with neuropsychiatric disorders presumably related to streptococcus. It is particularly noteworthy that there is no description of carditis in PANDAS since at least 60% of patients with SC do have heart lesions [25] and the ABGA are also cross-reactive with cardiac antigens [16].

In 1998 Swedo and colleagues proposed diagnostic criteria for PANDAS: OCD and/or tic disorder; pediatric onset; episodic clinical course; association with GABHS infection; presence of choreiform movements. Not only have these criteria not been validated but they have significant limitations. As already discussed in previous items, association with GABHS infection lacks specificity; and the criterion choreiform movements do not correspond to any recognized category of movement disorder. "Episodic clinical course" is so characteristic of TS and other idiopathic tic disorders that it has been included in their diagnostic criteria (DSM-IV).

## ■ Laboratory and Immunological Findings in Streptococcus Related Neuropsychiatric Disorders

In the previous section it has already been described that, by definition, all patients diagnosed with PANDAS have positive ASTO and/or anti-DNAse B. Another approach to the problem is to determine the percentage of patients who meet diagnostic criteria for idiopathic tic disorders that presents with laboratory evidence of GABHS infection. In summary, there is a proportion of patients with tic disorders that do present with positivity on studies of streptococcal infection. It must be stressed, however, that the positive and negative subset of patients are not clinically distinct.

Singer et al. [63] performed ELISA and WB studies to search for reactivity against basal ganglia antigens in patients with TS (41) and controls (39), comparing these results with clinical features and markers of streptococcal infection. On ELISA they found that the reactivity against putamen, but not caudate and globus pallidus, was greater in patients with TS. Antibodies against antigens of 83, 67, and 60 kDa were detected more frequently in the TS group. There was no correlation of these laboratory findings with clinical variables such as age of onset of tic, sudden onset of tic, tic severity and behavioral disorders (ADHD or OCD). However, the group of patients with higher titers of streptococcal markers (ASTO or antiDNAse B) included a significantly larger number of TS patients. The sensible conclusion of the authors is that the relation between the antiputamen antibody and clinical and streptococcal markers is, at best, equivocal.

Church et al. [49] studied 100 patients with TS, 50 children with other neurological disease, 40 children with uncomplicated streptococcal infection, 50 adults with neurological disease, and 50 healthy adults. On WB, the authors identified ABGA in 23%

of TS patients (the 60 kDa antigen was the most common target). With the exception of a higher frequency of ADHD in the ABGA negative group (50% *versus* 22%), there was no clinical difference between the two groups. There was, however, a correlation between elevation of ASTO (91%) and positivity for ABGA (91% among those who tested positive and 57% in the negative group). In summary, this study confirms the conclusions of Singer et al. [63] that, indeed, a subgroup of TS patients does have autoimmunity against the basal ganglia. Another implication, of value particularly to clinicians, is the lack of clinical markers capable of distinguishing ABGA positive patients. The data of Church and his colleagues also further strengthen the notion that markers of streptococcal infection are of little value to identify TS subjects ABGA positive, since 2/3 of those ABGA negative also have elevated ASTO.

Quite recently, employing ELISA and WB techniques Singer et al. [64] measured the titers of ABGA in 15 patients meeting criteria of PANDAS (they were recruited by Swedo's group) and 15 matched controls. On both techniques the authors failed to find any difference between the two groups in relation to antibodies against caudate, putamen and globus pallidus. Just when they performed discriminant analysis (a statistical method to assess mean binding patterns on WB), the authors noticed greater binding of the supernatant fraction of caudate in PANDAS patients. The conclusion of the authors is the lack of significant concentration of ABGA in PANDAS. This study can be criticized on the grounds of having included a small number of patients. If one believes that no more than 20% of TS patients do have a significant reactivity against basal ganglia [49], just 3 patients of this study are positive – a number probably insufficient to result in a statistically significant difference.

A German group has also investigated markers of streptococcal infection in TS patients. In their first study [65], they studied 13 chidren/teenagers with TS, 23 adults with TS, 17 schizophrenics, and age-matched controls. The frequency of elevated ASTO and/or antiDNAse B was higher in patients with TS, either adults or children/adolescents, in comparison with the psychotic group as well as the age matched controls. In a subsequent investigation, these authors refined their findings by studying antibodies against different fractions of the capsular M protein of Streptococcus [66]. Comparing 25 adults with TS with healthy controls, they found a higher mean optical density on ELISA for antibodies against M12 and M19. There was no difference with controls in relation to reactivity against proteins M1, M4 and M6. Using ELISA and WB, Morshed et al. [67] determined ASTO titers and the reactivity against several epitopes, among them neural antigens, in the sera of 81 TS patients, 27 SC patients, 52 subjects with autoimmune disorders and 67 normal controls. In comparison to controls, TS patients had higher ASTO titers and reactivity against neural antigens. However, the mean reactivity against neural antigens was lower in TS than in SC and patients with other autoimmune disorders. ASTO titers were, however, higher in the TS group than among the patients with other autoimmune disorders. In a similar line, Loiselle and colleagues [68] also assessed the relationship between antistreptococcal markers and clinical features in 41 children with TS and 38 controls with previous history of streptococcal infection. Anti-DNAse and ASTO titers were similar in the two groups. However, the authors found that more children with ADHD had elevated ASTO titers (64% *versus* 34% in patients without this disorder).

The interpretation of these studies is not simple. One of the obstacles is the lack of standardization of the laboratory methods employed by different investigators. This problem starts with significant discrepancies in the manner the data has been presented. As already discussed, the Queen Square group defined a positive/negative system of ELISA and WB readings based on a cutoff limit of mean plus two standard deviations of the optical density of controls. The investigators from Johns Hopkins, on the other hand, have decided to present the values of the optical density. The Yale group chose to create a a rank system ranging from 0 to 227 to present their results of ASTO and ELISA studies [67]. There are more fundamental technical differences, however. One of them is the use of different anatomical regions to collect antigens. Depending on the study, the choice has included caudate, putamen, globus pallidus, subthalamic nucleus. Another methodological issue is the use of different ways of obtaining the tissue preparations. Another possible technical problem is the use of brain from adults to obtain antigens to test antibodies present in a disease which is essentially confined to children and adolescents. Nevertheless, taking together these studies, it can be concluded that a proportion of TS patients greater than controls present with elevated titers of markers of streptococcal infection and ABGA. However, there is no firm correlation between these laboratory findings and clinical features.

Finally, at least three studies assessed the effects of infusion of sera of TS and/or PANDAS patients in the *striatum* of rodents. In the first, Hallett and colleagues [69] selected five TS patients with elevated titers of antibodies against a solubilized neuroblastoma cell membrane fraction. In comparison to controls, infusion of sera of these patients in the ventral *striatum* of rats resulted in significant increase in stereotypic behaviors. Taylor *et al.* [70] used a similar methodology but ABGA in the sera of TS patients were detected using IF technique and the site of infusion was more lateral in comparison to the previous study [69]. Nevertheless, the authors also found increased oral stereotypies. These results were challenged by a more recent study of Loiselle *et al.* [71]. These authors infused not only sera from nine TS patients and eight PANDAS subjects (all selected on the grounds of elevated optical density on an ELISA study for antibodies against putamen) but also antibodies against anti-M5 protein (a rheumatogenic streptococcal protein). Despite infusion into ventrolateral and ventral *striatum*, in none of the groups was observed any effect distinct from controls. In conclusion, these results indicate that more studies are needed before a firm statetement can be made about the potential of passive transfer of immune-mediated dysfunction of the basal ganglia.

## ■ Therapeutic Implications

One very important practical implication of the PANDAS hypothesis is the possibility of the use of antimicrobian agents and immunosuppressive treatments in these conditions. Despite the problems discussed in the previous sections surrounding the notion of GABHS infection as a cause of neuropsychiatric conditions other than CS, there have been many reports of attempts to manage patients with tics, OCD and other conditions. Unfortunately, most of these articles describe noncontrolled and/or open-label trials involving a limited number of patients followed up for short periods of time.

Before describing proposed treatments of PANDAS, it is necessary to keep in mind that even in SC, the prototype of neurological complication of GABHS, there is no definite proof of the therapeutic value of immunosuppression. Recently, we have reported the preliminary experience of the MDC-UFMG in treating SC patients refractory to conventional treatment (antibiotics, valproic acid, and neuroleptics). In this study, iv methyl-prednisolone followed by oral prednisone improved patients previously disabled by chorea and/or parkinsonism or dystonia induced by neuroleptics [20]. There are, however, obvious limitations to this trial: open-label nature, inclusion of just five patients, and the exceptional clinical features of the patients (persistent SC, refractoriness to conventional treatment).

In 1999, the NIH group described the treatment of 29 patients meeting their criteria of PANDAS [72]. The treatment arms were plasma exchange (10 subjects), intravenous immunoglobulin (9 patients), and placebo or sham plasma exchange in the remaining individuals. One month after receiving the active treatments patients were reported to have a 50% improvement of OCB and tics. Problems of this study (e.g., limited number of patients, short follow up and non-blinded design) led the author of an accompanying editorial to recommend caution in the interpretation of the results [73]. It is appropriate to remind the readers that even in adults plasma exchange and intravenous immunoglobulin are treatments carrying the potential to cause serious complications. Clearly, it is still lacking evidence demonstrating their safety and effectiveness in children with tics, OCD and others.

The same NIH group [74] described the negative results of the treatment of 37 PANDAS patients with oral penicillin V. This was a double-blind, balanced cross-over study where patients were followed up for eight months. Neither clinical features (tics and OCB) nor streptococcal markers changed with the two regimens. The authors suggested that the antibiotic dosage was not sufficient to modify the GABHS infection. Additional explanations for the negative findings are the small number of patients enrolled and the limitation of the inclusion criteria. Murphy and Pichichero [75] described, however, a different scenario. Along a three-year period they identified 12 school children meeting PANDAS criteria. Eradication of the streptococcus by antibiotics treatment was reported to follow improvement of tics and OCD. More boldly, there is one recent suggestion of treatment of PANDAS with tonsillectomy [76].

Currently on both sides of the Atlantic there are ongoing, well-designed (prospective and controlled) trials enrolling larger number of patients to test the safety and efficacy of these treatment modalities. Until the results of these studies are available, treatment of tics and related behavioral disorders with antibiotics or immunomodulatory therapies remains experimental and must not be incorporated into clinical practice.

We recently compared the pattern of response to dopamine receptor blockers in 100 SC patients and the same number of subjects with TS [77]. Despite the groups being matched by age and dosage of neuroleptics, 5% of patients with chorea developed parkinsonism, dystonia or both whereas these complications were not seen among the TS patients. This finding shows that the typical patient with tic disorder has a pattern of response to dopamine receptor blockers distinct from patients with neurologic complication of GABHS.

# Conclusion

GABHS infection can cause dysfunction of the basal ganglia resulting in abnormal movements and behavioral disorders which characterize SC. Despite recent advances in the understanding of the immune mechanisms present in SC, it still remains speculative that GABHS-induced ABGA are responsible for the generation of brain dysfunction in RF. The hypothesis that a similar pathogenic mechanism can account for a subset of patients with tics, other movement disorders, OCB and other behavior disturbances is appealing though unproved at this time.

**Acknowledgements:** *The author expresses his gratitude to Antonio Lúcio Teixeira Jr MD PhD for critical reading of the manuscript as well his collaboration in many of the studies cited in the text. It is also acknowledged the collaboration of Débora Palma Maia MD, Mauro César Quintão Cunningham MD and MD Fidel Castro Alves Meira in the investigations of Sydenham's chorea performed at the MDC-UFMG.*

# References

1. Bruetsch WL. Late cerebral sequelae of rheumatic fever. *Arch Int Med* 1944; 73: 472-6.
2. Chapman AH, Pilkey L, Gibbons MJ. A psychosomatic study of eight children with Sydenham's chorea. *Pediatrics* 1958; 21: 582-95.
3. Kondo K, Kabasawa T. Improvement in Gilles de la Tourette syndrome after corticosteroid therapy. *Ann Neurol* 1978; 4: 387.
4. Kiessling LS. Tic disorders associated with evidence of invasive group A beta-hemolytic streptococcal disease. *Dev Med Child Neurol Suppl* 1989; 59: 48.
5. Swedo SE, Rapoport JL, Cheslow DL, et al. High prevalence of obsessive-compulsive symptoms in patients with Sydenham's chorea. *Am J Psychiatry* 1989; 146: 246-9.
6. Swedo SE, Leonard HL, Schapiro MB, et al. Sydenham's chorea: physical and psychological symptoms of St Vitus dance. *Pediatrics* 1993; 91: 706-13.
7. Swedo SE. Sydenham's chorea. A model for childhood autoimmune neuropsychiatric disorders. *JAMA* 1994; 272: 1788-91.
8. Allen AJ, Leonard HL, Swedo SE. Case study: a new infection-triggered, autoimmune subtype of pediatric OCD and Tourette's syndrome. *J Am Acad Child Adolesc Psychiatry* 1995; 34: 307-11.
9. Giedd JN, Rapoport JL, Leonard HL, et al. Case study: acute basal ganglia enlargement and obsessive-compulsive symptoms in an adolescent boy. *J Am Acad Child Adolesc Psychiatry* 1996; 35: 913-5.
10. Swedo SE, Leonard HL, Mittleman BB, et al. Identification of children with pediatric autoimmune neuropsychiatric disorders associated with streptococcal infections by a marker associated with rheumatic fever. *Am J Psychiatry* 1997; 154: 110-2.
11. Greenberg BD, Murphy DL, Swedo SE. Symptom exacerbation of vocal tics and other symptoms associated with streptococcal pharyngitis in a patient with obsessive-compulsive disorder and tics. *Am J Psychiatry* 1998; 155: 1459-60.
12. Perlmutter SJ, Garvey MA, Castellanos X, et al. A case of pediatric autoimmune neuropsychiatric disorders associated with streptococcal infections. *Am J Psychiatry* 1998; 155: 1592-8.
13. Swedo SE, Leonard HL, Garvey M, et al. Pediatric autoimmune neuropsychiatric disorders associated with streptococcal infections: clinical description of the first 50 cases. *Am J Psychiatry* 1998; 155: 264-71.

14. Kurlan R. Tourette's syndrome and "PANDAS": will the relation bear out? Pediatric autoimmune neuropsychiatric disorders associated with streptococcal infection. *Neurology* 1998; 50: 1530-4.
15. Taranta A, Stollerman GH. The relationship of Sydenham's chorea to infection with group A streptococci. *Am J Med* 1956; 20: 1970.
16. Husby G, Van De Rijn U, Zabriskie JB, et al. Antibodies reacting with cytoplasm of subthalamic and caudate nuclei neurons in chorea and acute rheumatic fever. *J Exp Med* 1976; 144: 1094-110.
17. Bronze MS, Dale JB. Epitopes of streptococcal M proteins that evoke antibodies that cross-react with human brain. *J Immunol* 1993; 151: 2820-8.
18. Ayoub EM, Barrett DJ, Maclaren NK, Krischer JP. Association of class II human histocompatibility leukocyte antigens with rheumatic fever. *J Clin Invest* 1986; 77: 2019-26.
19. Feldman BM, Zabriskie JB, Silverman ED, Laxer RM. Diagnostic use of B-cell alloantigen D8/17 in rheumatic chorea. *J Pediatr* 1993; 123: 84-6.
20. Cardoso F, Maia D, Cunningham MC, Valença G. Treatment of Sydenham chorea with corticosteroids. *Mov Disord* 2003; 18: 1374-7.
21. Church AJ, Cardoso F, Dale RC, et al. Antibasal ganglia antibodies in acute and persistent Sydenham's chorea. *Neurology* 2002; 59: 227-31.
22. Singer HS, Loiselle CR, Lee O, et al. Antibasal ganglia antibody abnormalities in Sydenham chorea. *J Neuroimmunol* 2003; 136 (1-2): 154-61.
23. Wendlandt JT, Grus FH, Hansen BH, Singer HS. Striatal antibodies in children with Tourette's syndrome: multivariate discriminant analysis of IgG repertoires. *J Neuroimmunol* 2001; 119: 106-13.
24. Alexander GE, DeLong MR, Strick PL. Parallel organization of functionally segregated circuits linking basal ganglia and cortex. *Annu Rev Neurosci* 1986; 9: 357-81.
25. Cardoso F. *Infectious and transmissible movement disorders.* In: Jankovic J, Tolosa E, eds. *Parkinson's disease and movement disorders.* 4th ed. Baltimore: Williams and Wilkins, 2002: 930-40.
26. Giedd JN, Rapoport JL, Kruesi MJ, et al. Sydenham's chorea: magnetic resonance imaging of the basal ganglia. *Neurology* 1995; 45: 2199-202.
27. Kirvan CA, Swedo SE, Heuser JS, Cunningham MW. Mimicry and autoantibody-mediated neuronal cell signalling in Sydenham chorea. *Nat Med* 2003; 9: 914-20.
28. Church AJ, Dale RC, Cardoso F, et al. CSF and serum immune parameters in Sydenham's chorea: evidence of an autoimmune syndrome? *J Neuroimmunol* 2003a; 136: 149-53.
29. Teixeira Jr AL, Cardoso F, Souza ALS, Teixeira MM. Increased serum concentrations of monokine induced by interferon- (/CXCL9 and interferon- (-inducible protein 10/CXCL-10 in Sydenham's chorea patients. *J Neuroimmunol* 2004; 150 (1-2): 157-62.
30. Donadi EA, Smith AG, Louzada-Junior P, et al. HLA class I and class II profiles of patients presenting with Sydenham's chorea. *J Neurol* 2000; 247: 122-8.
31. Eisen JL, Leonard HL, Swedo SE, et al. The use of antibody D8/17 to identify B cells in adults with obsessive-compulsive disorder. *Psychiatry Res* 2001; 104: 221-5.
32. Harel L, Zeharia A, Kodman Y, et al. Presence of the D8/17 B-cell marker in children with rheumatic fever in Israel. *Clin Genet* 2002; 61: 293-8.
33. Kaur S, Kumar D, Grover A, et al. Ethnic differences in expression of susceptibility marker (s) in rheumatic fever/rheumatic heart disease patients. *Int J Cardiol* 1998; 64: 9-14.
34. Murphy TK, Benson N, Zaytoun A, et al. Progress toward analysis of D8/17 binding to B cells in children with obsessive compulsive disorder and/or chronic tic disorder. *J Neuroimmunol* 2001; 120: 146-51.
35. Jansen TL, Hoekstra PJ, Bijzet J, et al. Elevation of D8/17-positive B lymphocytes in only a minority of Dutch patients with post-streptococcal reactive arthritis (PSRA): a pilot study. *Rheumatology* 2002; 41: 1202-3.
36. Loiselle CR, Singer HS. Genetics of childhood disorders: XXXI. Autoimmune disorders, part 4: is Sydenham chorea an autoimmune disorder? *J Am Acad Child Adolesc Psychiatry* 2001; 40: 1234-6.

37. Cardoso F, Silva CE, Mota CC. Sydenham's chorea in 50 consecutive patients with rheumatic fever. *Mov Disord* 1997; 12: 701-3.
38. Nausieda PA, Grossman BJ, Koller WC, et al. Sydenham's chorea: an update. *Neurology* 1980; 30: 331-4.
39. Mercadante MT, Campos MC, Marques-Dias MJ et al. Vocal tics in Sydenham's chorea. *J Am Acad Child Adolesc Psychiatry* 1997; 36: 305-6.
40. Jankovic J. Differential diagnosis and etiology of tics. *Adv Neurol* 2001; 85: 15-29.
41. Cunningham MCQS. *Avaliação da fluência verbal em pacientes com Coréia de Sydenham*. Dissertação de Mestrado. Departamento de Morfologia, Pós-Graduação em Biologia Celular, ICB, UFMG, 2003.
42. Teixeira Jr AL, Meira FCA, Cardoso F. Migraine headache in patients with Sydenham's chorea. *Cephalagia* 2005 (in press).
43. Kwack C, Vuong KD, Jankovic J. Migraine headache in patients with Tourette syndrome. *Arch Neurol* 2003; 60: 1595-8.
44. Asbahr FR, Negrao AB, Gentil V, et al. Obsessive-compulsive and related symptoms in children and adolescents with rheumatic fever with and without chorea: a prospective 6-month study. *Am J Psychiatry* 1998; 155: 1122-4.
45. Mercadante MT, Busatto GF, Lombroso PJ, et al. The psychiatric symptoms of rheumatic fever. *Am J Psychiatry* 2000; 157: 2036-8.
46. Maia DP, Teixeira Jr AL, Cunningham MCQ, Cardoso F. Behavioral disorders in Sydenham's chorea. *Neurology* 2005 (Submitted).
47. Guidelines for diagnosis of rheumatic fever, Jones criteria, 1992 update. Special Writing Group of the Committee of Rheumatic Fever, Endocarditis, and Kawasaki Disease of the Council on Cardio-Vascular Disease of the Young of the American Heart Association. Guidelines for the diagnosis of rheumatic fever. *JAMA* 1992; 268: 2069-73.
48. Cardoso F, Vargas AP, Oliveira LD, et al. Persistent Sydenham's chorea. *Mov Disord* 1999; 14: 805-7.
49. Church AJ, Dale RC, Lees AJ, et al. Tourette's syndrome: a cross sectional study to examine the PANDAS hypothesis. *J Neurol Neurosurg Psychiatry* 2003; 74: 602-7.
50. Morita JY, Kahn E, Thompson T, et al. Impact of azithromycin on oropharyngeal carriage of group A Streptococcus and nasopharyngeal carriage of macrolide-resistant Streptococcus pneumoniae. *Pediatr Infect Dis J* 2000; 19: 41-6.
51. DiFazio MP, Morales J, Davis R. Acute myoclonus secondary to group A beta-hemolytic streptococcus infection: A PANDAS variant. *J Child Neurol* 1998; 13: 516-8.
52. Dale RC, Church AJ, Cardoso F, et al. Poststreptococcal acute disseminated encephalomyelitis with basal ganglia involvement and auto-reactive antibasal ganglia antibodies. *Ann Neurol* 2001; 50: 588-95.
53. Dale RC, Church AJ, Benton S, et al. Post-streptococcal autoimmune dystonia with isolated bilateral striatal necrosis. *Dev Med Child Neurol* 2002; 44: 485-9.
54. Dale RC, Church AJ, Surtees RA, et al. Post-streptococcal autoimmune neuropsychiatric disease presenting as paroxysmal dystonic choreoathetosis. *Mov Disord* 2002; 17: 817-20.
55. Martinelli P, Ambrosetto G, Minguzzi E et al. Late-onset PANDAS syndrome with abdominal muscle involvement. *Eur Neurol* 2002; 48: 49-51.
56. Ben-Pazi H, Livne A, Shapira Y, Dale RC. Parkinsonian features after streptococcal pharyngitis. *J Pediatr* 2003; 143: 267-9.
57. Dale RC, Church AJ, Surtees RA, et al. Encephalitis lethargica syndrome: 20 new cases and evidence of basal ganglia autoimmunity. *Brain* 2004; 127 (Pt 1): 21-33.
58. Kalita J, Misra UK, Pandey S, Dhole TN. A comparison of clinical and radiological findings in adults and children with Japanese encephalitis. *Arch Neurol* 2003; 60: 1760-4.
59. Cardoso F, Veado CC, de Oliveira JT. A Brazilian cohort of patients with Tourette's syndrome. *J Neurol Neurosurg Psychiatry* 1996; 60: 209-12.

60. Sokol MS. Infection-triggered anorexia nervosa in children: clinical description of four cases. *J Child Adolesc Psychopharmacol* 2000; 10: 133-45.
61. Mathew SJ. PANDAS variant and body dysmorphic disorder. *Am J Psychiatry* 2001; 158: 963.
62. Vojdani A, Campbell AW, Anyanwu E, et al. Antibodies to neuron-specific antigens in children with autism: possible cross-reaction with encephalitogenic proteins from milk, Chlamydia pneumoniae and Streptococcus group A. *J Neuroimmunol* 2002; 129 (1-2): 168-77.
63. Singer HS, Giuliano JD, Hansen BH, et al. Antibodies against human putamen in children with Tourette syndrome. *Neurology* 1998; 50: 1618-24.
64. Singer HS, Loiselle CR, Lee O, et al. Antibasal ganglia antibodies in PANDAS. *Mov Disord* 2004; 19: 406-15.
65. Muller N, Riedel M, Straube A, et al. Increased antistreptococcal antibodies in patients with Tourette's syndrome. *Psychiatry Res* 2000; 94: 43-9.
66. Muller N, Kroll B, Schwarz MJ, et al. Increased titers of antibodies against streptococcal M12 and M19 proteins in patients with Tourette's syndrome. *Psychiatry Res* 2001; 101: 187-93.
67. Morshed SA, Parveen S, Leckman JF, et al. Antibodies against neural, nuclear, cytoskeletal, and streptococcal epitopes in children and adults with Tourette's syndrome, Sydenham's chorea, and autoimmune disorders. *Biol Psychiatry* 2001; 50: 566-77.
68. Loiselle CR, Wendlandt JT, Rohde CA, Singer HS. Antistreptococcal, neuronal, and nuclear antibodies in Tourette syndrome. *Pediatr Neurol* 2003; 28: 119-25.
69. Hallett JJ, Harling-Berg CJ, Knopf PM, et al. Anti-striatal antibodies in Tourette syndrome cause neuronal dysfunction. *J Neuroimmunol* 2000; 111 (1-2): 195-202.
70. Taylor JR, Morshed SA, Parveen S, et al. An animal model of Tourette's syndrome. *Am J Psychiatry* 2002; 159: 657-60.
71. Loiselle CR, Lee O, Moran TH, et al. Striatal microinfusion of Tourette syndrome and PANDAS sera: failure to induce behavioral changes. *Mov Disord* 2004; 19: 390-6.
72. Perlmutter SJ, Leitman SF, Garvey MA, et al. Therapeutic plasma exchange and intravenous immunoglobulin for obsessive-compulsive disorder and tic disorders in childhood. *Lancet* 1999; 354: 1153-8.
73. Singer HS. PANDAS and immunomodulatory therapy. *Lancet* 1999; 354: 1137-8.
74. Garvey MA, Perlmutter SJ, Allen AJ, et al. A pilot study of penicillin prophylaxis for neuropsychiatric exacerbations triggered by streptococcal infections. *Biol Psychiatry* 1999; 45: 1564-71.
75. Murphy ML, Pichichero ME. Prospective identification and treatment of children with pediatric autoimmune neuropsychiatric disorder associated with group A streptococcal infection (PANDAS). *Arch Pediatr Adolesc Med* 2002; 156: 356-61.
76. Heubi C, Shott SR. PANDAS: pediatric autoimmune neuropsychiatric disorders associated with streptococcal infections – an uncommon, but important indication for tonsillectomy. *Int J Pediatr Otorhinolaryngol* 2003; 67: 837-40.
77. Teixeira AL, Cardoso F, Maia DP, Cunningham MC. Sydenham's chorea may be a risk factor for drug induced parkinsonism. *J Neurol Neurosurg Psychiatry* 2003; 74: 1350-1.

# Stereotypies in autistic and other childhood disorders

**Joseph Jankovic**

*Parkinson's Disease Center and Movement Disorders Clinic, Dpt of Neurology, Baylor College of Medicine, Houston, Texas, USA*

Stereotypies may be defined as involuntary or involuntary (in response to or induced by inner sensory stimulus or unwanted feeling), coordinated, patterned, repetitive, rhythmic, seemingly purposeless, movements or utterances [1, 2]. Typical motor stereotypies include body rocking, head nodding, head banging, hand waving, repetitive and sequential finger movements, lip smacking, and chewing movements; phonic stereotypies include grunting, moaning, and humming. Stereotypies are usually either continuous, such as seen in patients with tardive dyskinesia, mental retardation, or autism, or they are intermittent, as in stereotypic tics in patients with Tourette syndrome (TS). Mannerisms, which are gestures peculiar or unique to the individual, may at times seem stereotypical (patterned), but they are usually not continuous. There is often an overlap between stereotypies and self-injurious behavior, such as biting, scratching, and hitting [3-5].

In addition to motor and phonic, stereotypies can be classified as either simple (*e.g.* foot tapping, body rocking) or complex (*e.g.* complicated rituals, sitting down and arising from chair). Stereotypies can also be described according to distribution of the predominant site of involvement (orolingual, hand, leg, truncal). The term stereotypy should be used to describe a phenomenological, not as etiological, category of hyperkinetic movement disorders. However, recognition of stereotypy as a distinct movement disorder can logically lead from a phenomenological to an etiological diagnosis *(Table I)*. It is well-known that stereotypies often accompany a variety of behavioral disorders such as anxiety, obsessive-compulsive disorders (OCD), TS, schizophrenia, autism, mental retardation, akathisia, restless legs syndrome, and a variety of neurodegenerative disorders, including fronto-temporal dementia [6]. Thus, stereotypy is a motor-behavioral disorder found most frequently in patients who are in the borderland between neurology and psychiatry.

## Pathophysiology of Stereotypies

There is no clear anatomical-clinical correlation for stereotypies, although it is believed that both cortical and subcortical structures are involved. While dysfunction in the basal ganglia has been implicated in the pathogenesis of certain stereotypies, some studies have also provided evidence for the role of the mesolimbic system, particularly the nucleus accumbens-amygdala pathway, in the pathogenesis of stereotypical movements. Stereotypies with or without associated obsessive-compulsive behavior have been observed in patients with structural lesions in different anatomical areas, including bilateral lesions of the medial frontoparietal cortices [7, 8] and cerebellum [9].

Stereotypical behavior is common in animals in lower species up to and including the primates, and are particularly common in farm and zoo animals housed in restraining environments with low stimulation [5, 10]. Self-injurious behavior, observed in 14% of housed monkeys, may be viewed as a form of stereotypy [11]. Therefore, stereotypy has been viewed as either a self-generating sensory stimulus or a motor expression of underlying tension and anxiety. The repetitive and ritualistic behavior displayed by some animals has been used as an experimental model of OCD. Indeed, studies of animal and human stereotypies have provided important insights into relationships between motor function and behavior. Some veterinarian scientists have even suggested changing the nomenclature of stereotypies to obsessive-compulsive behaviors, but there is little evidence to indicate that the stereotypic behavior observed in animals is driven by underlying obsessions and represent a compulsive behavior [10, 12].

Most studies of stereotypical behavior in experimental animals have focused on the role of dopaminergic systems in the basal ganglia and limbic structures. Intrastriatal injection of dopamine and systemic administration of both pre-synaptically active dopaminergic drugs, such as amphetamine, and post-synaptically active dopamine agonists, such as apomorphine, in rats produce dose-related repetitive sniffing, gnawing, licking, biting, rearing, head bobbing, grooming and other stereotyped learned activities.

The observation that self-biting behavior induced by dopaminergic drugs in 6-hydroxydopamine rats and monkeys with a unilateral lesion in the ventral medial tegmentum can be blocked by a selective $D_1$ antagonist SCH 23390 suggests that self-injurious behavior is mediated primarily by the $D_1$ receptors [4]. Selective dopamine receptor agonists and antagonists have been used in experimental models to study different effects of $D_1$ and $D_2$ receptors on stereotypical behavior. SKF 38393, a $D_1$ agonist, produced no stereotypic behavior in normal rats, but it did enhance stereotypy induced by apomorphine, a mixed $D_1$ and $D_2$ agonist [13]. This suggests that the $D_2$ dopamine receptors mediate stereotypical behavior, and that activation of the $D_1$ receptors potentiates these $D_2$-mediated effects. Additional evidence for the role of $D_2$ dopamine receptors in the pathogenesis of stereotypies is the observation that upregulation of $D_2$ receptors (e.g. with haloperidol, a selective $D_2$ antagonist), but not of $D_1$ receptors (e.g. with SCH 23390, a selective $D_1$ antagonist), enhanced apomorphine-induced stereotypies [14]. Drug-induced models of stereotypy, however, may not accurately reflect spontaneous or disease-related repetitive

**Table I. Etiologic Classification of Stereotypies.**

- Physiological
    - Normal child development
    - Stress-related
    - Self-gratifying behavior
    - Sensory deprivation, including restraining, blindness, deafness
- Pathological
    - Mental retardation
    - Autism (including Kanner's infantile autism, Asperger syndrome)
    - Rett syndrome
    - Neuroacanthocytosis
    - Schizophrenia
    - Catatonia
    - Obsessive-compulsive disorder
    - Tourette syndrome
    - Tardive and other dyskinesias
    - Akathisia
    - Restless legs syndrome
    - Frontotemporal dementia
    - Epileptic automatism
    - Psychogenic

behaviors. Using several selective dopaminergic agonists (apomorphine, SKF81297, and quinpirole) as well as intrastriatal administration of the $D_2$ receptor antagonist raclopride to study stereotypic behaviors in the deer mouse model of spontaneous and persistent stereotypy, showed that spontaneously emitted and drug-induced stereotypies may have different mechanisms [15]. Nevertheless, these studies suggest that the striatal dopaminergic system is significantly involved in stereotypic behaviors. Oral and forelimb stereotypies can be induced in the rat with injections of amphetamine into the ventrolateral striatum [16] and certain genes can be activated in the striasomes with these drugs when administered orally [17]. These studies provide further support for a basal ganglia involvement in stereotypies. Although there is experimental evidence from rodent and primate studies to support the notion that differential activation of striosomes in the basal ganglia plays an important role in pathophysiology of stereotypies [18], some recent studies found that motor stereotypies do not require enhanced activation of striosomes [19].

Besides the classic neurotransmitters, evidence is accumulating in support of involvement of neuropeptides as modulators of stereotypical behavior. For example, microinjection of cholecystokinin and neurotensin into the medial nucleus accumbens markedly potentiated apomorphine-induced stereotypy [20]. Since injection of these peptides into the striatum had no effect on the apomorphine-induced stereotypy, these studies provide additional evidence for the involvement of the limbic system in the pathogenesis of this movement disorder. Improvement in self-injurious behavior observed in autistic children after administration of the opiate blockers naloxone and naltrexone has been interpreted as evidence for the role of endogenous opiates (*e.g.* beta-endorphins) in this abnormal behavior [21]. Additional support for the role of endorphins in self-injurious and stereotypical behavior is the finding of elevated plasma and cerebrospinal fluid levels of beta-endorphins in autistic patients with these behavioral abnormalities [21]. More recently, the emphasis has shifted to the serotonin system, supported by the observation that certain animal behaviors improve with serotonin uptake inhibitors [22].

## ■ Physiological Stereotypies

Certain stereotypies, such as tapping of the feet, adduction-abduction and crossing-uncrossing and other repetitive movements of the legs may be part of a repertoire of movements seen in otherwise normal individuals. In infants and children there seems to be a progression of normal stereotypies [23]. For example, thumb and hand sucking in infancy is later replaced by body rocking, head rolling and head banging. Some infants demonstrate head stereotypies that resemble bobble-head doll syndrome, sometimes associated with ataxia, but without any other neurologic deficit and normal subsequent development [9]. A review of 40 "normal" children, aged 9 months to 17 years, with complex hand and arm stereotypies, such as flapping, shaking, clenching, posturing and other "ritual" movements, showed that the movements can be temporarily suppressed in nearly all when cued [24]. Although the children were classified as "normal" 25% had co-morbid ADHD and 20% had learning disability, probably due to referral bias since this group is also known for their work in TS. This was supported by relatively high family history of stereotypies (25%) and tics (33%). A variety of stereotypies can be observed in children [25, 26] and young adults [27] without any other neurological deficits. We have observed otherwise normal children with persistent head stereotypies similar to the bobble-head syndrome, but without abnormal neuroimaging studies. Stereotypies may also occur during development of otherwise normal children who are congenitally blind [28] or deaf [29]. Patients with Williams syndrome, a hypersociable behavior associated with hemizygous deletion in chromosome band 7q11.23, including the gene for elastin, also can present with slow, complex, persistent head stereotypies [30]. Head banging is seen in up to 15% of normal children [31]. Some girls exhibit stereotypic crossing and extending of legs which actually represents a self-gratifying or masturbatory behavior [32]. Otherwise normal children can also develop bruxism, nail biting, trichotillomania, and other stereotypical behaviors. These behaviors have been often attributed to underlying generalized anxiety disorder or OCD. However, when stereotypy is accompanied by other behavioral and neurological findings, it usually indicates the presence of a serious underlying neurological and/or psychiatric disorder *(Table I)*.

## ■ Mental Retardation

It is beyond the scope of this chapter to review the current notions about the clinical features and pathogenesis of mental retardation, but the reader is referred to some recent reviews of this topic [33]. In one study of 102 institutionalized mentally retarded people, mean age 35 (range 21-68) years, 34% exhibited at least one type of stereotypy (rhythmic movement 26%, bizarre posturing 13%, object manipulation 7%, and others) [34]. In another study 100 individuals with severe or profound intellectual disability were randomly selected and followed for 26 years [35]. Their behavior was recorded through carer and psychiatrist ratings using the Modified Manifest

Abnormality Scale of the Clinical Interview Schedule. The follow-up evaluations found that stereotypies, emotional abnormalities, eye avoidance, and other behavioral symptoms persist. Although there seems to be an inverse correlation between stereotypies and IQ, stereotypical behavior may be seen even in the mildly retarded. In some mental retardation disorders, typically Lesch-Nyhan syndrome, stereotypies are associated with self-injurious behavior. Supersensitivity of $D_1$ receptors, possibly in response to abnormal arborization of dopamine neurons in the striatum, has been postulated as a possible mechanism of self-injurious behavior in Lesch-Nyhan syndrome [36].

## ■ Autism

Autism is a type of pervasive developmental disorder (PDD), sometimes referred to as autistic spectrum disorders, with onset during infancy or childhood, characterized by impairment in reciprocal social and interpersonal interactions, impairment in verbal and non-verbal communication, markedly restricted repertoire of activities and interests, and stereotyped movements [37]. Earlier studies have suggested that about 0.1% of all children are autistic [38], but more recent epidemiological studies have estimated that the prevalence of autistic disorders and related PDD to range between 0.3% [39] and 0.6% [40]. In children and adults with autism of any cause, stereotypies and other self-stimulatory activities constitute the most recognizable symptoms. Typical stereotypies seen in autistic individuals include facial grimacing, staring at flickering light, waving objects in front of the eyes, producing repetitive sounds, arm flapping, rhythmic body rocking, repetitive touching, feeling and smelling of objects, jumping, walking on toes, and unusual hand and body postures. The motor manifestations are often associated with insensitivity or excessive sensitivity to sensory stimuli including pain and extremes of temperature, preoccupations with perceptual sensations such as lights or odors, insistence on preservation of sameness, and absence of fear or other emotional reactions. Self-stimulatory and self-injurious behaviors such as self-biting and head banging, are also common. In addition to these and other behavioral and developmental abnormalities, some autistic individuals have isolated areas of remarkable and sometimes spectacular mental skills-the so-called Savant syndrome [41, 42].

There are many causes of autism, including the fragile X syndrome and a variety of eponymically classified types such as Kanner, Heller, Asperger, Down and Rett syndromes [43]. Asperger syndrome is one of the most common forms of autism, found in 1-3/1000 children [44]. Characterized by social isolation in combination with odd and eccentric behavior, Asperger syndrome shares many features with infantile autism. Several studies have indeed noted an overlap in various clinical and demographic characteristics between Asperger syndrome and infantile autism [45, 46]. In one study of 23 patients, the Asperger children seemed to have relatively poor motor skills, had a stiff and awkward gait (without arm-swing), and their speech development was delayed, although they acquired better expressive speech as compared with infantile autism. In contrast to infantile autism, Asperger syndrome usually does not become fully manifest until 30-36 months of age, but some may have first symptoms in infancy. A study of 7 patients with the combination of Asperger syndrome and TS showed

MRI evidence of cortical and subcortical abnormalities in 5 of these patients [47]. Because Asperger children are generally less cognitively impaired, it has been suggested that this syndrome merely represents a mild variant of autism. We studied eight patients with Asperger syndrome and an additional four with other forms of PDD referred to our Movement Disorders Clinic for evaluation of tics [43]. All patients exhibited stereotypic movements; in addition seven had tics and six of these met inclusion diagnostic criteria for TS. Of the six patients with clinical features of both Asperger syndrome and TS, three had severe congenital sensory deficits, suggesting that sensory deprivation contributes to the development of adventitious movements in this population. Besides Asperger, other autistic children also show features of TS [48].

Dysfunction of the frontal-parietal cortex, neostriatun, thalamus, and cerebellum has been suggested in autistic patients by various cerebral metabolic and imaging studies. MRI studies have found left frontal and brainstem atrophy in some autistic patients [49], but other studies have failed to find any characteristic abnormalities on MRI scans of autistic children [50]. More recent MRI studies have found white matter enlargement in patients with autism [51]. The pathogenesis of autism is still unknown, but one hypothesis suggests that in autistic children the normal high brain serotonin synthesis capacity is somehow disrupted during early development [52], which may explain the beneficial effects of selective serotonin uptake inhibitors in some patients with autism [53].

In patients with mental retardation and autism, irrespective of etiology, stereotypies are often associated with self-injurious behavior. This is particularly true for patients with body-rocking movements, a stereotypy most often associated with self-hitting [54]. While head banging and other self-injurious behavior may occur in normal children, this type of behavior is usually abnormal and is particularly common in patients who also exhibit stereotypical behavior.

Some studies in autistic children reported that stereotypy interfered with learning suggesting that treatment of stereotypies in patients with autism facilitates learning [55] and implied that controlling stereotypic behavior was a necessary precondition for learning. Drugs that block postsynaptic dopamine and serotonin receptors, such as risperidone, have been found to be effective in the treatment of tantrums, aggression, and self-injurious behaviors in patients with autistic disorders [56, 57]. These benefits, however, must be weighed against potential side effects such as sedation, weight gain and parkinsonism. Other agents used in the treatment of autistic disorders include CNS stimulants, anticonvulsants, naltrexone, lithium, anxiolytics, and other treatments, but well controlled, double-blind studies are lacking [58].

## ■ Rett Syndrome

Rett syndrome is a disorder occurring almost exclusively in girls and manifested clinically by stereotypic movements and other movement disorders [59,60]. The prevalence has been reported to range between 1:10,000 and 1:28,000 [61]. In contrast to infantile autism and mental retardation, Rett patients tend to have normal development until 6-18 months of age; this is then followed by gradual regression of both motor and language skills. Usually between the ages of 9 months and 3 years there is a gradual social withdrawal and psychomotor regression with loss of acquired communication skills. Acquired finger and hand skills are gradually replaced by stereotypical hand movements, including hand clapping, wringing, clenching, washing, patting, rubbing, picking, and mouthing *(Figure 1)*. Additionally, Rett girls often exhibit body-rocking movements and shifting of weight from one leg to the other. Although most girls with Rett are able to walk they tend to walk on toes, their gait is usually broad-based and apraxic, and associated with retropulsion and loss of balance. Other motor disturbances include respiratory dysregulation with episodic hyperventilation and breath holding, bruxism, ocular deviations, dystonia, myoclonus, athetosis, tremor, jerky truncal and gait ataxia and parkinsonian findings. In a study of 32 Rett patients, ages 30 months to 28 years, we suggested that the occurrence of the different motor disorders seemed to be age-related [62]. The hyperkinetic disorders were more common in younger girls while bradykinetic disorders seemed more prominent in the older patients.

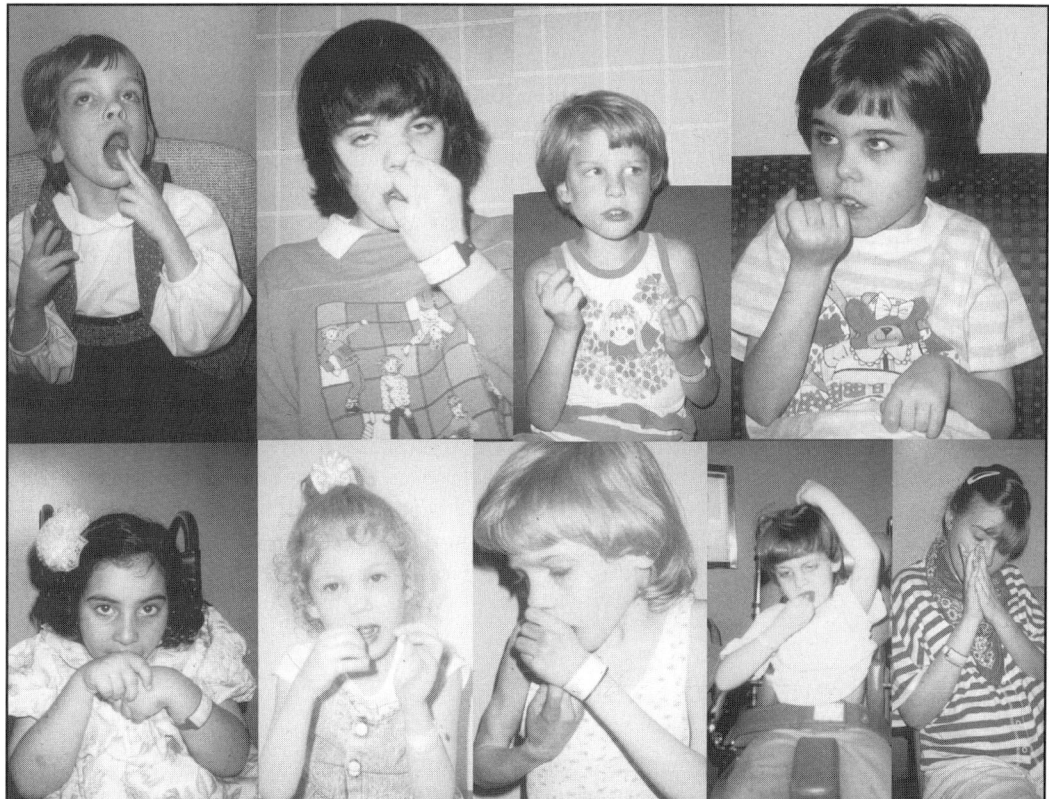

**Figure 1.** A collage of typical hand and mouthing stereotypies exhibited by girls with Rett syndrome.

The pathophysiological basis of the motor disturbances in Rett syndrome has not been fully elucidated. MRI studies have shown generalized brain and bilateral caudate atrophy [63]. Electroencephalographic recordings show age-related progressive deterioration characterized by slowing, loss of normal sleep characteristics and the appearance of epileptiform activity. In a few postmortem examinations of Rett brains, besides marked reduction in both gray- and white-matter volume, particularly involving the caudate nucleus [64], some studies also found spongy degeneration of cerebral and cerebellar white matter, deposition of lipofuscin, and depigmentation of *substantia nigra* and *locus coeruleus* [65]. The various neuropathological findings have been interpreted as a failure in the proper development or maintenance of synaptic connections. Since there is no evidence of a neurodegenerative process there is a possibility of a therapeutic intervention that may not only alter the symptoms but also favorably modify the natural course of the disease.

The major advance in understanding the biology of Rett syndrome has come with the discovery of a gene that is responsible for most, but not all cases of Rett phenotype. Since the initial discovery of the gene in 1999 [66], loss-of-function mutations of the X-linked gene encoding methyl-CpG binding protein 2 (MeCP2) have been found to be responsible for more than 80% of Rett cases [67]. The phenotypic spectrum of MeCP2 mutations is broadening and it includes not only the classical Rett syndrome but also Rett variants, mentally retarded males and autistic children [68]. The function of MeCP2 protein is still unknown, but is expressed ubiquitously in neurons and binds primarily, but not exclusively, to methylated DNA, and it is thought to regulate gene expression, chromatin composition, and chromosomal architecture and may be important for maintenance of neuronal chromatin during late development and in adulthood. The MeCP2 is expressed exclusively in neurons at the time when the neurons are starting to form synapses. In the cerebellum, the Purkinje cells which are born early, strongly express MeCP2 soon after birth, but granule cells that mature later do not express the protein until several weeks after birth. Thus, the protein is not turned on until it is needed for the formation of synapses. Furthermore, selective knock out of the gene in mice results in a Rett-like phenotype, including a reduction in brain atrophy and neuronal dystrophy. Rett syndrome appears to be a disorder of synapse formation and proliferation. A broad range of associated with MeCP2 mutations have been described involving not only girls and women, but also males and include a variety of autistic spectrum disorders, such as the Angelman syndrome, learning disability, mental retardation, and fatal encephalopathy [60]. Although stereotypies are sometimes present in patients with TS, we excluded mutations in the MeCP2 gene in our population of patients with TS [69].

## ■ Schizophrenia and Catatonia

Various stereotypies were described in schizophrenic patients long before neuroleptics were first introduced for the treatment of psychotic disorders. Since stereotypies in untreated childhood schizophrenia have not been well studied, the discussion of this topic is beyond the scope of this review [70].

## ■ Obsessive-Compulsive Disorder and Tic Disorders

Stereotypies can be encountered in various tic disorders, including TS and neuroacanthocytosis, both of which can be also associated with OCD. TS will be discussed elsewhere in this volume and, therefore, only a brief discussion of other tic disorders and OCD follows. Also, reader is referred to recent reviews on this topic [2, 71, 72].

Progression from a hyperkinetic to a bradykinetic movement disorder, as seen in Rett syndrome, may be also encountered in neuroacanthocytosis, another disorder manifested by stereotypical and self-injurious (e.g. lip and tongue biting) behavior. Symptoms usually first begin in the 3rd and 4th decade, but may start during childhood, with lip and tongue biting followed by orolingual ("eating") dystonia, motor and phonic tics, generalized chorea, distal and body stereotypies, parkinsonism, vertical ophthalmoparesis, and seizures. Other features include cognitive and personality changes, dysphagia, dysarthria, amyotrophy, areflexia, evidence of axonal neuropathy, and elevated serum creatine kinase without evidence of myopathy. Besides movement disorders other associated features included: dysarthria, absent or reduced reflexes, dementia, psychiatric problems such as depression, anxiety and obsessive-compulsive disorder, dysphagia, seizures, muscle weakness and wasting, and elevated creatine phosphokinase. MR volumetry and FDG PET show striatal atrophy in patients with neuroacanthocytosis [73].

Although autosomal dominant, X-linked recessive, and sporadic forms of neuroacanthocytosis have been reported, the majority of the reported families indicate autosomal recessive inheritance. Genomewide scan for linkage in 11 families with autosomal recessive inheritance showed a linkage to a marker on chromosome 9q21, indicating a single locus for the disease. Sequencing has identified a polyadenylation site with a protein with 3096 amino acid residues, which has been named "Chorein", and subsequent studies have identified multiple mutations in the *CHAC* gene [74].

Another psychiatric disorder frequently accompanied be stereotypic movements is OCD [72]. Foot tapping, crossing and uncrossing the legs, and tapping fingers on a chair arm, and similar stereotypic behaviors may be associated with obsessive-compulsive symptoms [27]. Once considered a rare psychiatric disorder, recent epidemiological studies indicate that the lifetime prevalence of OCD is approximately 2.5% [75]. Compulsions may be difficult to differentiate from stereotypies. In contrast to stereotypies, compulsions are usually preceded by or associated with feelings of inner tension or anxiety and a need to perform the same act repeatedly in the same manner. Examples of compulsions are ritualistic hand washing, repetitively touching the same place, evening up, arranging and checking doors, locks and appliances. Reports of focal striatal lesions giving rise to severe OCD and the frequent association of OCD with basal ganglia disorders such as TS, Parkinson's disease and Sydenham's chorea [8, 76] provide additional support for the link between abnormal behavior, such as OCD, and extrapyramidal dysfunction [77, 78].

# ■ Tardive Dyskinesia

Repetitive and patterned movements, phenomenologically identical to stereotypy, are characteristically seen in patients with tardive dyskinesia [79]. All types of movement disorders, including parkinsonism, tremor, chorea, dystonia, tics, myoclonus and stereotypy, can result from the use of dopamine receptor blocking drugs (neuroleptics) both acutely and chronically (tardive). The most typical form of tardive dyskinesia, the orofacial-lingual-masticatory movement, is one of the best examples of a stereotypic movement disorder [80]. Tardive dystonia tends to occur more frequently in younger patients, although it is quite rare in children. Tardive stereotypy is more typically observed in middle-aged or elderly patients, particularly women, and this is a very rare complication in children. We described a one-year-old girl who developed orofacial-lingual stereotypy at age 2 months after a 17-day treatment with metoclopramide for gastroesophageal reflux [81]. The stereotypy, documented by sequential videos, persisted for at least 9 months after the drug was discontinued. This patient, perhaps the first documented case of tardive dyskinesia in an infant, draws attention to the possibility that this disorder is frequently unrecognized in young children.

Akathisia, a combination of complex stereotypies, such as hair and face rubbing, picking at clothes, crossing and uncrossing of legs, adduction-abduction and up-and-down pumping of legs, arising and sitting down, marching in place, pacing and shifting weight, and feelings of restlessness, is typically a manifestation of tardive dyskinesia, but may be also seen in patients with Parkinson's disease, and various forms of mental retardation and autism [82]. In some individuals, particularly those who abuse amphetamines or cocaine and in patients with Parkinson's disease taking levodopa, certain stereotypic behaviors, called "punding" are seen [83, 84]. These include compulsive sorting of objects, nail polishing, shoe shining, hair dressing, and intense fascination with repetitive handling and examining of mechanical objects, such as picking at oneself or taking apart watches and radios or sorting and arranging of common objects, such as lining up pebbles, rocks, or other small objects. This stereotypic behavior has not been previously described in children, even in those taking CNS stimulants for ADHD, although no studies specifically designed to study punding in children has been reported.

With the advent of atypical neuroleptics, the incidence of tardive dyskinesia is decreasing, but its frequency in children has not been well studied. Campbell and colleagues [85], in their 15-year-long prospective double blind, placebo-controlled study of autistic children exposed to haloperidol reported that tardive dyskinesia developed in 9 of 118 children (7.6%) [85]. We analyzed five studies of tardive dyskinesia involving 392 children, ages 2.3 to 18 years, with multiple psychiatric diagnoses, autism, and mental retardation [86]. Tardive dyskinesia developed in 50 of the 392 (12.7%) patients, but these were not designed as epidemiological studies and, therefore, the true incidence and prevalence of tardive dyskinesia is unknown.

The most important step in the management of tardive dyskinesia is prevention; dopamine receptor blocking drugs, particularly the typical neuroleptics, should be used only if other drugs do not adequately control the behavior or neurological disorder, such as TS. Atypical antipsychotics may be better alternative medications with less risk of causing tardive dyskinesia and should be considered whenever possible. Drugs found to be useful in the treatment of tardive dyskinesia include clonazepam and other benzodiazepines and dopamine depletors such as tetrabenazine [87, 88]. Beta-blockers, clonidine, gabapentin, and opioids have also been found effective in some patients with akathisia. Botulinum toxin injections are usually effective in the treatment of focal or segmental tardive dystonia [89].

# References

1. Jankovic J. *Stereotypies*. In: Marsden CD, Fahn S, eds. *Movement Disorders*. 3rd ed. Butterworth Heinemann, London: 1994: 503-17.
2. Jankovic J. *Tics and stereotypies*. In: Freund, Jeannerod, Hallett, Leiguarda, eds. *Higher-Order Motor Disorders*, Oxford University Press, Oxford, UK: 2005 (in press).
3. Jankovic J, Sekula SL, Milas D. Dermatological manifestations of Tourette's syndrome and obsessive-compulsive disorder. *Arch Dermatol* 1998; 134: 113-4.
4. Schroeder SR, Oster-Granite ML, Berkson G, et al. Self-injurious behavior: gene-brain-behavior relationships. *Ment Retard Dev Disabil Res Rev* 2001; 7: 3-12.
5. Lutz C, Well A, Novak M. Stereotypic and self-injurious behavior in rhesus macaques: a survey and retrospective analysis of environment and early experience. *Am J Primatol* 2003; 60: 1-15.
6. Nyatsanza S, Shetty T, Gregory C, et al. A study of stereotypic behaviours in Alzheimer's disease and frontal and temporal variant frontotemporal dementia. *J Neurol Neurosurg Psychiatry* 2003; 74: 1398-402.
7. Sato S, Hashimoto T, Nakamura A, Ikeda S. Stereotyped stepping associated with lesions in the bilateral medial frontoparietal cortices. *Neurology* 2001; 51: 711-3.
8. Kwak C, Jankovic J. Tourettism and dystonia after subcortical stroke. *Mov Disord* 2002; 17: 821-5.
9. Hottinger-Blanc PM, Ziegler AL, Deonna T. A special type of head stereotypies in children with developmental (?cerebellar) disorder: description of 8 cases and literature review. *Eur J Paediatr Neurol* 2002; 6: 143-52.
10. Garner JP, Meehan CL, Mench JA. Stereotypies in caged parrots, schizophrenia and autism: evidence for a common mechanism. *Behav Brain Res* 2003; 145: 125-34.
11. Novak MA. Self-injurious behavior in rhesus monkeys: New insights into its etiology, physiology, and treatment. *Am J Primatol* 2003; 59: 3-19.
12. Low M. Stereotypies and behavioural medicine: confusions in current thinking. *Aust Vet J* 2003; 81: 192-8.
13. Koller WC, Herbster G. D1 and D2 dopamine receptor mechanisms in dopaminergic behaviors. *Clin Neuropharmacol* 1988; 11: 221-31.
14. Chipkin RE, McQuade RD, Iorio LC. D1 and D2 dopamine binding site up-regulation and apomorphine-induced stereotypy. *Pharmacol Biochem Behav* 1987; 28: 477-82.
15. Presti MF, Gibney BC, Lewis MH. Effects of intrastriatal administration of selective dopaminergic ligands on spontaneous stereotypy in mice. *Physiol Behav* 2004; 80: 433-9.
16. Canales JJ, Gilmour G, Iversen SD. The role of nigral and thalamic output pathways in the expression of oral stereotypies induced by amphetamine injections into the striatum. *Brain Res* 2000; 856: 176-83.
17. Canales JJ, Graybiel AM. A measure of striatal function predicts motor stereotypy. *Nature Neurosci* 2000; 3: 377-83.
18. Saka E, Graybiel AM. Pathophysiology of Tourette's syndrome: striatal pathways revisited. *Brain Dev* 2003; 25 (suppl 1): S15-9.

19. Glickstein SB, Schmauss C. Focused motor stereotypies do not require enhanced activation of neurons in striosomes. *J Comp Neurol* 2004; 469: 227-38.
20. Blumstein LK, Crawley JN, Davis LG, Baldino F. Neuropeptide modulation of apomorphine-induced stereotyped behavior. *Brain Res* 1987; 404: 293-300.
21. Sandman CA. β-endorphin disregulation in autistic and self-injurious behavior: a neurodevelopmental hypothesis. *Synapse* 1988; 2: 193-9.
22. Hugo C, Seier J, Mdhluli C, et al. Fluoxetine decreases stereotypic behavior in primates. *Prog Neuropsychopharmacol Biol Psychiatry* 2003; 27: 639-43.
23. Castellanos FX, Ritchie GF, Marsh WL, Rapoport JL. DSM-IV stereotypic movement disorder: persistence of stereotypies of infancy in intellectually normal adolescents and adults. *J Clin Psychiatry* 1996; 57: 116-22.
24. Mahone EM, Bridges D, Prahme C, Singer HS. Repetitive arm and hand movements (complex motor stereotypies) in children. *J Pediatr* 2004; 145: 391-5.
25. Castellanos FX, Giedd JN, Hamburger SD, et al. Brain morphometry in Tourette's syndrome: The influence of co-morbid attention-deficit/hyperactivity disorder. *Neurology* 1996; 47: 1581-3.
26. Tan A, Salgado M, Fahn S. The characterization and outcome of stereotypical movements in non-autistic children. *Mov Disord* 1997; 12: 47-52.
27. Niehaus DJ, Emsley RA, Brink P, Stein DJ. Stereotypies: prevalence and association with compulsive and impulsive symptoms in college students. *Psychopathology* 2000; 33: 31-5.
28. Troster H. Prevalence and functions of stereotyped behaviors in non-handicapped children in residential care. *J Abnorm Child Psychol* 1994; 22: 79-97.
29. Bachara GH, Phelan WJ. Rhythmic movement in deaf children. *Percept Mot Skills* 1980; 50 (3 Pt 1): 933-4.
30. Doyle TF, Bellugi U, Korenberg JR, Graham J. "Everybody in the world is my friend" hypersociability in young children with Williams syndrome. *Am J Med Genet* 2004; 124A: 263-73.
31. Sallustro A and Atwell CW. Body rocking, head banging, and head rolling in normal children. *J Pediatr* 1978; 93: 704-8.
32. Mink JW, Neil JJ. Masturbation mimicking paroxysmal dystonia or dyskinesia in a young girl. *Mov Disord* 1995; 10: 518-20.
33. Nokelainen P, Flint J. Genetic effects on human cognition: lessons from the study of mental retardation syndrome. *J Neurol Neurosurg Psychiatry* 2002; 72: 287-96.
34. Dura JR, Mullick JA, Rasnake LK. Prevalence of stereotypy among institutionalized non-ambulatory profoundly mentally retarded people. *AM M Ment Defic* 1987; 91: 548-9.
35. Thompson CL, Reid A. Behavioural symptoms among people with severe and profound intellectual disabilities: a 26-year follow-up study. *Br J Psychiatry* 2002; 181: 67-71.
36. Jankovic J, Caskey TC, Stout JT, and Butler I. Lesch-Nyhan syndrome: a study of motor behavior and CSF monoamine turnover. *Ann Neurol* 1988; 23: 466-9.
37. Bodfish JW, Parker DE, Lewis MH, Sprague RL, Newell KM. Stereotypy and motor control: differences in the postural stability dynamics of persons with stereotyped and dyskinetic movement disorders. *Am J Ment Retard* 2001; 106: 123-34.
38. Sugiyama T and Abe T. The prevalence of autism in Nagoya, Japan: a total population study. *J Autism Dev Dis* 1989; 19: 87-96.
39. Yeargin-Allsopp M, Rice C, Karapurkar T, et al. Prevalence of autism in a US metropolitan area. *JAMA* 2003; 289: 49-55.
40. Chakrabarti S, Fombonne E. Pervasive developmental disorders in preschool children. *JAMA* 2001; 285: 3093-9.
41. Miller LK. The savant syndrome: intellectual impairment and exceptional skill. *Psychol Bull* 1999; 125: 31-46.
42. Treffert DA. The Savant syndrome and autistic disorder. *CNS Spectrums* 1999; 4: 57-60.

43. Ringman JM, Jankovic J. Occurrence of tics in Asperger's syndrome and autistic disorder. *J Child Neurol* 2000; 15: 394-400.
44. Gillberg C. The borderland of autism and Rett syndrome: five case histories to highlight diagnostic difficulties. *J Autism Dev Disord* 1989; 19: 545-59.
45. Gillberg IC, Gillberg C. Asperger syndrome in 23 Swedish children. *Dev Med Child Neurol* 1989; 31: 520-31.
46. Szatmari P, Bremner R, Nagy J. Asperger syndrome: a review of clinical features. *Can J Psychiatry* 1989; 34: 554-60.
47. Berther ML, Bayes A, Tolosa ES. Magnetic resonance imaging in patients with concurrent Tourette's disorder and Asperger's syndrome. *J Am Acad Child Adolesc Psychiatry* 1993; 32: 633-9.
48. Rapin I. Autism spectrum disorders: relevance to Tourette syndrome. *Adv Neurol* 2001; 85: 89-101.
49. Hashimoto T, Tayama M, Mori F, et al. Magnetic resonance imaging in autism: preliminary report. *Neuropediatrics* 1989; 20: 142-6.
50. Kleiman MD, Neff S, Rosman NP. The brain in infantile autism: are posterior fossa structures abnormal? *Neurology* 1992; 42: 753-60.
51. Herbert MR, Ziegler DA, Makris N, et al. Localization of white matter volume increase in autism and developmental language disorder. *Ann Neurol* 2004; 55: 530-40.
52. Chugani DC, Chugani HT. PET: mapping of serotonin synthesis. *Adv Neurol* 2000; 83: 165-71.
53. DeLong RG. Autism: New data suggest a new hypothesis. *Neurology* 1999; 52: 911-6.
54. Rojahn J. Self-injurious and stereotypic behavior of non-institutionalized mentally retarded people: prevalence and classification. *Am J Ment Defic* 1986; 91: 268-76.
55. Koegel RL, Covert A. The relationship of self-stimulation to learning in autistic children. *J Appl Behav Anal* 1972; 5: 381-7.
56. Research Units on Pediatric Psychopharmacology Autism Network. Risperidone in children with autism and serious behavioral problems. *N Engl J Med* 2002; 347: 314-21.
57. Gagliano A, Germano E, Pustorino G, et al. Risperidone treatment of children with autistic disorder: effectiveness, tolerability, and pharmacokinetic implications. *J Child Adolesc Psychopharmacol* 2004; 14: 39-47.
58. Owley T. The pharmacological treatment of autistic spectrum disorders. *CNS Spectrum* 2002; 7: 663-69.
59. Fitzgerald PM, Jankovic J, Glaze DG, Schultz R, Percy AK. Extrapyramidal involvement in Rett's syndrome. *Neurology* 1990; 40: 293-5.
60. Percy AK. Rett syndrome: Current status and new vistas. *Neurol Clin N Am* 2002: 20: 1125-41.
61. Kozinetz CA, Skender ML, MacNaughton N, et al. Epidemiology of Rett syndrome: a population-based registry. *Pediatrics* 1993; 91: 445-50.
62. Fitzgerald PM, Jankovic J, Percy AK. Rett syndrome and associated movement disorders. *Movement Disorders* 1990b; 5: 195-203.
63. Reiss AL, Faruque F, Naidu S, et al. Neuroanatomy of Rett syndrome: a volumetric imaging study. *Ann Neurol* 1993; 34: 227-37.
64. Subramaniam B, Naidu S, Reiss AL. Neuroanatomy in Rett syndrome: cerebral cortex and posterior fossa. *Neurology* 1997; 2: 399-407.
65. Hagberg BA. Rett syndrome: clinical peculiarities, diagnostic approach, and possible cause. *Pediatr Neurol* 1989; 5: 75-83.
66. Amir RE, Van den Veyver IB, Wan M, Tran CQ, Francke U, Zoghbi HY. Rett syndrome is caused by mutations in X-linked MECP2, encoding methyl-CpG-binding protein 2. *Nat Genet* 1999; 23: 185-8.
67. Akbarian S. The neurobiology of Rett syndrome. *Neuroscientist* 2003; 9: 57-63.

68. Neul JL, Zoghbi HY. Rett syndrome: A prototypical neurodevelopmental disorder. *Neuroscientist* 2004; 10: 118-28.
69. Rosa AL, Jankovic J, Ashizawa T. Screening for Mutations in the MECP2 (Rett Syndrome) Gene in Gilles de la Tourette Syndrome. *Arch Neurol* 2003; 60: 502-3.
70. Ihara M, Kohara N, Urano F, et al. Neuroleptic malignant syndrome with prolonged catatonia in a dopa-responsive dystonia patient. *Neurology* 2002; 59: 1102-4.
71. Jankovic J. *Differential diagnosis and etiology of tics.* In: Cohen DJ, Jankovic J, Goetz CG, eds. Tourette Syndrome, *Adv Neurol*, vol. 85. Philadelphia: Lippincott Williams and Wilkins, 2001: 15-29.
72. Jenike MA. Obsessive-compulsive disorder. *N Engl J Med* 2004; 350: 259-65.
73. Jung HH, Hergerberg M, Kneifel S, et al. McLeod syndrome: A novel mutation, predominant psychiatric manifestations, and distinct striatal imaging findings. *Ann Neurol* 2001; 49: 384-92.
74. Rampoldi L, Dobson-Stone C, Rubio JP, et al. A conserved sorting-associated protein is mutant in chorea- acanthocytosis. *Nat Genet* 2001; 28: 119-20.
75. Snider LA, Swedo SE. Pediatric obsessive-compulsive disorder. *JAMA* 2000; 284: 3104-6.
76. Church AJ, Cardoso F, Dale RC, et al. Antibasal ganglia antibodies in acute and persistent Sydenham's chorea. *Neurology* 2002; 59: 227-31.
77. Cummings JL. Frontal sub-cortical circuits and human behaviour. *Arch Neurol* 1993; 50: 873-80.
78. Rosario-Campos MC, Leckman JF, Mercadante MT, et al. Adults with early-onset obsessive-compulsive disorder. *Am J Psychiatry* 2001; 158: 1899-903.
79. Jankovic J. Tardive syndromes and other drug-induced movement disorders. *Clin Neuropharmacol* 1995; 18: 197-214.
80. Miller LG, Jankovic J. Neurological approach to drug-induced movement disorders: a study of 125 patients. *South Med J* 1990b; 83: 525-35.
81. Mejia N, Jankovic J. Metoclopramide-induced tardive dyskinesia in an infant. *Mov Disord* 2005; 20: 86-9.
82. Bodfish JW, Newell KM, Sprague RL, Harper VN, Lewis MH. Akathisia in adults with mental retardation: development of the Akathisia Ratings of Movement Scale (ARMS). *Am J Ment Retard* 1997; 101: 413-23.
83. Evans AH, Katzenschlager R, Paviour D, et al. Punding in Parkinson's disease: its relation to the dopamine dysregulation syndrome. *Mov Disord* 2004; 19: 397-405.
84. Voon V. Repetition, repetition, and repetition: compulsive and punding behaviors in Parkinson's disease. *Mov Disord* 2004; 19: 367-70.
85. Campbell M, Armenteros JL, Malone RP, Adams PB, Eisenberg ZW, Overall JE. Neuroleptic-related dyskinesias in autistic children: a prospective, longitudinal study. *J Am Acad Child Adolesc Psychiatry* 1997; 36: 835-43.
86. Mejia N, Jankovic J. Tardive dyskinesia in children. 2005 (submitted) b.
87. Hunter CB, Vuong KD, Jankovic J. Tetrabenazine in the treatment of movement disorders in children. *Mov Disord* 2004; 19 (Suppl 9): S422.
88. Jankovic J, Beach J. Long-term effects of tetrabenazine in hyperkinetic movement disorders. *Neurology* 1997; 48: 358-62.
89. Jankovic J. Botulinum toxin in clinical practice. *J Neurol Neurosurg Psychiatry* 2004; 75: 951-7.

# Functional (psychogenic) movement disorders in childhood

**Robert Surtees**

*Neurosciences Unit, Institute of Child Health, University College London, London, United Kingdom*

Very little is known about functional movement disorders in childhood and adolescence that is open to scientific scrutiny. Neurological disorders believed functional in origin comprise 4-7% of all referrals to paediatric neurology services [1, 2]. Of these, approximately 12% have a motor disorder [1], but the proportion with a movement disorder is not known. However, functional movement disorders in children appear rare [3, 4].

By contrast, psychogenic movement disorders have been extensively studied in adults [5]. In adults the incidence is around 3% of all movement disorders and their prevalence varies with the type of movement disorder; for instance psychogenic dystonia is rare [6], but psychogenic myoclonus is common [7]. The study of psychogenic movement disorders in adults has led to the delineation of clinical clues that increase suspicion that the movement disorder is psychogenic in origin (*Tables I, II and III*; modified from Fahn [8]). Here I will present 5 brief illustrative cases of children and adolescents presenting with a functional movement disorder and, by way of contrast, one brief case of a child with an undiagnosed primary dystonia, previously thought to be functional in origin. I will then discuss the terminology (psychogenic and functional), therapeutic approach and outcome.

## ■ Illustrative Cases

### Case 1

A 12 year old girl presented with a sudden onset of being unable to walk. At the age of 6 years she had had a sudden onset of an abnormal head position and difficulties using her dominant hand. At the time there was a questionable response to treatment with carbidopa/laevodopa. Investigations then (including mutation analysis of the GTP-cyclohydrolase 1 gene) were all negative and the symptoms spontaneously resolved after approximately 7 months. She remained well for the next 6 years. Examination at the age of 12 showed dystonic posturing of the non-dominant hand as the

**Table I. Clinical clues from the history that increase suspicion that a movement disorder is psychogenic in origin.**

- Abrupt onset
  - May follow minor injury
- Rapid progression to maximal severity
- Nonprogressive course
  - Characteristics may change with time
  - Paroxysmal exacerbations
- Spontaneous remissions
- Other medically unexplained symptoms

**Table II. Clinical clues from the examination that increase suspicion that a movement disorder is psychogenic in origin.**

- Inconsistency
- Incongruity
- Other abnormal movements
  - Shaking
  - Slowness
  - Bizarre gait
  - Excessive startle
- Other nonorganic sensory or motor signs

**Table III. Clinical clues from the examination of specific movement disorders that increase suspicion that the movement disorder is psychogenic in origin.**

- Tremor
  - Decreases with distraction
  - Increases with attention
  - Frequency can be entrained
  - Absent finger tremor
- Dystonia
  - Begins with fixed posture

only abnormality when seated at rest. Attempts to passively flex her hips or passively extend her knees or to get her to stand caused immediate, sustained and extreme plantar flexion of both feet. Biochemical, immunological, genetic and brain structural investigations (along the lines of [9]) showed no abnormality. Cognitive assessment showed mild to moderate global learning difficulties. Treatment included a change in school and cognitive-behavioural therapy and there was a sudden remission six months after the second presentation. Despite continuing psychological support and treatment she has developed a pattern of relapsing and remitting symptoms with inconsistent and incongruous signs. A diagnosis of functional dystonia was made.

## Case 2

A 14 year old boy had a sudden onset of tremor affecting his dominant arm and preventing him writing. This remitted for 2 months during the school summer vacation. The tremor relapsed when he returned to school. On examination within 2 weeks of the tremor relapse, he had a variable tremor of the right arm and hand, but not involving the fingers. The tremor varied in intensity being more marked when attention was drawn to it, and also varied in frequency. He was also noted to have dystonic head and neck tics (as did his father) and an obsessive personality. He was being bullied at school and he thought that the tremor was "all in my mind". After discussion of the nature of functional tremor, his symptoms remitted. The tic-disorder was noted but not otherwise commented on.

## Case 3

This 14 year old girl had a sudden onset of abnormal head and dominant arm posture and an inability to stand or walk without the support of another person. She had a previous history of physical and emotional abuse, had long-standing challenging behaviour and was in the care of the Social Services. On examination she had fixed posturing of her right arm and a fixed torticollis. Lower limb muscular tone and tendon reflexes were normal, but she showed "give-way" muscular weakness in all groups tested. She was unable to stand or walk without the light support of another person. Magnetic resonance imaging of her brain showed cerebellar hypoplasia. Biochemical, immunological and genetic investigations were normal. She was admitted for inpatient psychiatric treatment but deteriorated and developed all the features of the pervasive refusal syndrome [10].

## Case 4

At the age of 12 years, some months after an episode of left otitis media, this boy developed paroxysm of excruciating left facial pain. Infective, brain structural and angiographic and ear, nose and throat investigations were all negative. His father, to whom he was particularly close, had recently left the family. A diagnosis of atypical facial pain was made and he was treated with amitriptyline and cognitive and behavioural therapy. The paroxysms of pain decreased in frequency and he continued to attend school and do well there. At the age of 14 years, following a paroxysm of facial pain, he became depersonalised, breathless and fell to the floor. On recovery, after some minutes, he had developed difficulty with walking and had lost sensation in both arms from shoulder to wrist and both legs from hip to ankle. On examination he had a bizarre, monoplegic gait with his right leg held stiffly extended and externally rotated at the hip. He had circumferential loss of all sensory modalities in both arms from shoulder to wrist and both legs from hip to ankle. Muscle tone and power were normal as were deep tendon reflexes. The gait disorder and disordered sensation remitted with rehabilitation and cognitive and behaviour therapy.

## Case 5

This 12 year girl has congenital ataxia and moderate learning difficulties caused by a cerebellar malformation. She also has had a cadaveric renal transplant because of chronic renal failure secondary to nephronophthisis. Two years previously she had had an episode of transient generalised dystonia, thought to be a post-infectious autoimmune phenomenon and associated with circulating antibasal ganglia antibodies. She presented with a sudden onset of dominant arm tremor. Antibasal ganglia antibodies were again positive. A diagnosis of autoimmune basal ganglia disease was made and she was treated symptomatically with first trihexyphenidyl and later with carbamazepine. Despite this her tremor worsened, spread to involve both arms and her trunk and she became unable to perform any acts of daily living without assistance. At this stage examination showed a highly variable tremor affecting her right arm, but not her fingers, at rest. The tremor was not evident when she was distracted but increased in amplitude when attention was drawn to it. The frequency of the tremor could be entrained. A diagnosis of a functional tremor was made and the condition explained to the patient and her family. The tremor remitted following two sessions of cognitive behavioural therapy.

## Case 6

This 13 year girl has undiagnosed congenital sensorineural deafness and mild learning difficulties. At the age of 10 years she developed task-specific dystonia of her dominant arm affecting her writing. Extensive brain structural, immunological, biochemical and genetic investigation was negative. A trial of laevodopa/carbidopa was ineffective. The dystonia remitted spontaneously for a 3 month period but relapsed at the age of 11 years and spread to involve the non-dominant arm. Prior to this relapse, her father and her brother had left the family home. A diagnosis of a functional movement disorder was made (because of bizarre movements, period of spontaneous remission and the relapse occurring at a time of psychological stress) and treatment was started with a selective serotonin re-uptake inhibitor and cognitive and behavioural therapy. However, the dystonia progressed and she developed axial involvement by the age of 13 years. Examination at this time showed a generalised dystonia affecting the left more than the right arm, a hyperlordosis and scoliotic movements concave towards the left. She had a dystonic writer's cramp on the right and an elevating left arm controlled by a sensory trick. There was no clear involvement of the legs, but she had a positive Babinski sign on walking. A diagnosis of an idiopathic (not associated with the common deletion in *DYT1* gene) generalised dystonia was made and she was started on trihexyphenidyl.

## Discussion of cases

These cases were seen in a specialist, quaternary movement disorder clinic over the past three years suggesting an incidence of around 3%, very similar to the incidence in adult series. The children were all seen in their teenage or immediate pre-teen years, although one (case 1) first developed symptoms at 6 years of age. All of the children with a functional movement disorder had pre-existing neurological or psychological problems (learning difficulties 2, abuse at home or school 2 (and suspected in case 1 also), tic-disorder 1 and medically unexplained symptoms 1). Interestingly case 6, who has an idiopathic dystonia, also had a pre-existing neurological disorder. With the exception of the children with functional tremor, all had extensive investigations to exclude structural, biochemical, immunological and genetic causes of their movement disorder. This suggests that functional tremor is more easily diagnosed on clinical grounds than the other functional movement disorders. All of the children with functional movement disorders had clinical features suggestive of the diagnosis *(see tables)*. A cognitive and behavioural approach to treatment, in the setting of an assessment by a multidisciplinary team which included a clinical psychologist, physiotherapist, occupational therapist, neurologist and a psychiatrist, proved helpful to all children except case 3. However, only those children with a relatively brief duration of symptoms (a few months) were cured; although the others, with the exception of case 3, were all rehabilitated back to a normal school and home life.

These findings suggest that early diagnosis should be possible in functional movement disorders in children, where specific psychological intervention offer the prospect of cure. In long-established disease, most children can be rehabilitated although symptoms persist.

## ■ Terminology

The concept of functional movement disorders implies that the disease origins do not lie in an organic neurological disease, but rather in a subconscious psychological domain. That is, these disorders are caused by abnormal brain function and not by abnormalities of the biophysical substrate of the brain. Many different terms have been used to describe these disorders that reflect their perceived origin and the prevalent linguistic culture. Thus, "hysterical", "psychosomatic", "stress-related", "medically unexplained", "conversion", "psychogenic" and "functional" have all been used. The preferred term used should be acceptable to the child and his or her parents, describe the nature of the disorder and lead to a discussion of the symptoms and their cause.

An imaginative study from Edinburgh, Scotland, calculated the degree of offensiveness of these labels in adults attending a general neurology clinic [11]. They found that the label "functional" was least likely to cause offence (for the time being at least). In addition, the use of this label implies abnormal functioning of the central nervous system but avoids debate about the biological, psychological and social contributions to the disorder; and leads the way to a transparent explanation of the symptoms to the child and parent. However, in adult practice the term psychogenic is currently preferred. Thus here, I have used functional when discussing children and psychogenic when discussing adults.

## ■ Management

A clear explanation of the nature of the disorder, understandable by both the child and his or her parents, is an essential first step in management. Firstly, I stress that there has been no damage to the brain but the symptoms have been produced by abnormal brain function. This implies that there is the potential for recovery. Often an analogy is needed to improve understanding. Examples given by children and parents in roughly ascending sophistication are: a car that is working properly but whose driver doesn't know where to go; an out-of-tune musical instrument; a computer with software problems. Then, I introduce the idea that the cause of the brain dysfunction is emotional in origin; but also that we often do not identify a definite triggering stressor. It is also important to state explicitly that we do not think that the child is mad or putting on their symptoms. It is important that the child and parents understand the multidisciplinary approach to assessment and treatment and that the child will be followed up by the neurologist until there is full recovery.

Almost always, the management of functional movement disorders in childhood is multidisciplinary. Assessment will normally involve input from Neurology, Nursing, Psychiatry, Clinical Psychology, Social Work, Occupational Therapy and Physiotherapy. Treatment normally consists of two parallel approaches: rehabilitation (in particular a prompt return to school as soon as the child shows improvement) and cognitive and behavioural therapy. If a coexisting medical or psychiatric condition is also diagnosed and amenable to treatment, this should also be treated. Underlying psychological and social problems, where identified, should also be addressed and ameliorated where possible; this may also involve the child's school.

## ■ Outcome

There have been very few scientific studies of the outcome of children with functional neurological disorders. One study found that with treatment over 70% of the children improved, although over 50% of the children still had the same (or more rarely different) symptoms [1]. Another study of children with astasia-abasia (a functional inability to stand or walk) found that most recovered over a prolonged period of treatment, but around 30% continued to have symptoms [12].

There have been no studies on the outcome of functional movement disorders in childhood. Personal experience suggests that almost all children improve with psychological support and the use of cognitive and behavioural techniques to control their symptoms; however, unless symptoms are of short duration, they are rarely cured.

**Acknowledgement:** *I would like to thank the children and their parents who have taught me so much about movement disorders in childhood.*

## References

1. Spierings C, Poels PJ, Sijben N, Gabreels FJ, Renier WO. Conversion disorders in childhood: a retrospective follow-up study of 84 inpatients. *Dev Med Child Neurol* 1990; 32 (10): 865-71.
2. Thomas NH. Somatic presentation of psychogenic disease in child neurologic practice. *Neurology* 2002; 58 (Suppl 3): A28.
3. Ozekmekci S, Apaydin H, Ekinci B, Yalcinkaya C. Psychogenic movement disorders in two children. *Mov Disord* 2003; 18 (11): 1395-7.
4. Kirsch DB, Mink JW. Psychogenic movement disorders in children. *Pediatr Neurol* 2004; 30 (1): 1-6.
5. Miyasaki JM, Sa DS, Galvez-Jimenez N, Lang AE. Psychogenic movement disorders. *Can J Neurol Sci* 2003; 30 (Suppl 1): S94-100.
6. Pringsheim T, Lang AE. Psychogenic dystonia. *Rev Neurol* (Paris) 2003; 159 (10 Pt 1): 885-91.
7. Monday K, Jankovic J. Psychogenic myoclonus. *Neurology* 1993; 43 (2): 349-52.
8. Fahn S. *Psychogenic movement disorders*. In: Marsden CD, Fahn S, editors. *Movement disorders 3*. Oxford: Butterworth-Heinemann Ltd, 1994: 359-72.
9. Assmann B, Surtees R, Hoffmann GF. Approach to the diagnosis of neurotransmitter diseases exemplified by the differential diagnosis of childhood-onset dystonia. *Ann Neurol* 2003; 54 (Suppl 6): S18-S24.

10. Lask B, Britten C, Kroll L, Magagna J, Tranter M. Children with pervasive refusal. *Arch Dis Child* 1991; 66 (7): 866-9.
11. Stone J, Wojcik W, Durrance D, et al. What should we say to patients with symptoms unexplained by disease? The "number needed to offend". *BMJ* 2002; 325 (7378): 1449-50.
12. Stickler GB, Cheung-Patton A. Astasia-abasia. A conversion reaction. Prognosis. *Clin Pediatr (Phila)* 1989; 28 (1): 12-6.

# Index

## A

Action dystonia 35, 57, 215.

ADHD 131, 237-240, 250, 256.

Alternating hemiplegia 59, 65, 70, 147, 149-150, 153, 155, 157-158.

Anti-Hu 123-124, 128, 133-134.

Apneic episodes 151.

Arginine glycine amidinotransferase deficiency 223, 229, 230.

Asperger syndrome 249, 251-252, 259.

Ataxia 2, 22-24, 28, 61, 70, 96, 97-98, 117, 121-122, 132-138, 140-146, 148-149, 155, 174, 203-207, 210-211, 224, 250, 253, 263.

Ataxia-telangiectasia 32, 59, 117, 137, 139, 140, 143-146.

Ataxia with oculomotor apraxia 138, 140, 145.

Athetosis 2, 63, 69-70, 149, 152, 164-165, 176, 178-179, 187, 203, 205, 210, 217.

Autism 1, 9, 13, 16-17, 25, 70, 189, 232, 239, 246-247, 249, 251-252, 256-259.

Autonomic dysfunction 92, 187-188, 190-192.

Autosomal dominant ataxias 141.

Autosomal Recessive Ataxias 137.

Azathioprine 129-131, 136.

## B

B12 deficiency 29, 30.

Ballismus 2, 12, 165, 203, 224.

Basal ganglia 14, 18, 22, 28, 34, 44, 59, 62-63, 68-69, 82, 88, 89, 99, 100-102, 104-107, 111-113, 144, 159-165, 167-183, 190, 203, 205, 210-211, 224, 232-236, 238-239, 240-241, 243-245, 248-249, 255, 263.

Behavior problems 205-206.

Benign hereditary chorea 115, 117, 119.

Benign myoclonus of early infancy 20-21, 28.

Benign neonatal sleep myoclonus 19, 27-28.

Benign paroxysmal torticollis 24, 29.

## C

Catatonia 249, 254, 260.

Cervical dystonia 46-48, 50, 55, 58, 60, 62, 64, 68, 141-142, 167.

Chediak-Higashi syndrome 107, 113.

Chorea 2, 4, 7-8, 12, 14, 15, 17, 65-66, 72, 96, 97, 98, 102, 110, 115-119, 138-145, 163-165, 167, 174, 176-178, 180, 187-188, 203, 205, 207, 210, 217, 224, 231-238, 242, 244-246, 255-256, 260.

Choreoathetosis 64, 67, 112, 142, 148-150, 153-155, 164, 168, 174, 179, 187-188, 206-208, 218, 245.

Complex movement disorder 2, 13.

Creatine deficiency 78, 223-224, 226-230.

## D

Dancing eyes syndrome 121, 133.

Deep brain stimulation 77-78, 81-82, 85.

Dentatorubral-pallidoluysian atrophy 59, 138, 141, 145, 174, 183.

Dopa-responsive dystonia 16, 32, 35, 51-52, 58, 60, 68, 78, 94, 106, 109, 191, 201, 213, 214, 218, 222, 260.

Dyskinetic cerebral palsy 1, 6, 13-14, 179.

Dystonia 2, 4, 7, 10-11, 14-17, 21-22 25, 28-29, 31-37, 39-55, 57-59, 60-85, 91-98, 100, 104-106, 108-114, 116-118, 138-146, 148, 150, 154, 158, 161, 163-165, 168-169, 172-173, 176-180, 187-188, 192, 194-196, 198, 200, 203, 205, 207, 210, 213, 215-219, 221-222, 232, 236, 238, 242, 245, 253, 255-258, 261-264, 266-267.

Dystonia musculorum deformans 39, 52, 59, 68, 84.

Dystonia plus syndrome 31-33.

DYT13 45-46, 54, 58, 68.

DYT 1 Dystonia 39.

DYT2 45-46, 54, 58.

DYT4 45-46, 58.

DYT6 45-46, 58, 60.

## E

Encephalitis lethargica 100-102, 106, 112, 238-239, 245.

Epileptic automatism 249.

Essential laryngeal tremor 11.

Essential palatal tremor 11.
Essential tremor 1, 7, 11-12, 16-17, 21, 84, 87-88, 90, 180.

# F

Familial nocturnal alternating hemiplegia 153.
Focal dystonia 36, 41, 47, 51, 59-60, 62-63, 65-66, 69, 94, 167.
Fragile X syndrome 251.
Friedreich's ataxia 137, 139, 143-145.
Functional movement disorders 261, 264-266.

# G

Globus pallidus stimulation 73.
Glutaric acidemia 59.
GM1 and GM2 gangliosidosis 59.
Group A beta-hemolytic streptococcus (GABHS) 231.
Guanidinoaceteate methyltransferase deficiency 223.

# H

Hallervorden-Spatz syndrome 59, 99, 111, 170, 175, 181.
HARP 97, 99, 105-106, 111.
Hartnup's disease 59.
Head banging 13, 17, 29, 247, 250-252, 258.
Hemiplegic migraine 24, 65, 152, 154-157.
Hereditary essential myoclonus 117.
HIV infection 100, 111, 160-161, 177.
Homocystinuria 59, 99, 111, 155.
Huntington's disease 32, 59, 72, 78, 96, 106, 109, 117, 119, 162, 174, 183, 236.
Hyperekplexia 191.
Hyperphenylalaninemia 213-215, 222.

# I

Immunoglobulin 100, 130, 136, 242, 246.
Immunomodulation 129-130.
Inherited ataxia 137, 141.

## J

Japanese B encephalitis 99, 106, 111, 163, 177, 238, 245.
Jitteriness 11.
Juvenile neuronal ceroid lipofuscinosis 59, 99, 105-106, 111.

## K

Kinetic tremor 87, 137, 139.
Kinsbourne syndrome 121, 135, 136.

## L

L-amino acid decarboxylase deficiency 185, 193, 194.
L-DOPA-responsive dystonia 67, 139, 142, 145, 195-196, 200, 222.
L-dopa responsive progressive encephalopathy 195.
Lesch-Nyhan syndrome 32, 59, 251, 258.

## M

Machado-Joseph disease 32, 59, 97, 110, 141, 145.
Mannerisms 247.
Masturbatory behavior 250.
Metachromatic leukodystrophy 32, 59.
Methylmalonic aciduria 59.
Midazolam Withdrawal Syndrome 27.
Mitochondrial cytopathy 72, 79, 98.
Myoclonic dystonia 61, 68, 117, 119, 138, 145.
Myoclonus 2, 4, 7-8, 12, 17, 20, 27, 35, 43, 61, 72, 78, 82, 98, 119, 121-122, 126, 128, 130, 132-136, 139, 141-143, 145, 150, 163, 167, 187, 188, 203, 205, 207, 209-210, 232, 238, 245, 253, 256, 261, 266.
Myoclonus-dystonia 31-32, 35, 41, 49, 52-53, 55, 58, 67, 78, 82, 85.

## N

Neuroacanthocytosis 59, 97, 110, 249, 255.
Neuroblastoma 20, 27, 121-123, 126-128, 130, 132-136, 234, 241.
Neuromuscular disorder 191, 196.
Neuronal intranuclear inclusion body disease 98, 106.
Niemann-Pick type C 32, 59, 98, 106.

## O

Obsessive-compulsive behavior 101, 231, 236, 248.

Obsessive-compulsive disorder 122, 231, 243-244, 246-247, 249, 255, 257, 260.

Oculogyric crisis 95, 101, 151, 187-188, 193-194, 196-197, 215, 217, 219, 236.

Oppenheim dystonia 39, 58.

Opsoclonus-myoclonus syndrome 121, 132-136.

## P

PANDAS 102, 112, 232, 237-243, 245-246.

Pantothenate kinase-associated neurodegeneration 31-32, 78, 170, 181.

Paraneoplastic antibodies 123.

Parkin mutations 92-95, 106-109, 114.

Parkinsonism 13-14, 17, 32, 35, 51, 53, 57-59, 64, 67, 78, 84, 91-102, 104-114, 139, 142-143, 146, 163, 167-170, 174-177, 179-181, 184, 187-189, 195-196, 200-201, 212, 215-216, 232, 238, 242, 246, 252, 255-256.

Parkinsonism (Juvenile) 59, 78, 84, 91-92, 94, 96, 98, 100, 104-105, 107-110, 112, 114, 178, 190.

Paroxysmal dyskinesias 17, 22-23, 28, 154-155.

Paroxysmal Tonic Upgaze 22.

Postural tremor 47, 90, 95, 137, 139, 143.

Primary torsion dystonia 31-32, 35, 52-55, 68, 73, 85.

Psychogenic movement disorders 261, 266.

Ptosis 24, 188, 191, 196, 217.

## R

Restless legs syndrome 247, 249.

Rett Syndrome 13, 25, 32, 59, 66, 70, 249, 252-255, 259-260.

Rigid-hypokinetic syndrome 2, 4, 7, 12, 14.

Rituximab 129-130, 132, 136.

## S

Schizophrenia 190, 231, 247, 249, 254, 257.

Secondary dystonia 31, 57, 69, 71, 79-83.

Segawa disease (or Segawa syndrome) 8, 32, 35, 190, 214.

Segmental dystonia 37, 41, 45, 47, 57, 165.

Self-gratifying 249-250.

Self-stimulation 25-26, 259.

Sepiapterin reductase 186, 213-214, 219, 222.

Shuddering attacks 21, 28.

Shuddering spells 11.

Spasmus nutans 11.

Spastic diplegia 61.

Spastic paraplegia 95, 195, 197, 201, 215.

Spinocerebellar ataxia 32, 96, 110, 138, 140, 142, 145-146.

SSPE 100, 111.

Status dystonicus 71-76.

Stereotactic thalamotomy 75.

Stereotypies 1-2, 4, 7, 13, 25, 29, 144, 146, 241, 247-258.

Succinate semialdehyde dehydrogenase deficiency 203, 211.

Sydenham's chorea 17, 117, 163, 177, 231-232, 235, 237, 243-246, 255, 260.

Systemic lupus erythematosus 106, 112, 161, 178.

## T

Tardive dyskinesia 62, 68, 205, 211-212, 247, 256-257, 260.

Tetrahydrobiopterin deficiencies 213, 222.

Tic disorders 15-16, 236, 239, 243, 246, 255.

Tics 2-14, 18, 21, 25, 49, 97, 102, 118, 141, 232, 236, 238, 241-243, 245, 247, 250, 252, 255-257, 259-260, 263.

Todd's paralysis 154.

Tourette Syndrome 3, 9-10, 15-16, 18, 231, 236, 243, 245-247, 249, 259-260.

Transient idiopathic dystonia in infancy 21, 28.

Transient movement disorders 19, 27.

Tremor 2, 4, 7, 11, 12, 14, 21, 26-28, 32-33, 40-41, 47, 65, 68, 87-92, 95-96, 98, 102, 104, 110, 114, 116, 118-119, 137-143, 145-146, 148, 150, 154, 163, 167-169, 174, 176, 180, 187-188, 196, 203, 215-217, 219, 253, 256, 262-264.

Triose-phosphate isomerase deficiency 59.

Tyrosine hydroxylase deficiency 35, 106, 109, 191, 195, 200-201, 215, 217, 221-222.

## V

Vitamin E deficiency 138, 145.

## W

Whipple's disease 107, 113.
Williams syndrome 250, 258.
Wilson's disease 31-32, 45-46, 59, 78, 95-96, 106-107, 109, 162, 169, 174, 183.
Writer's cramp 31, 40-41, 49, 51, 55, 59-62, 68-69, 138, 264.

Achevé d'imprimer par Corlet, Imprimeur, S.A.
14110 Condé-sur-Noireau
N° d'Imprimeur : 82518 - Dépôt légal : juin 2005

*Imprimé en France*